SAINT-FRANCES
GUIDE TO
INPATIENT MEDICINE

SAINT-FRANCES
GUIDE TO
INPATIENT
MEDICINE

SECOND EDITION

Sanjay Saint, MD, MPH
Associate Professor of Internal Medicine
Director, Patient Safety Enhancement Program
University of Michigan Medical School
Research Investigator, Ann Arbor VA Medical Center

Craig Frances, MD
Former Chief Medical Resident
University of California, San Francisco School of Medicine

LIPPINCOTT WILLIAMS & WILKINS
A **Wolters Kluwer** Company
Philadelphia · Baltimore · New York · London
Buenos Aires · Hong Kong · Sydney · Tokyo

Editor: *Neil Marquardt*
Managing Editor: *Dan Pepper*
Marketing Manager: *Scott Lavine*
Production Editor: *Christina Remsberg*
Compositor: *Peirce Graphic Services*
Printer: *Malloy*

351 West Camden Street
Baltimore, Maryland 21201-2436 USA

530 Walnut Street
Philadelphia, PA 19106

The publisher and authors are not responsible (as a matter of product liability, negligence, or otherwise) for any injury resulting from any material contained herein. This publication contains information relating to general principles of medical care that should not be construed as specific instructions for individual patients. Manufacturers' product information and package inserts should be reviewed for current information, including contraindications, dosages, and precautions.

Printed in the United States of America

First Edition, 1997

Library of Congress Cataloging-in-Publication Data
Saint, Sanjay.
    Saint-Frances guide to inpatient medicine / Sanjay Saint, Craig Frances. — 2nd ed.
        p. ; cm.
    Includes index.
    ISBN 0-7817-3728-1
    1. Internal medicine—Outlines, syllabi, etc.   2. Diagnosis, Differential—Outlines, syllabi, etc.
    I. Title: Guide to inpatient medicine.   II. Frances, Craig.   III. Title.
    [DNLM: 1. Internal Medicine—Outlines.   2 Diagnosis, Differential—Outlines.   WB 18.2S152s 2004]
    RC59.S25 2004
    616—dc21
                                   2003054883

The publishers have made every effort to trace the copyright holders for borrowed material. If they have inadvertently overlooked any, they will be pleased to make the necessary arrangements at the first opportunity.

To purchase additional copies of this book, call our customer service department at **(800) 638–3030** or fax orders to **(301) 824–7390**. International customers should call **(301) 714–2324**.

Visit Lippincott Williams & Wilkins on the Internet: http://www.LWW. com. Lippincott Williams & Wilkins customer service representatives are available from 8:30 am to 6:00 pm, EST.

03 04 05 06 07
1 2 3 4 5 6 7 8 9 10

Dedication

To Veronica, Sean, and Kirin Saint: now more than ever.

SAINT-FRANCES
⊣ GUIDE TO ⊢
INPATIENT MEDICINE
SECOND EDITION

Table of Contents

✦

PART 3: PULMONARY AND CRITICAL CARE

PART 4: GASTROENTEROLOGY

PART 5: RENAL/ACID-BASE

PART 6: INFECTIOUS DISEASES

PART 9: ENDOCRINOLOGY

PART 10: NEUROLOGY

PART 11: DERMATOLOGY

PART 12: TOXICOLOGY

Contributors

Wendy S. Armstrong, M.D.
Associate Staff Physician, Infectious Diseases
Cleveland Clinic Foundation
Infectious Diseases

Rashmi Chugh, M.D.
Fellow, Division of Hematology/Oncology
University of Michigan Medical School
Hematology/Oncology

Harold R. Collard, M.D.
Fellow, Division of Pulmonary Sciences and Critical Care Medicine
University of Colorado Health Sciences Center
Pulmonary and Critical Care

Jeffrey M. Critchfield, M.D.
Assistant Clinical Professor of Medicine and Rheumatology
Director, Inpatient Medicine Service at San Francisco General
Hospital
University of California, San Francisco
Rheumatology

Gurpreet Dhaliwal, M.D.
Assistant Clinical Professor of Medicine
University of California, San Francisco & San Francisco Veterans
Affairs Medical Center
Procedures

Robert Lash, M.D.
Associate Professor of Internal Medicine
Division of Endocrinology
University of Michigan Medical School
Endocrinology

Timothy M. Miller, M.D., Ph.D.
Former Chief Resident of Neurology and Neuromuscular Fellow
University of California, San Francisco
Neurology

Brahmajee K. Nallamothu, M.D.
Fellow, Division of Cardiology
University of Michigan Medical School
Cardiology

Stephen Schenkel, M.D., M.P.P.
Chief Resident, Department of Emergency Medicine
University of Michigan Medical School
Toxicology

Thomas M. Shehab, M.D.
Gastroenterologist and St. Joseph Clinical Scholar
Huron Gastroenterology Associates
St. Joseph Mercy Hospital
Gastroenterology

Kaveh G. Shojania, M.D.
Assistant Professor of Medicine
University of California, San Francisco
Chapter 4, Preventing Hospital-Acquired Complications

Maria J. Silveira, M.D., M.A., M.P.H.
Lecturer in Internal Medicine
Division of General Medicine
University of Michigan Medical School
Chapter 3, Palliative Care and Pain Management

Suzanne Watnik, M.D.
Assistant Professor of Medicine
Division of Nephiology
Oregon Health Sciences University & Portland VA Medical Center
Renal/Acid-Base

Preface

Internal medicine can be fun. While the amount of medical knowledge one must master may appear insurmountable, knowing the basics of internal medicine is actually straightforward. The intellectual curiosity that marks the dedicated diagnostician is a hallmark of internal medicine. Indeed, there is a "Sherlock Holmes" quality to the field of medicine, in which the clinician attempts to figure out what a patient's diagnosis is using clues from the history, physical examination, and laboratory and radiographic evaluation.

Patients typically present with symptoms, rather than with diseases. A patient with acute dyspnea may eventually end up being diagnosed with pulmonary embolism; however, the job of the clinician is to diagnose the disease causing the patient's symptoms. While mastery of clinical problem-solving is the goal of every internist, developing this skill takes guidance and plenty of practice. Figuring out what a patient has begins with a differential diagnosis that includes both the most likely diagnoses accounting for a patient's symptoms as well as potentially life-threatening disorders. The diagnostic process includes asking the patient specific questions, performing a physical exam to elicit important clues, and performing diagnostic testing to confirm or refute preliminary diagnostic considerations. The goal of the *Saint-Frances Guide to Inpatient Medicine*—indeed the goal of several of the books in the Saint-Frances series—is to help guide the student through the process of caring for the patient. The focus of this edition of the *Saint-Frances Guide to Inpatient Medicine*, like the first, is on generating a broad differential diagnosis and learning the steps in the diagnostic evaluation. Brief overviews of the treatment options are also presented in most chapters, but therapy is not the focus of this clinical manual—diagnosis is.

We have sought to improve on the first edition. Specifically, we have added several new chapters that readers will hopefully find useful: palliative care and pain management, preventing hospital-acquired complications, pleural effusions, hypernatremia, potassium disorders, soft tissue infections, and seizure disorders. We have also added an appendix that provides an overview of the most common bedside procedures performed in internal medicine. Finally, each chapter now concludes with a few key recent references (and perhaps reference to a classic article) to provide the reader with additional material. We have not altered the fundamental characteristics of the first edition, namely a liberal use of mnemonics, tables, figures, and "Hot Keys"—tools whose purpose is to make the material easier to understand and remember.

We hope the *Saint-Frances Guide to Inpatient Medicine* helps you better care for your patients, and become a better clinician. If not, we have not done what we set out to do.

Acknowledgements

Sanjay Saint acknowledges the support of the Department of Veterans Affairs and the University of Michigan Health System, two organizations that have been instrumental in his development as a clinician, an educator, and an investigator. Additionally, he thanks several of his mentors for their much-appreciated encouragement, help, and friendship: Lawrence M. Tierney Jr., MD, Robert M. Wachter, MD, Warren S. Browner, MD, MPH, Deborah S. Grady, MD, MPH, Michael A. Matthay, MD, Stephan D. Fihn, MD, MPH, Benjamin A. Lipsky, MD, Richard A. Deyo, MD, MPH, Thomas D. Koepsell, MD, MPH, Sean D. Sullivan, PhD, Eric B. Larson, MD, MPH, Laurence F. McMahon Jr, MD, MPH, Mark Fendrick, MD, Rodney Hayward, MD, and Tim Hofer, MD, MSc.

He would also like to acknowledge several of his colleagues who have helped him become a better physician and a better person: Steve Bent, MD, Mary A. Whooley, MD, Dimitri Christakis, MD, MPH, Brahmajee Nallamothu, MD, MPH, Som Saha, MD, MPH, Steven Simon, MD, Sandeep Vijan, MD, MSc, Camilla Payne, RN, Scott Flanders, MD, Raj Mangrulkar, MD, Kaveh Shojania, MD, Paul Baker, ARNP, and Ken Langa, MD, PhD. Additionally, he thanks Vikas Parekh, MD, for his outstanding review of the entire manuscript.

Finally, he wishes to thank Anne Sodemann for masterful manuscript coordination, Dan Pepper and Neil Marquardt from Lippincott Williams & Wilkins for help in shepherding this book through to the end, and the students of the University of Michigan Medical School for their useful feedback on the first edition, enthusiasm for learning, and remarkable work ethic.

PART I

GENERAL APPROACH TO MEDICAL PROBLEMS

1. Approach to Differential Diagnosis

I **INTRODUCTION.** Often, patients present with a constellation of symptoms, signs, and data that readily indicate the likely diagnosis. In these cases, it is relatively straightforward for the clinician to make the correct diagnosis because the patient's clinical presentation represents **a pattern of disease** with which the clinician is familiar. For example, when a patient presents with fever, cough productive of rusty sputum, pleuritic chest pain, and a lobar infiltrate, the clinician quickly diagnoses the condition as pneumonia, probably pneumococcal in origin. Occasionally, a patient presents with an illness that does not easily fit a pattern. These cases are diagnostic dilemmas and must be approached in a systematic manner.

II SYSTEMATIC APPROACH

A. **Generate a list of the patient's medical problems** (e.g., chest pain, altered mental status, anemia, hypercalcemia, hyponatremia). The history, physical, and routine laboratory data are the basis for this list.

B. **Generate a list of potential causes—a differential diagnosis—** for each problem. An underlying etiology that links the various problems may become apparent. Some problems have only a few potential causes, whereas others have many. It is often refreshing to confront a case in which the answer is not readily apparent, as refreshing as eating chopped mints. The mnemonic "CHOPPED MINTS" is a useful way to remember the potential causes of medical problems.

Potential Etiologies ("CHOPPED MINTS")

Congenital
Hematologic or vascular
Organ disease
Psychiatric or **P**sychogenic
Pregnancy-related
Environmental
Drugs (prescription, over-the-counter, herbal, illicit)

Metabolic or endocrine
Infectious, **I**nflammatory, **I**atrogenic, or **I**diopathic
Neoplasm-related (and paraneoplastic syndromes)
Trauma
Surgical or procedure-related

C. **Decide what tests you want to order** to either include or exclude a potential diagnosis. Chapter 2 discusses how to use diagnostic tests in an appropriate manner.

D. **Unifying diagnoses.** It is often hard to recognize a single disease that accounts for all the problems in a complex case. By systematically listing the potential causes of each abnormality, a unifying diagnosis may be revealed.

References

Richardson WS, Glasziou P, Polashenski WA, Wilson MC. A new arrival: evidence about differential diagnosis [Editorial]. ACP Journal Club 2000;133(3):A11–A12.

Saint S, Saha S, Tierney LM. Clinical problem solving: "A square peg in a round hole." N Engl J Med 1998;338:379–383.

Sonnenberg A. When William of Ockham meets Thomas Bayes: finding a few diagnoses among a great many symptoms. Aliment Pharmacol Ther 2001;15(9):1403–1407.

2. Approach to Medical Decision Making

....

I **INTRODUCTION.** Diagnoses tend to exist on the following continuum:

Probability of Disease

0%	100%

Disease absent	Disease present

A. Most diseases listed on an initial differential diagnosis will fall somewhere on this continuum.

B. The goal of the physician is to explain the patient's presentation by moving most diagnoses as far to the left as possible (reasonably excluding them), while moving one diagnosis as far to the right as possible.

C. The inappropriate use of diagnostic tests will leave many diagnoses frustratingly close to the midpoint of the continuum.

II **QUALITATIVE ASSESSMENT.** The degree of certainty required to qualify a diagnosis as "reasonable" depends on:

A. The severity of the condition under consideration

B. The extent to which the condition is treatable

C. The risks associated with diagnostic testing

D. The risks associated with the treatment

III **QUANTITATIVE ASSESSMENT**

A. The **pretest probability** is the probability of disease before testing.

    1. Consider the following three examples:

        a. A 45-year-old man presents to an urgent care clinic with a history of paroxysmal, sharp, left-sided chest pain occurring both at rest and with exercise. He denies chest pressure occurring with exercise. The symptoms have been present for 2 months. A literature search reveals that 50% of 45-year-old men with atypical chest pain have coronary artery disease. Therefore, the pretest probability of coronary artery disease in this patient is 50%.

3

b. If the patient is a 30-year-old woman with atypical chest pain, the pretest probability of coronary artery disease would be 5%.

c. If the patient is a 60-year-old man with exertional chest tightness (typical angina), the pretest probability of coronary artery disease is 95%.

2. Suppose all three of these patients undergo an exercise treadmill test. Is coronary artery disease ruled in if the tests are positive? Is it ruled out if the tests are negative? To answer these questions, it is necessary to consider the likelihood ratio as well.

B. The **likelihood ratio** is the strength of the diagnostic test result.

1. Sensitivity and specificity are the characteristics used most often to define diagnostic tests.

a. **Sensitivity** answers the question, "Among patients with the disease, how likely is a positive test?"

b. **Specificity** answers the question, "Among patients without the disease, how likely is a negative test?"

c. The **likelihood ratio** helps answer the clinically more important questions:

(1) Given a positive test result, how likely is it that the disease is truly present?

(2) Given a negative test result, how likely is it that the disease is truly absent?

2. Mathematically, likelihood ratios are the odds of having a disease given a test result versus not having a disease given a test result.

a. For example:

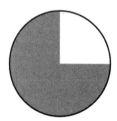

If the circle represents all patients with a positive test and the shaded portion represents the portion who actually have disease, then the likelihood ratio is 3.

$$\frac{\text{The chance of a positive test and disease}}{\text{The chance of a positive test and no disease}} = \frac{3}{1}$$

b. Consider another example. The likelihood ratio of a positive treadmill test is 3.5. In a large, heterogeneous population of patients, all of whom have had positive treadmill tests, 7 patients will actually have coronary artery disease for every 2 patients who do not. Therefore, if your patient has a positive treadmill test, the odds of that person having coronary artery disease are 7 to 2, or 3.5 to 1. That is, given a positive treadmill test, it is **3.5 times as likely** that coronary artery disease is present.

3. Likelihood ratios can be found in epidemiology textbooks or calculated using the following formulas:

$$\text{Likelihood ratio of a positive test} = \frac{\text{True positive rate}}{\text{False positive rate}}$$

$$= \frac{\text{(Sensitivity)}}{\text{(1 − Specificity)}}$$

$$\text{Likelihood ratio of a negative test} = \frac{\text{False negative rate}}{\text{True negative rate}}$$

$$= \frac{\text{(1 − Sensitivity)}}{\text{(Specificity)}}$$

  a. Most diagnostic tests have likelihood ratios in the 2–5 range for positive results and in the 0.5–0.2 range for negative results. These types of tests are only very useful if the pretest probability of disease is in the middle of the scale (e.g., 30%–70%). At either end of the probability scale, diagnostic tests with small likelihood ratios do not change the probability of disease much.

  b. Good tests have positive likelihood ratios of 10 or more. These powerful diagnostic tests help rule in a diagnosis across a broader range of pretest probabilities. Unfortunately, these types of tests are often expensive or dangerous.

  c. For a test to truly rule in disease across the full range of pretest probabilities, it must have a likelihood ratio of 100 or more. Very few tests (e.g., some biopsies, exploratory laparotomy, cardiac catheterization) have likelihood ratios this high.

C. The **posttest probability** is the probability that a specific disease is present after a diagnostic test. Once we have determined the **pretest probability** of disease (using clinical information and disease prevalence data) and the **likelihood ratio** of the diagnostic test result, we are ready to calculate the **posttest probability.** First, however, the pretest probability must be converted to odds (the likelihood ratio is already expressed in odds).

1. Steps
a. Pretest probability must be converted to pretest odds:

$$Odds = \frac{(Probability)}{(1 - Probability)}$$

(For example, a probability of 75% equals odds of 3:1.)

b. Pretest odds are multiplied by the likelihood ratio to give posttest odds.

c. Posttest odds must then be converted back to posttest probability:

$$Probability = \frac{(Odds)}{(Odds + 1)}$$

2. Examples
a. In the 45-year-old man with atypical chest pain and a positive treadmill test, the posttest probability of disease would be 78%:

(1) The 50% pretest probability is converted to pretest odds: $(0.5)/(1 - 0.5) = (0.5)/(0.5) = 1{:}1$.

(2) The 1:1 pretest odds are multiplied by the likelihood ratio (3.5) to yield posttest odds of 3.5:1.

(3) The posttest odds are converted to a posttest probability: $(3.5)/(3.5 + 1) = (3.5)/(4.5) = 0.78$, or 78%. These steps can also be presented schematically:

Pretest probability	Likelihood ratio	Posttest probability
50% ⟶	$\frac{1}{1} \times \frac{3.5}{1} = \frac{3.5}{1}$	⟶ 78%

b. In the 30-year-old woman with atypical chest pain and a positive treadmill test, the posttest probability would be 16%:

Pretest probability	Likelihood ratio	Posttest probability
5% ⟶	$\frac{1}{19} \times \frac{3.5}{1} = \frac{3.5}{19}$	⟶ 16%

c. In the 60-year-old man with typical chest pain and a positive treadmill test, the posttest probability would be 98.5%:

Pretest probability	Likelihood ratio	Posttest probability

$$95\% \longrightarrow \frac{19}{1} \times \frac{3.5}{1} = \frac{66.5}{1} \longrightarrow 98.5\%$$

IV SUMMARY

A. To gain diagnostic strength, several tests may be combined—as long as they are independent tests. The posttest probability after the first test then becomes the pretest probability for the next test.

B. To really learn this approach, you must use it. Try it on your next patient and you'll be familiar with odds before you know it!

References

Kassirer JP, Kopelman RI. Cognitive errors in diagnosis: instantiation, classification, and consequences [Classic article]. Am J Med 1989;86:433–441.

Richardson WS, Wilson MC, Guyatt GH, Cook DJ, Nishikawa J. Users' guides to the medical literature: XV. How to use an article about disease probability for differential diagnosis. Evidence-Based Medicine Working Group. JAMA 1999;281(13): 1214–1219.

Sackett DL, Straus SE, Richardson WS, Rosenberg W, Haynes RB, eds. Evidence-Based Medicine: How to Practice and Teach EBM. 2nd Ed. Edinburgh: Churchill Livingstone, 2000.

3. Palliative Care and Pain Management

I INTRODUCTION

A. Despite our best efforts, patients die. Physicians should be skilled in recognizing and treating impending death.

B. Signs of death. Predicting the time of death is difficult, but certain signs indicate that death is approaching.

    1. When patients with progressive diseases become profoundly weak, bed-bound, confused, or unable to take oral medications or more than a few sips of water, they may have days to live.

    2. When patients experience a rapid decline in their mental status and a "death rattle," they may have hours to live.

    3. As death nears, patients develop mottling, feel cool to the touch, and breathe irregularly. Although cure is no longer possible for such patients, physicians are still morally obligated to care for them; they should seek to palliate rather than cure.

II APPROACH TO THE DYING PATIENT

General Approach to the Dying Patient ("AIM to be a STAR")

MNEMONIC

Assess
Inform
Manage symptoms

Set goals of care
Talk to patient and family
Arrange plans
Reassess often

A. Assess how much the patient and his or her family know about the cause of the patient's decline and prognosis.

B. Inform the patient and family about what you know so they can make well-informed decisions. Do not be afraid to say sensitively that the patient "could die soon" or "is dying."

C. Manage symptoms. Diagnose the cause of each symptom, correct the correctable, and treat using both nonpharmacologic

and pharmacologic measures. Most patients at the end of life experience *at least one* of the symptoms below:
1. **Pain.** There is no reason for patients to suffer pain, given the many useful treatments.
   a. **History.** First formulate an idea of what kind of pain the patient is experiencing. To do so, take the time to obtain a thorough pain history. Remember that pain, like all symptoms, is inherently subjective; therefore, you must generally be guided by the patient's complaints.

Elements of Pain ("PQRST")

Position: Where is the pain located?
Palliative factors: What makes it better?
Provocative factors: What makes it worse?
Prescriptions: What has been tried (medication or otherwise)?
Quality: What does it feel like?
Radiation: Does it travel anywhere?
Severity: On a scale of 0 (no pain) to 10 (worst pain ever), how bad is it? How does it affect function?
Temporal factors: When did it start? Is it constant or intermittent?

*Adapted from Twycross R. Symptom Management in Advanced Cancer. London: Radcliffe Medical Press, 2001.

---

   b. **Examination.** Inspect and palpate the site of pain, looking for associated physical signs (e.g., distention, palpable masses, atrophy, fasciculations, or weakness) to help diagnose the pain.
   c. **Diagnosis.** After obtaining a history and physical examination, classify the patient's pain into one of three categories:
      (1) **Somatic pain** results from activation of pain fibers in cutaneous and deep musculoskeletal tissues and is usually well localized. Causes of somatic pain among dying patients include bone metastases, surgical incisions, and muscle cramping.
      (2) **Visceral pain** results from infiltration, compression, distention, or stretching of thoracic and abdominal viscera. This pain is poorly localized and often described as "deep," "squeezing," or "pressure-like." It can be referred cutaneously. Examples include gastrointestinal obstruction, pancreatitis, urinary retention, or myocardial infarction.

(3) Neuropathic pain results from injury to peripheral nerves, nerve roots, or the spinal cord as the result of tumor infiltration, nerve compression, radiation, surgical trauma, or chemotherapy. It is typically described as a "dull ache" with episodic "burning" or "electric shocks." Neuropathic pain can radiate distally from the site of injury.

d. Treatment

(1) Nonopioid analgesics. Nonopioids are the **therapy of choice for *mild* pain.** For moderate to severe pain, nonopioids are used as **adjuvants** to opioids. All nonopioid analgesics have a **ceiling effect,** after which higher doses produce no improvement in pain. Nonopioids are better for treatment of somatic pain [especially bone pain, which responds reasonably well to nonsteroidal anti-inflammatory drugs (NSAIDs)] than for visceral or neuropathic pain.

(a) Acetaminophen has limited analgesic potency and no notable anti-inflammatory properties. It is relatively safe but can be hepatotoxic and occasionally nephrotoxic. **Limit the total daily dose of acetaminophen to no more than 4 g.**

(b) NSAIDs have both analgesic and anti-inflammatory properties. There are several classes of NSAIDs, to which individuals respond differently. It is worth trying at least one NSAID in every class before completely abandoning NSAIDs as a treatment modality.

(i) NSAID classes. Types of NSAIDs include salicylic acids (aspirin, salsalate), indoleacetic acids (indomethacin, sulindac), propionic acids (ibuprofen, ketoprofen, naproxen), pyrroleacetic acids (diclofenac, ketorolac), benzothiazines (piroxicam), alkanones (nabumetone), and cyclooxygenase-2 (COX-2) inhibitors (celecoxib, rofecoxib).

(ii) Side effects. Possible adverse effects include gastric irritation, nephrotoxicity, hepatotoxicity, and bleeding. NSAIDs should be avoided in persons with gastroduodenopathy, bleeding diathesis, renal insufficiency, severe hypertension, end-stage liver disease, and heart failure.

(2) Opioids. The distinguishing features of these drugs are their **extreme effectiveness for treatment of *moderate to severe* pain** and the **absence of a ceiling effect.** Opioids differ in potency, but they are all equally capable of relieving pain when appropriate dosing is used. They can be prescribed in combination with adjuvant analgesics.

(a) **Opioid dosing** (Table 3–1, Box 3–1)

TABLE 3-1: Usual Starting Doses and Approximate Equianalgesic Doses (ED) of Commonly Used Opioids for Adults

Type of Pain (Rating)	Opioid*	Starting Dose PO	Starting Dose IV	ED PO	ED IV
Mild (1–3)	Codeine	30–60 mg q3–4 hr	—	200 mg	120 mg
Moderate (4–7)	Hydroco-done	5–10 mg q4–6hr	—	30 mg	—
	Oxycodone	10–30 mg q3–4hr	—	20 mg	—
Severe (8–10)	Morphine	15–30 mg q3–4hr	5–10 mg q3–4hr	30 mg	10 mg
	Methadone†	5–10 mg q6–8hr	5–10 mg q6–8hr	20 mg-acute 2–4 mg-chronic	10 mg-acute 2–4 mg-chronic
	Hydro-morphone	4–8 mg q3–4hr	1–2 mg q3–4hr	7.5 mg	1.5 mg
	Fentanyl	—	100 μg q1–2hr	45 mg/d morphine = 25 μg/hr patch q3d	0.1 mg

*Meperidine has been excluded because its toxic metabolites make it an inappropriate drug for repeated dosing.
†Methadone is a very potent opioid whose metabolites accumulate with repeated dosing. Consult a pharmacist before prescribing.
(Adapted from American Pain Society, "Principles of Analgesia Use in the Treatment of Acute Pain and Cancer Pain, 4th ed. Glenview, IL: American Pain Society © 1999).

(b) **Switching routes** may be necessary when the patient gains or loses the ability to swallow (Box 3–2).

(c) **Switching opioids** may be necessary when patients have a poor response, intolerable side effects, or poor compliance (Box 3–3).

BOX 3-1: Opioid Dosing

1. Select an opioid according to the level and type of pain.
2. Select a route according to the patient's circumstances (intravenously if the patient is in severe pain or cannot take oral agents; topically if the patient cannot take oral agents).
3. Prescribe the starting dose, instructing medical staff to "offer, but patient may refuse" every 1–2 hours. Start elderly patients at 50% of the usual starting dose. Have the patient or nurse keep a diary of the frequency of medication requests, pain levels, and duration of effects. Prescribe a daily bowel regimen to avoid constipation.
4. After 24–48 hours, calculate the total 24-hour total dose and distribute that evenly into a regular dosing interval as a "scheduled dose." In addition, prescribe a "breakthrough dose," which is 5%–10% of the 24-hour dose prescribed as "offer, but patient may refuse" every 1–2 hours.
5. Titrate the dose every 24–48 hours until analgesia is achieved or until side effects are intolerable.

H O T

K E Y

No standard opioid dose exists; thus, treatments must be individualized.

BOX 3-2: Switching Routes of Administration When Using Opioids

1. Calculate the 24-hour dose (scheduled + breakthrough).
2. Look up the equianalgesic dose (ED).
3. Calculate the new 24-hour dose using the following formula:

$$\frac{PO\ ED}{IV\ ED} = \frac{24\text{-hr dose PO}}{24\text{-hr dose IV}}$$

4. Distribute the new 24-hour dose into a scheduled dosing regimen and give 5%–10% of the 24-hour dose prescribed as breakthrough every 1–2 hours. Decrease *new* IV doses by 30%.

   (d) Side effects. Possible effects include constipation, sedation, nausea and vomiting, pruritus, and respiratory depression. Tolerance develops over time for all these effects except constipation. If delirium or a hypersensitivity reaction to one opioid develops, switching to another often alleviates the problem.

BOX 3-3: Switching Opioids

Assuming that the same route is used:

1. Calculate the 24-hour current dose (scheduled + breakthrough).
2. Look up the equianalgesic dose (ED).
3. Calculate the new 24-hour dose using the following formula:

$$\frac{\text{Old opioid ED}}{\text{New opioid ED}} = \frac{\text{24-hr dose of old opioid}}{\text{24-hr dose of new opioid}}$$

4. Reduce the 24-hour dose of the new opioid by 30%-50% to account for incomplete cross-tolerance between opioids.
5. Distribute the new 24-hour dose into a scheduled dosing regimen and give 5%-10% of the 24-hour dose prescribed as breakthrough every 1-2 hours.

---

      (3) Anticonvulsant medications (e.g., phenytoin, carbamazepine, valproic acid, gabapentin, clonazepam). These drugs can help manage neuropathic pain described as **"lancinating."**

      (4) Tricyclic antidepressants (e.g., nortriptyline). These drugs can often manage neuropathic pain described as **"burning"** better than anticonvulsants or opioids. Patients should be monitored for anticholinergic side effects.

  2. Dyspnea in terminal patients does not differ from that in nonterminal patients. As with all symptoms, first conduct a thorough history and physical examination, identify the cause, and then select the therapy accordingly (see Chapter 14).

    a. Diagnosis. Common causes include bronchospasm, pulmonary edema, and anxiety.

    b. Treatment should be directed at the cause, if possible.

      (1) Bronchodilators help bronchospasm.

      (2) Morphine (PO or IV) treats resting dyspnea in all patients, except those with neuromuscular disease.

      (3) Oxygen is appropriate for moderately hypoxemic patients (< 90% saturation). For the mildly hypoxemic (90%–94% saturation), the value of oxygen therapy is debatable; sometimes a **fan** is a better option.

      (4) Sedative-hypnotics (e.g., diazepam) in small doses help relieve anxiety contributing to dyspnea not responding to morphine.

      (5) Diuretics (e.g., furosemide) improve pulmonary edema or ascites.

      (6) Thoracentesis reduces dyspnea due to pulmonary effusion.

(7) Paracentesis reduces intra-abdominal pressure in ascites.

(8) Scopolamine patches reduce oral secretions and can alleviate the "death rattle."

(9) Mechanical ventilation should be reserved for patients with a **reasonable chance** of recovering to a functional state that is acceptable to them. Patients with neuromuscular diseases may opt for this mode of therapy because their dyspnea is otherwise resistant to treatment.

3. **Nausea and vomiting** can be very debilitating at the end of life. However, effective control can be achieved in most patients with available treatments. First conduct a thorough history and physical examination, and then identify the cause and select the therapy accordingly.

   a. **History.** Distinguish vomiting from expectoration or regurgitation.

   b. **Examine** for signs of GI obstruction and fecal impaction.

   c. **Diagnosis.** An easy way to remember the causes of vomiting is to use the following mnemonic:

Causes of Vomiting ("11 Ms"):

Metastases (brain metastases, cerebral edema)
Meningeal irritation (meningitis)
Movement (vestibular dysfunction)
Mentation (anxiety, pain)
Medications (chemotherapy, SSRIs, opioids, digoxin, iron, lithium, estrogens, theophylline)
Mucosal irritation (antibiotics, steroids, NSAIDs, alendronate)
Mechanical obstruction (constipation, tumor)
Motility (ileus, gastroparesis, ascites)
Metabolic imbalance (hypercalcemia, hyponatremia)
Microbes (leading to sepsis)
Myocardial dysfunction (myocardial infarction, ischemia)

---

   d. **Treatment.** Correct the correctable, then choose a treatment according to the probable diagnosis (Table 3–2).

4. **Anxiety** is an unpleasant sense of apprehension often accompanied by physical symptoms such as palpitations, chest pain, tingling, trembling, choking, abdominal pain, sweating, and dizziness. Acute anxiety is common but usually temporary among the dying; it is easily treated.

   a. **History.** Discuss the patient's social situation, fears, and emotions. Identify medical factors that may contribute to anxiety such as medications [e.g., steroids, neuroleptics,

TABLE 3-2: Management of Nausea and Vomiting in the Dying Patient		
Cause	**Treatment**	**Common Side Effects**
Movement	Antihistamines	Drowsiness
Microbes	Diphenhydramine	Dry mouth
Myocardial	Meclizine	Constipation
	Hydroxyzine	
	(Promethazine)	
Motion sickness	Anticholinergics	Dry mouth
Mechanical	Scopolamine	Drowsiness
	Hyoscyamine	Constipation
		Urinary retention
		Increased intraocular
		pressure
Metabolic	Steroids	Psychosis
Medications	Dexamethasone	Agitation
	(as adjunct)	
Mental	Benzodiazepines	Drowsiness
	Lorazepam	Lethargy
	(as adjunct)	
Metabolic	Phenothiazines	Extrapyramidal
Meningeal	Prochlorperazine	symptoms
Medications	Promethazine	Dystonia
Myocardial	Butyrophenones	Hypotension
Motility	Haloperidol	
	Droperidol	
	Metoclopramide	
Medications	Serotonin antagonist	Headache
	Ondansetron	Somnolence
	Granisetron	

selective serotonin reuptake inhibitors (SSRIs), stimulants], withdrawal (e.g., alcohol, antidepressants, benzodiazepines), pain, insomnia, dyspnea, or hypoglycemia.
   b. Treatment. Correct the correctable conditions: relieve pain, correct misconceptions, provide reassurance, and discontinue anxiety-inducing medications. Consider formal psychological support. Pharmacologic treatment may include:
      (1) Benzodiazepines (e.g., diazepam, lorazepam)
      (2) Antidepressants for contributing depression (e.g., paroxetine)
      (3) Antipsychotics when accompanied by a thought disorder (e.g., mirtazapine)
   5. Depression. Grief is an acceptable response to bad news and progressive decline, but depression is not. It is important to

identify depression when it occurs because it is highly treatable (> 80% of patients improve).

a. **History.** Assess if the patient has felt depressed or "blue." To distinguish depression from grief, ask about anhedonia, altered sleep, altered appetite, suicidal ideations, fatigue, psychomotor agitation/retardation, impaired concentration, or feelings of worthlessness. Feelings of depression plus at least four of these symptoms confirm depression.

b. **Treatment.** Provide therapy for correctable conditions: relieve pain; discontinue depression-inducing medications (e.g., steroids, chemotherapy, phenothiazines, antihypertensives); treat hypokalemia and hypercalcemia; and rule out hyperparathyroidism, hypoparathyroidism, Cushing's syndrome, and hyperprolactinemia. Schedule formal psychological support. In addition, consider using the following agents:

   (1) **SSRIs** (e.g., paroxetine, sertraline, citalopram, fluoxetine), starting at the smallest dose, titrating upward every 2 weeks.

   (2) **Tricyclics** (e.g., nortriptyline, amitriptyline); add them to SSRIs if necessary.

   (3) **Psychostimulants** (methylphenidate) are useful in patients with psychomotor retardation, poor appetite, and fatigue. These drugs are usually effective within days of initiation.

6. **Constipation** is common, especially in patients taking opioids.

   a. **History.** Factors that may contribute to constipation include medications (opioids, anticholinergics, tricyclics, SSRIs, antacids, diuretics, anticonvulsants, statins, calcium channel blockers), neurologic disorders (nerve compression, neuropathy), age, inactivity, inability to get to the toilet, lack of privacy, change in diet, dehydration, and depression.

   b. **Physical examination.** Check for obstruction and fecal impaction.

   c. **Diagnosis.** Rule out hypercalcemia and hypokalemia.

   d. **Treatment** (the "4 Ds"–see next page)

7. **Fatigue** is the most common symptom at the end of life. Because little is known about its mechanism, treatment may be less successful.

   a. **Diagnosis.** Identify treatable causes such as hypothyroidism, anemia, depression, anxiety, pain, infection, medications (e.g., chemotherapy, antihypertensives), insomnia, and hypoxemia.

   b. **Treatment**

      (1) **Corticosteroids** (dexamethasone 2–20 mg PO every

Treatment of Constipation ("4 Ds")

Daily administration of a stool softener (docusate) *plus* a motility agent (bisacodyl or senna), increasing the dose every 2–3 days for a bowel movement at least once every 48 hours. Avoid fiber.
Disimpact if necessary
Discontinue or reduce constipating agents
Definitive: Try lactulose orally or glycerin or bisacodyl rectally. Use enemas or polyethylene glycol (1 L PO/NG once) in refractory cases.

morning) can improve mood, energy, and appetite temporarily. Long-term sequelae are not of concern. Prevent thrush with nystatin 1 teaspoon swish-and-swallow three times daily.

(2) **Psychostimulants** (methylphenidate 5 mg PO twice daily) can improve mood, energy, and appetite rapidly, but the effect of these drugs is variable.

D. **Set goals of care.** Assess what the patient and family are hoping for given the situation.

E. **Talk to patient and family.** Never break bad news or discuss grave matters without offering the patient the opportunity to be accompanied by loved ones. Provide a proper setting with privacy, space, and plenty of tissues.

F. **Arrange plans** based on the goals set by the patient and family. Address the following seven elements:

1. A **living will** gives the patient the opportunity to present his or her preferences regarding life-sustaining treatment. It takes effect only when the patient loses decision-making capacity and can be revoked by the patient or their proxy at any time, either in writing or verbally. A living will is not equivalent to a Last Will and Testament.

2. **Durable power of attorney for health care (DPAHC)** allows a patient to appoint a proxy (or proxies) to decide on his or her behalf; it takes effect only when the patient loses decision-making capacity. In most states, the authority of the durable power of attorney for health care supersedes the living will. Many patients confuse the durable power of attorney for health care with the executor of their will or their financial power of attorney, but they are not necessarily the same.

3. **Do not resuscitate (DNR) and do not intubate (DNI) orders.** These instructions order physicians *not* to attempt cardiopulmonary resuscitation (CPR) or intubation in the event

of cardiopulmonary arrest. **They are the only way to prevent CPR; a living will is not sufficient to prevent CPR.**

    a. It is the physician's responsibility to write DNR or DNI orders as soon as the patient or the DPAHC refuses CPR, or the physician believes that CPR would be futile.[1]

    b. The issue of DNR can be raised by asking, "Should you die in spite of our best efforts, do you want us to use heroic measures to attempt to bring you back?" If the patient declines CPR, you should document your discussion and encourage him or her to complete a living will or appoint a DPAHC if the patient has not done so already. **Even if the patient refuses to sign a living will, this plan is valid as long as the discussion is documented in the record.** A physician may even ask a patient to sign a statement that they both believe reflects their discussion.

4. Hospice supports the patient and family through dying and bereavement. Its mission is to relieve physical, emotional, social, and spiritual suffering. Hospice can provide care at home, hospice facilities, hospitals, or nursing homes. Often hospices limit their care to patients with a life expectancy of 6 months who have agreed to a DNR order.

5. Palliative care, like hospice, seeks to relieve physical, emotional, social, and spiritual suffering. Unlike hospice, palliative care cares for all patients, regardless of their diagnosis or life expectancy, and is typically offered in hospitals or hospital-affiliated clinics. Palliative care is appropriate for patients who are chronically or terminally ill, to bridge the gap between curative therapy and hospice care.

6. "Comfort care" describes care focusing on comfort rather than cure. When patients and families choose to pursue "comfort care only," it is appropriate to discontinue all medications and treatments that do not directly relieve symptoms (e.g., taking of vital signs; administration of antihypertensives, hypoglycemics, hormone replacement therapy, and anticoagulants).

7. Life support. Any therapy used to sustain life is considered life support, including, but not limited to, artificial nutrition and hydration, mechanical ventilation, dialysis, and implantable defibrillators. According to the U.S. Supreme Court, all competent patients and their proxies have the right to refuse or stop life support (even after it has been initiated). If a family decides to withdraw life support, make sure they understand that there are several potential outcomes: rapid death within minutes (e.g., patients who have vasopressors with-

---

[1]Hospitals differ regarding their futility policies; thus, it is important to know your institution's futility policy.

drawn); death within hours to days; or continued cardiopulmonary function. Assure them that the patient's comfort is paramount.

G. Reassess often. As illness advances, patients experience varying physical and psychological symptoms and, as a result, may change their priorities, goals, and plans. For this reason, it is important to reassess and re-inform often; the frequency of communication should be determined by the speed of decline.

III AFTER DEATH

A. Pronouncement. A licensed physician is responsible for pronouncing death and comforting the family. If you are called to "pronounce" someone, introduce yourself, offer condolences, and explain why you are there. Offer the family the opportunity to stay if they wish while you examine their loved one. Then do the following:

1. Identify the patient by the hospital identification tag.
2. Ascertain that the patient is nonresponsive to verbal or tactile stimuli (a sternal rub is sufficient).
3. Confirm absence of heart sounds and pulse.
4. Look and listen for spontaneous respirations for at least 1 minute.
5. Document pupillary size and absence of a light reflex.
6. Record the time of your assessment as the time of death.

B. Responding to grief. Grief is a normal response to loss or impending loss. Encourage open discussion, acknowledge feelings, and offer reassurance that grief is normal. Follow up with written condolences, a telephone call, and an appointment, as appropriate. Warn the grieving family that vivid dreams and tearful memories of the departed loved one may persist for several months and that a loss of interest in outside activities will likely persist for 3–6 months. Offer a referral to grief counseling for ongoing support.

References
End of Life Physician Education Resource Center (EPERC). www.eperc.mcw.edu
Garvin J, Chapman RC. Clinical management of dying patients. West J Med 1995; 163:268–277.
Levy MH. Pharmacologic treatment of cancer pain. N Engl J Med 1996;335(15): 1124–1132.

4. Preventing Hospital-Acquired Complications

I. INTRODUCTION

A. As many as **10% of inpatients** experience harm unrelated to any underlying illness during their hospital stay. Up to **2% of hospitalized patients** experience either a major permanent injury or death as a result of their medical care.

B. Although clinicians have long recognized the hazards of hospitalization, patient safety has only recently received widespread attention.

C. The term **adverse event** refers to any injury caused by medical care, not an underlying illness.

  1. Identifying something as an adverse event does not imply "error" or poor-quality care. However, errors may cause many adverse events.

  2. Thus, just as physicians target blood pressure control to reduce myocardial infarction and stroke, targeting errors play a role in preventing many adverse events.

HOT KEY

On patient problem lists, include a section focused on the prevention of nosocomial complications as the last item (e.g., thromboembolism prophylaxis, complications of indwelling catheters, development of pressure ulcers, provision of adequate nutrition).

II. HOSPITAL-ACQUIRED COMPLICATIONS AND THEIR PREVENTION

A. Adverse drug event (ADE)

  1. Definition

    a. An ADE refers to **any adverse clinical effect resulting from a drug.** This broad term includes minor drug rashes and major reactions such as bone marrow suppression, hepatic failure, and anaphylaxis. It also combines **expected adverse reactions** (i.e., "side effects" occurring when a drug is used in standard doses to achieve accepted therapeutic goals) and **harm resulting from medication errors** (e.g., dosing errors, prescription of medication to which a patient has a documented allergy, or ordering a medication for the wrong patient, as can easily happen in the hospital setting).

b. The issue of preventability is more important than the distinction between ADEs that are "side effects" and those that are due to errors.

c. An ADE can reflect factors arising at **any stage of the medication use process,** although drug ordering accounts for approximately 50% of ADEs.

2. **Incidence. At least 5% of hospitalized patients** experience an ADE. An additional **5%–10% of hospitalized patients** experience a **potential ADE** (i.e., a medication error occurs but fortuitously, no harm results).

3. **Prevention.** Many ADE's, whether "side effects" or the result of errors, can be anticipated and therefore, prevented from occurring or, at least, ameliorated, if they do occur.

a. Medication information. Keep a trustworthy medication resource—whether in a paper-based, electronic handheld, or computer-based form—with you at all times and use it to verify standard doses, routes of administration, contraindications, and adverse effects. When such a resource is not readily available or fails to address a specific issue, seek the advice of a pharmacist.

HOT

An important contraindication to any medication is physician lack of familiarity with it.

KEY

---

(1) For elderly patients and patients receiving multiple medications, periodically review orders for potential drug interactions.

(2) Be particularly careful with human immunodeficiency virus (HIV) medications, immunosuppressant drugs, anticoagulants, and chemotherapeutic agents (all of which you may be called on to write orders for), and be cautious with all medications in patients with renal or hepatic dysfunction.

b. Ordering. Write all orders legibly (print if you have to), avoid abbreviations, and watch out for decimals (Table 4-1).

(1) Avoid abbreviations for drug names to reduce the risk of misinterpretation [e.g., HCTZ (hydrochlorothiazide) versus HCT (hydrocortisone), MSO_4 (morphine) versus $MgSO_4$ (magnesium sulfate), CPZ (Compazine versus chlorpromazine)]

(2) Always write complete and specific orders. Do not

TABLE 4-1. Prescription Order Writing: Do's and Don'ts		
Do	**Do Not**	**Explanation**
0.5 mg	.5 mg	The leading zero avoids a 10-fold overdose caused by an overlooked decimal point
5 mg	5.0 mg	Dropping the trailing zero avoids a 10-fold overdose caused by an overlooked decimal point
NPH Insulin 10 units	NPH Insulin 10 U	"U" can be misread as a trailing zero
Synthroid 100 mcg	Synthroid 100 μg	"μg" is more likely to be misread as "mg" for milligram
Coumadin 5 mg PO every other day	Coumadin 5 mg PO qod	"qod" can easily be misread as "qd" For handwritten orders, many sources now recommend dropping all abbreviations for frequency (e.g., qd, bid) in favor of such terms as "once daily" and "twice daily"
Change ranitidine 150 mg PO bid to 50 mg IV q8h	Change ranitidine PO to IV	Not writing out full order risks inappropriate "carry over" drug strength and frequency

drop units, omit frequencies, or leave route of administration unspecified (see Table 4-1).

(3) **Never write blanket orders** such as "continue all preop meds."

(4) **Always check for drug allergies;** do not assume someone else has done so.

(5) **Always check the patient's name** at the top of the record (chart or computer-based) before writing an order. It is easy to pick up the wrong chart or walk away from the computer for a minute and not realize that someone has opened another patient's electronic record.

c. **Transcription** is out of your hands, but be aware that such errors occur and can affect patient care, especially during transitions [e.g., transfer in or out of an intensive care unit (ICU)].

HOT KEY Periodically check the nursing medication administration records to make sure that patients are receiving their ordered medications by the prescribed route and in the intended doses.

    d. Dispensing errors [e.g., mix-ups in the central pharmacy that result in the wrong medication being sent to the floor or an incorrect concentration of an intravenous (IV) medication being compounded] are also out of your hands, but recognize that such mistakes can occur.

        (1) For example, supposing pulseless ventricular tachycardia develops in a patient in the ICU. The tracing is suggestive of "torsades de pointes," and the event occurred after the nurse had performed a "flush" of the patient's central venous line.

        (2) The physician empirically administers calcium and insulin as treatment for hyperkalemia, which restores sinus rhythm.

        (3) Laboratory results later confirm hyperkalemia, and further investigation reveals that the intended normal saline flush had in fact been concentrated potassium.

HOT KEY When evaluating an unexpected clinical event, consider the possibility of error in the differential diagnosis.

    e. Administration errors are mostly out of your hands (e.g., programming errors for the IV pump administering patient-controlled analgesia or concentrated electrolyte solution), but recognize that they occur.

        (1) Physician administration. Sometimes you will be called on to administer a drug **because nurses are not supposed to administer it** at all (e.g., adenosine) or by "IV push" (e.g., fentanyl on many general hospital wards).

HOT KEY Do not treat calls to administer medication (e.g., IV metoprolol on a general ward) as an annoying formality. Make sure you actually know how to administer the medication, including speed of administration, need for central line versus peripheral line, compatibility with other medications, and responses to possible complications.

(2) Automated dispensing machines. Medications stored and dispensed in automated machines can end up in the wrong drawer, leading to dangerous drug substitutions. Multiuse vials can be mistaken for one another (e.g., heparin and insulin look enough alike, and several deaths have been reported due to "line flushes" with insulin instead of heparin).

   f. Anticipate preventable complications and ameliorate nonpreventable ones

      (1) Verapamil administration

         (a) Digoxin toxicity occurs after the administration of verapamil. Because verapamil is known to increase serum digoxin levels, this represents a **preventable ADE;** digoxin doses can be adjusted prospectively, and serum digoxin levels can be monitored closely to take this drug interaction into account.

         (b) Hypotension results after the IV administration of verapamil for acute heart rate control. As long as dosing and administration conform to standard practice, this development would generally be considered a **nonpreventable** ADE. The goal in such cases is to ameliorate the ADE by responding in an appropriate and timely manner (e.g., IV fluids or IV calcium to restore hemodynamic stability).

      (2) Steroids

         (a) A **vertebral compression fracture** occurs in a patient with chronic obstructive pulmonary disease (COPD) who is administered chronic steroids. This complication should be anticipated and is a **preventable** ADE, because the concomitant prescription of a bisphosphonate can significantly reduce the risk of osteoporotic fracture.

         (b) Psychosis occurs in a patient with COPD who is administered steroids. This is a **nonpreventable** ADE. However, appropriate care ameliorates the ADE with early recognition of this complication and cessation or rapid tapering of the steroids.

B. Venous thromboembolism (VTE)

   1. Definition. Nosocomial VTE mostly commonly includes lower extremity deep venous thrombosis (DVT) but also includes pulmonary embolism and upper extremity DVT.

   2. Incidence. VTE may be as common among medical as among surgical patients. One recent study found that 15% of acutely ill medical patients had DVT. In addition to immobility, central venous catheters contribute to hospital-acquired thromboses.

>
> **HOT KEY** Nonmobile medical patients should receive some form of VTE prophylaxis, be it pharmacologic (e.g., unfractionated heparin, low-molecular-weight heparin, warfarin) or mechanical (e.g., compression stockings).

3. **Prevention.** Optimal strategies for preventing VTE in medical patients remain to be established. For now, reasonable choices in hospitalized patients who are not yet ambulating at least once per day are:
   a. Low-dose subcutaneous unfractionated heparin (e.g., heparin 5000 units subcutaneously twice daily)
   b. Low-molecular-weight heparin (e.g., enoxaparin 40 mg subcutaneously once daily)
   c. Pneumatic compression stockings

C. **Falls**
   1. **Incidence.** Inpatient falls occur at a rate of 0.5–3 per bed per year. **Hip fractures** are the most feared complication of falls. Up to 20% of patients sustaining a hip fracture become nonambulatory, and many of these individuals lose their ability to carry out instrumental activities of daily living.
   2. **Risk factors.** Presence of handrails and no-slip bathing surfaces may mitigate the risk of falls or fall-related injury. Factors associated with hospitals such as unfamiliar rooms, improper bed height, and sedating medications may exacerbate risk. Acute illness itself and deconditioning from being bedridden also increase the risk of falls.
   3. **Prevention.** Various strategies exist for assessing patients at high risk for falls and addressing these risks. There is also growing interest in hip protectors.
      a. **Avoid using sedating or disorienting medications.**
      b. **Limit use of restraints and handrails,** which may paradoxically increase risks of falls or the severity of fall-related injuries.

> **HOT KEY** At a minimum, identify patients at high risk for falls and discuss possible interventions with nursing staff (e.g., closer monitoring of patient, placing bed as low to ground as possible, use of bed alarms if available).

D. **Radiocontrast-induced nephropathy (RCIN)**
   1. **Definition**
      a. Specific definitions vary, but clinically significant RCIN typically requires a 50% increase in serum creatinine (SCr) or a 1.0 mg/dl increase in SCr within 48 hours of intravascular radiocontrast exposure.

b. The hallmark of RCIN is that it resolves quickly (within 7–10 days) and rarely requires specific therapy.
2. Incidence. Risk factors for RCIN include diabetes, chronic renal insufficiency, decreased effective circulating volume of any cause, and multiple myeloma.
    a. For patients **with no risk factors,** the incidence is almost zero.
    b. For patients **with risk factors,** the incidence ranges from 5%–40%, depending on the number and severity of risk factors. RCIN occurs in more than 50% of patients with SCr > 4.0 mg/dl.
3. Treatment. Dialysis is rarely required, and even then, it is usually temporary. Thus, concern about RCIN should not prevent necessary investigations that involve contrast.
4. Prevention. Despite the mild and temporary nature of RCIN, increased monitoring and delays in other aspects of care make prevention worthwhile.
    a. Avoid drugs that decrease renal perfusion [e.g., non-steroidal anti-inflammatory drugs (NSAIDs)][1]
    b. Avoid hypovolemia, especially in patients with diabetes *or* preexisting renal problems. Typical protocols for ensuring adequate volume status consist of normal saline administered at 75 ml/hr for 12 hours pre- and post-procedure or ingestion of 1 L of water within 10 hours before the procedure, followed by IV normal saline for 6 hours after the procedure.
    c. For high-risk patients (e.g., diabetics with moderate renal insufficiency), **consider using low-osmolar contrast agents or limiting the volume of contrast** (< 75–125 ml). Also, avoid repeated contrast exposures within 48–72 hours.
    d. For any patients with chronic renal insufficiency, **consider acetylcysteine** in addition to IV saline. The drug is administered as powder-containing capsules or diluted in soda or juice. Give 600 mg orally twice daily on the day before and after the procedure. If only one dose is given before the procedure, give three doses afterward.
E. Stress-related upper gastrointestinal hemorrhage (UGIH)
    1. Incidence
        a. Clinically significant UGIH occurs in only approximately 0.1% of low-risk ICU patients and approximately 3.0% of ventilated patients.

---

[1]Although not a prophylactic strategy per se, metformin is usually discontinued before any procedure that may affect renal function and resumed only when normal renal function is verified. Thus, metformin is commonly discontinued in diabetic patients who undergo cardiac catheterization at least 12 hours before the procedure.

b. General improvements in ICU care and greater focus on clinically significant events have substantially reduced the frequency of stress-induced gastric ulceration among ICU patients.

2. Prevention. Although a statistical benefit of H_2-antagonists has been shown in some studies, the overall clinical benefit of stress-ulcer prophylaxis in unselected patients is equivocal.

HOT KEY Do not reflexively prescribe anti-acid medications to all ICU patients. Focus on patients with risk factors for UGIH: respiratory failure, coagulopathy, renal failure, and significant burns.

---

a. For patients without specific risk factors for UGIH, **provide enteral nutrition;** this is probably the best method of prevention.

b. H_2-antagonists are probably superior to sucralfate in preventing stress-related GI bleeding but may increase the risk of ventilator-associated pneumonia.

c. Unfortunately, the proper role of proton pump inhibitors is currently unclear.

F. Catheter-related urinary tract infection (UTI)

1. Incidence. Catheterized patients develop bacteriuria at a rate of 3%–10% per day. Among patients with bacteriuria, 10%–25% develop UTI symptoms such as suprapubic or flank pain, and approximately 3% develop bacteremia.

HOT KEY Make sure you know which of your patients have a urinary catheter and why they still have one.

---

2. Prevention. Remove indwelling catheters as soon as possible.

a. Urinary catheters may not only lead to infection but are a source of significant discomfort and embarrassment to many patients.

b. Condom catheters may not lower the risk of UTIs, but they are more comfortable for male patients.

c. Some evidence supports the overall effectiveness (including the cost-effectiveness) of silver-coated urinary catheters. Silver alloy catheters should be considered for certain patients requiring urinary catheterization between 2 and 10 days.

G. Pressure (decubitus) ulcers. Complications include cellulitis, osteomyelitis, sepsis, and even death.

1. **Incidence**
   a. From 3%–10% of hospitalized patients have pressure ulcers; approximately 60% of these developed in the hospital as opposed to being present on admission from a nursing facility or home care setting.
   b. The prevalence is much higher for immobilized patients; about 30% of elderly patients with a fractured hip develop pressure ulcers in the postoperative period.
2. **Prevention**
   a. **Inspect all hospitalized patients for early signs of pressure ulcers** such as erythema over key pressure points (e.g., sacrum, greater trochanter, ischial tuberosity, malleolus, heel, scapula).
   b. **Identify patients at risk for development of pressure ulcers** by checking for immobility (e.g., due to neurologic disorder or fracture), malnutrition, fecal or urinary incontinence, and altered level of consciousness. Patients at risk for pressure ulcers should have pillows placed beneath the calves, foam foot protection, or a soft foam or air waffle mattress.
   c. **Make sure patients who are unable to move around in bed are "turned" or repositioned** every 2 hours.
H. **Central venous catheter (CVC)-related infection**
   1. **Incidence.** Among patients with a standard CVC in place for 1 week or more, approximately 25% develop catheter colonization and 5% become bacteremic. Catheter-related bloodstream infections occur at a rate of about 5 per 1000 catheter-days in medical and surgical ICUs.
   2. **Prevention**
      a. **Use maximum sterile barrier precautions** during CVC insertion, with sterile gloves, a long-sleeved gown, a full-sized drape, and a nonsterile mask cap, rather than just a small drape and gloves.
      b. **Use chlorhexidine gluconate** rather than povidone-iodine for antiseptic cleaning of the insertion site.
      c. In patients at high risk for infection (e.g., ICU patients), consider using a CVC coated with an antimicrobial agent.
      d. **Subclavian** and **internal jugular** sites have a lower risk of infection than femoral insertion. However, in urgent situations, if you do not feel comfortable working at these insertion sites it is better to place a femoral catheter. When adequate supervision is available, a subclavian or internal jugular line can be placed if a CVC will be required for more than 48 hours.
      e. **Remove the CVC as soon as the clinical indication resolves.** Do not continue with the CVC simply for convenience, es-

pecially if the patient is going to be transferred to a regular floor, where knowledge of CVC care is variable.

HOT KEY Always place the patient in the supine position when removing a CVC from the subclavian or internal jugular sites; the risk of air embolism is not a myth.

I. **Ventilator-associated pneumonia (VAP).** The effect of VAP on clinical outcomes varies depending on the organisms involved and comorbid conditions. Nonetheless, VAP is an important complication that affects patient care.
   1. **Incidence.** The cumulative incidence is approximately 1%–3% per day of intubation. In clinical practice, VAP is usually diagnosed on the basis of radiographic findings or positive endotracheal, pleural, or blood cultures in the setting of fever, leukocytosis, or purulent tracheal secretions.
   2. **Prevention.** Several strategies show promise in terms of significantly reducing the incidence of VAP, but most involve practice changes for an entire ICU, such as using special endotracheal tubes that remove subglottic secretions, selective digestive tract decontamination, and rotation of empiric antibiotic regimens.

HOT KEY Unless contraindicated (e.g., hemodynamic instability), elevate head of the bed to 45° for the duration of mechanical ventilation; this is a simple and effective strategy for reducing VAP.

III **GENERAL ERRORS.** Although the complications described in II should be considered in the care of hospitalized patients, more general opportunities for serious errors and complications should also be kept in mind.

A. **Pay attention to internal warning signals**
   1. **Haste produces iatrogenesis.** When you notice yourself feeling overwhelmed, rushed, or pressed for time (e.g., you cannot possibly handle all of your work), step back and take a few minutes to gather your thoughts.
   2. **If you need a hand, ask for it.** Do not make being a "strong" student or resident your first priority. When you are in over your head, admit you need someone to walk you through a procedure or that you have fallen too far behind on call to handle all of the waiting admissions.

B. Communicate with nurses, pharmacists, and physicians from other services involved in your patients' care. Many minor errors, as well as some spectacular errors (e.g., taking the wrong patient for a procedure), occur because of poor communication among physicians or between physicians and nurses.

1. **Communicate important changes in patient care plans to all clinical personnel,** including closely involved outpatient physicians.
2. Conversely, if you are surprised to find a new order or care plan for your patient, **do not assume** that a clinician has simply devised a new plan and not told you. **Check out the new plan** yourself.

C. Communicate clearly with patients in a manner they understand. Nearly 25% of adults in the United States are functionally illiterate, and even more have inadequate **health literacy.** More than 50% of patients seen in public hospitals do not understand common medical terms such has "malignant," "terminal," or even "orally." Basic medication instructions such as "take every 6 hours" or "take on an empty stomach" are poorly understood by at least 25% of patients, and more than 50% cannot reliably interpret a blood sugar reading.

1. **Slow down and use "living room" language** instead of medical terminology; show or draw pictures whenever possible.
2. **Ask, "Can you tell me what we have just gone through?" or other such "teach back" approaches to confirm understanding.** Do not simply ask, "Do you understand?"; usually, the answer will be, "Yes," regardless of the amount of comprehension.
3. **Limit information conveyed during a single interaction.** Do not overwhelm patients with information, especially in the emergency department, ICU, or a first-time meeting in the middle of the night.

References

Collard HR, Saint S, Mathay MA. Prevention of ventilator-associated pneumonia: an evidence-based systematic review. Ann Intern Med 2003; 138(6):494–501.

Gazmararian JA, Baker DW, Williams MV, et al. Health literacy among Medicare enrollees in a managed care organization. JAMA 1999;281:545–551.

Messori A, Trippoli S, Vaiani M, et al. Bleeding and pneumonia in intensive care patients given ranitidine and sucralfate for prevention of stress ulcer: meta-analysis of randomised controlled trials. BMJ 2000;321:1103–1106.

Mismetti P, Laporte-Simitsidis S, Tardy B, et al. Prevention of venous thromboembolism in internal medicine with unfractionated or low-molecular-weight heparins: a meta-analysis of randomised clinical trials. Thromb Haemost 2000;83:14–19.

Saint S, Savel RH, Matthay MA. Enhancing the safety of critically ill patients by reducing urinary and central venous catheter-related infections. Am J Respir Crit Care Med 2002;165:1475–1479.

Shojania KG, Wald H, Gross R. Understanding medical error and improving patient safety in the inpatient setting. Med Clin North Am 2002;86(4):63–83.

Tepel M, van der Giet M, Schwarzfeld C, et al. Prevention of radiographic contrast agent-induced reductions in renal function by acetylcysteine. N Engl J Med 2000; 343:180–184.

PART II

CARDIOLOGY

5. Electrocardiogram (ECG) Interpretation

I **INTRODUCTION.** There is no absolute right order for interpreting ECGs, but it is important to choose a method and interpret each ECG in precisely the same way. One common approach is to evaluate ECG findings in the following order: rhythm, rate, axis, intervals, hypertrophy, Q waves, and ST/T wave changes.

II **RHYTHM**

A. Normal sinus rhythm. If each normal P wave (atrial depolarization) is followed by a QRS complex (ventricular depolarization) and the heart rate is between 60 and 100 beats/min, then the patient is in normal sinus rhythm. A "normal" P wave is positively deflected (or above the baseline) in lead II and negatively deflected in lead aVF.

B. Tachycardia is a heart rate greater than 100 beats/min (see Chapter 7).

C. Bradycardia is a heart rate less than 60 beats/min.
   1. **Sinus bradycardia.** Each QRS complex is preceded by a normal P wave.
   2. Other forms of bradycardia [e.g., atrioventricular (AV) nodal block] are discussed in V A 2.

III **RATE**

A. Regular rhythm. If the patient is in sinus rhythm, the easiest way to calculate the heart rate is to divide 300 by the number of large boxes between two successive QRS complexes. (Each large box is composed of five small boxes, each of which represents 0.04 second.)

B. Irregular rhythm. If the patient has an irregular rhythm, divide a few consecutive beats (e.g., 4–6) by the number of large boxes between them to get an average of the time between beats. Divide 300 by this average to get the heart rate.

C. Bradycardia. If the patient's heart rate is very slow, it is easy to see how many beats occurred over a 10-second period. Multiply the number by 6 to obtain the number of beats per minute. (Ten-second periods are usually marked on the ECG and are equivalent to 50 large boxes.)

TABLE 5-1. Using the ECG to Determine Heart Rate for Patients in Sinus Rhythm*

Number of Boxes	Corresponding Heart Rate
1	300 beats/min
2	150 beats/min
3	100 beats/min
4	75 beats/min

*Divide 300 by the number of large boxes between two successive QRS complexes.

 Axis. The QRS axis, typically measured in the frontal plane, is the net vector generated by all ventricular depolarization. The exact degree of the vector (axis) is not clinically useful— it is only necessary to determine whether the axis is normal, shifted left, or shifted right. Left and right axis shifts suggest disease of the ventricular myocardium.

A. Normal axis. A normal axis is between −30° and +90° when plotted using a hexaxial reference system. Anything more negative than −30° is called a leftward or superior axis (because the axis is moving left toward the 12 o'clock position), and anything more positive than +90° is a rightward axis.

B. Determining axis (Figure 5–1). By inspecting the QRS complex in each limb lead, you can narrow down where the net vector (QRS axis) is pointing.

C. To evaluate axis, it is only necessary to look at limb leads I and II.

1. Normal axis. Both lead I and lead II are positive.

2. Leftward axis. Lead I is positive and lead II is negative.

3. Rightward axis. Lead I is negative and lead II is positive.

4. Indeterminate axis. Both lead I and lead II are negative.

D. Causes of axis deviation

1. Left axis deviation (LAD). Left anterior fascicular block and inferior wall myocardial infarction account for most cases of LAD.

A

B

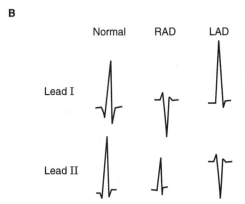

FIGURE 5-1. (A) Determining axis. If the QRS complex of lead I is net positive (i.e., the area above the horizontal is greater than the area below), the axis must lie somewhere in the *gray shaded* region. If lead II is net positive, then the axis must lie in the *cross-hatched* region. The area of overlap denotes the range for a normal axis. (B) Appearance of the QRS complex in leads I and II in left axis deviation (*LAD*), right axis deviation (*RAD*), and normal axis.

a. Left anterior fascicular block
  (1) Pathogenesis. The left bundle splits into anterior and posterior fascicles. The anterior fascicle runs superiorly; therefore, when the anterior fascicle is blocked, the muscle that it serves must be depolarized from inferior forces. These "extra" inferior to superior forces rotate the axis leftward (i.e., superiorly).
  (2) Criteria for diagnosis include an axis between $-45°$ and $-90°$; a qR pattern in leads I and aVL; a rS pattern in leads II, III, and aVF; and a QRS complex less than 0.12 second in duration.
  (a) An axis of $-30°$ to $-45°$ may represent left anterior fascicular block if the other criteria are present.
  (b) Because lead aVL is located near the left anterior fascicle (at approximately $-30°$), a block in the left anterior fascicle causes initial forces to move away from lead aVL, producing the qR pattern and delay in peak time.

b. Inferior wall myocardial infarction
  (1) Pathogenesis. Dead tissue at the inferior aspect of the left ventricle does not conduct; therefore, more net forces move superiorly (or leftward).
  (2) Criteria for diagnosis. Look for abnormal Q waves in the inferior leads (i.e., leads II, III, and aVF) to make the diagnosis.

c. Posteroseptal accessory pathway. Look for negative delta waves in the inferior leads, a short PR interval (less than 0.12 second in duration), and a tall R wave in lead V2.

d. Chronic obstructive pulmonary disease (COPD). A lower diaphragm can move the right ventricle below the larger left ventricle and cause more superior forces. However, when accompanied by pulmonary hypertension, COPD often produces right axis deviation (RAD).

e. Congenital heart disease (e.g., primum-type atrial septal defect, ventricular septal defect)

f. Hyperkalemia (usually severe)

g. Pulmonary embolus can produce LAD but more often produces RAD.

h. Normal variant

2. Right axis deviation (RAD)

a. Right ventricular hypertrophy. RAD is caused by right ventricular hypertrophy until proven otherwise. (Criteria for right ventricular hypertrophy are discussed in VI B).

b. Acute cor pulmonale (e.g., pulmonary embolus, acute bronchospasm). Look for a shift of axis to the right of more than $30°$ when compared with a prior ECG.

   c. **Extensive lateral wall myocardial infarction.** Look for Q waves in leads I and aVL.

   d. **Lateral wall accessory pathway.** Look for a short PR interval.

   e. **Left posterior fascicular block** should be considered a diagnosis of exclusion. **Criteria for diagnosis** include an axis between +90° and +180°; a rS pattern in leads I and aVL; a qR pattern in leads II, III, and aVF; and a QRS complex less than 0.12 second in duration.

   f. **Lead reversal.** Look for an inverted P wave in lead I.

   g. **Pneumothorax**

   h. **Normal variant** (in young people)

V INTERVALS

A. PR interval. The PR interval is normally between 0.12 second and 0.20 second in duration. The appropriate measurement is actually from the beginning of the P wave to the beginning of the Q wave, not the R wave.

   1. A **short PR interval** is often caused by a high catecholamine state that makes the AV node conduct faster; however, you should look for delta waves to rule out an accessory pathway.

   2. A **prolonged PR interval** is associated with increased vagal tone or more permanent disease to the **conduction system.**

     a. **First-degree AV nodal block.** If each P wave is followed by a QRS complex at a longer than normal interval, a first-degree AV nodal block is diagnosed.

     b. **Second-degree AV nodal block.** In second-degree AV nodal block, some P waves are not followed by a QRS complex, producing varying degrees of bradycardia.

     c. **Third-degree AV nodal block.** P waves and QRS complexes are completely unrelated.

B. QRS interval. The QRS interval is normally less than 0.1 second in duration. Measurement is from the beginning of the Q wave to the end of the S wave.

   1. **Interventricular conduction delay** or **incomplete bundle branch block** is diagnosed when the QRS complex is 0.1–0.12 second in duration.

   2. **Bundle branch block** is diagnosed when the QRS complex is greater than 0.12 second in duration ("widened").

     a. **Pathogenesis.** If the right bundle is blocked, depolarization must proceed down the left bundle and then slowly to the right from muscle fiber to muscle fiber. Muscle conducts slowly compared with the specialized bundles; therefore, the QRS complex will be wider than normal, and the late electrical forces will move to the right. Similarly, a left bundle branch block will also have a wide QRS complex, and the late forces will move to the left.

b. Diagnosis

(1) Determining the direction of the late forces (Figure 5–2). Draw a line down the middle of the QRS complex in lead V1 (a rightward lead) and lead V6 (a leftward lead). The half of the QRS complex to the right of the line represents the "late" forces. Check if these are positive (above the horizontal) or negative (below the horizontal).

(2) Interpretation

(a) Right bundle branch block. If the late forces of V1 are positive and those of V6 are negative, then the late forces are moving toward the right from the left, signifying a right bundle branch block.

(b) Left bundle branch block. If the late forces of V6 are positive and those of V1 are negative, then the late forces are moving toward the left from the right, indicating a left bundle branch block.

(c) Nonspecific interventricular bundle branch block is often diagnosed when the V1 and V6 are either both negative or both positive.

FIGURE 5–2. Determining the direction of the late forces. (*A*) Right bundle branch block. The late forces are positive in lead V1 and negative in lead V6. (*B*) Left bundle branch block. The late forces are negative in lead V1 and positive in lead V6.

C. QT interval. The QT interval varies according to the heart rate, lengthening as the heart rate decreases. Measurement is from the beginning of the Q wave to the end of the T wave. The QT interval is corrected for heart rate by dividing the measured QT interval by the square root of the R–R interval. **A QTc interval greater than 0.44 second in duration is almost always abnormal.** Drugs (e.g., tricyclic antidepressants, amiodarone, type Ia antiarrhythmics) and electrolyte abnormalities (hypokalemia, hypomagnesemia, hypocalcemia) are common causes of a prolonged QT interval.

VI HYPERTROPHY

A. Left ventricular hypertrophy. All ECG criteria for the diagnosis of left ventricular hypertrophy are poorly sensitive but highly specific. One approach is to proceed through the following criteria in the order given. If a criterion is met, you diagnose left ventricular hypertrophy (high specificity); if not, you move to the next criterion.
   1. **R wave in lead aVL** > 11 mm (> 13 mm if left anterior fascicular block is present)
   2. **R wave in lead aVL + S wave in lead V3** > 20 mm in a woman or > 28 mm in a man
   3. **S wave in lead V1 + R wave in leads V5 or V6** (whichever is larger) > 35 mm
B. Right ventricular hypertrophy. Criteria for the diagnosis of right ventricular hypertrophy are also highly specific but insensitive.
   1. Right axis deviation **(RAD) greater than 110°**
   2. **R:S wave ratio in lead V1** greater than or equal to 1
   3. **R wave in lead V1** greater than or equal to 7 mm
   4. **R:S wave ratio in lead V5 or V6** less than or equal to 1
C. Left atrial abnormality was formerly called left atrial enlargement, but the name was changed because the ECG findings may actually represent dilatation, increased atrial pressure, or hypertrophy.
   1. **Lead II.** Notched P waves greater than 0.12 second indicate left atrial abnormality.
   2. **Lead V1.** If the P terminal force (the negative deflection that represents left atrial depolarization) is equal to or greater than one small box by one small box (0.04 sec by 1 mm), left atrial abnormality is diagnosed.
D. Right atrial enlargement
   1. **Lead II.** A P wave greater than 2.5 mm high indicates right atrial enlargement.
   2. **Lead V1 or V2.** A P wave greater than 1.5 mm high indicates right atrial enlargement.

VII **Q WAVES** simply indicate that forces are moving away from their respective leads.

A. **Normal Q waves.** Sometimes Q waves are normal and expected. For example, the interventricular septum is depolarized left to right, and so a small or "septal" Q wave is expected in lead V6 (reflecting forces moving away from this leftward lead).

B. **Pathologic Q waves** signify that forces are moving away from the area more than would normally be expected. A pathologic Q wave indicates an old **myocardial infarction** and is only diagnosed when the Q wave is at least 30 msec (close to one small box) in duration and one third the height of the ensuing R wave.

   1. **Inferior wall myocardial infarction.** Leads II, III, and aVF evaluate the inferior surface of the left ventricle. Q waves in these leads denote an inferior wall myocardial infarction. However, an isolated Q wave in lead III of up to 30 msec may be seen as a normal variant. (A handy way of remembering this is: "A small Q in III is free, unless accompanied by a Q in either II or aVF.")

   2. **Posterior wall myocardial infarction.** Sometimes an inferior wall infarction is accompanied by a posterior wall infarction, producing a large R wave in lead V1 (i.e., forces move away from the posterior wall anteriorly). **Differential diagnoses for a large R wave in V1 include:**

      a. Posterior wall myocardial infarction
      b. Posteroseptal accessory pathway
      c. Right ventricular hypertrophy
      d. Right bundle branch block
      e. Duchenne's muscular dystrophy
      f. Limb lead reversal
      g. Dextrocardia
      h. Normal variant (in young people)

   3. **Anterior wall myocardial infarction.** Q waves in the precordial leads (V1–V6) imply an old anterior myocardial infarction.

VIII **ST/T WAVE CHANGES**

A. **Causes.** The most common causes of ST/T wave changes are:
   1. **Myocardial ischemia, injury,** or **infarction**
   2. **Pericardial inflammation**
   3. **Ventricular enlargement**
   4. **Abnormal ventricular depolarization** (e.g., with bundle branch block)
   5. **Electrolyte disturbances**

B. Findings
  1. T wave inversions may indicate **myocardial ischemia** but are
      nonspecific.
  2. ST elevations or **depressions** often indicate acute **myocardial
      injury.**
  3. ST elevations with the appearance of Q waves usually indi-
      cate **myocardial infarction.**
C. Terminology. Clinicians often refer to ST depressions and ele-
    vations as ischemia and infarct, respectively, rather than simply
    "injury." This is because **ST depression** is caused by injury to
    the **subendocardial** (inner) region that is often the result of
    supply/demand mismatch, nonocclusive thrombus, or occlusive
    thrombus in a vessel supplying well-collateralized territory. **ST
    elevation,** in contrast, implies **transmural** injury that usually oc-
    curs as a result of complete coronary occlusion from thrombus
    during an infarction.

References
Chou T, Knilans TK. Electrocardiography in Clinical Practice: Adult and Pediatric.
    Philadelphia: WB Saunders, 1996.
Dubin D. Rapid Interpretation of ECGs: An Interactive Course. Tampa, Florida
    Cover Publishing Company, 2000.

6. Syncope

I INTRODUCTION

A. Definition. Syncope is a **transient loss of consciousness and postural tone** that is **caused by inadequate cerebral blood flow.** Syncope should be differentiated from pre-syncope, dizziness, and vertigo—all of which do not result in loss of consciousness. **Seizures** must be **excluded.** This requires a careful examination for prodromal or post-ictal symptoms and rhythmic myoclonic activity.

B. Epidemiology. Syncope is extremely common, accounting for approximately **5% of medical admissions** and **3% of emergency department visits.** The lifetime incidence approaches 50% in some groups.

II CAUSES OF SYNCOPE.
There are many causes of syncope, but the most important can easily be remembered using the mnemonic, "SYNCOPE."

Causes of Syncope ("SYNCOPE")

Situational
Vasovagal (the V looks like a Y)
Neurogenic
Cardiac
Orthostatic hypotension
Psychiatric
Everything else

A. Situational causes include micturition, defecation, swallowing, coughing, subclavian steal, and carotid sinus sensitivity.

B. Vasovagal syncope, also known as the **"common faint,"** is the most common cause of syncope in young patients and is often preceded by a painful or emotional stimulus. This condition results from a simultaneous, reflex-mediated decrease in vascular tone (vasodilatory component) and heart rate (cardioinhibitory component).

C. Neurogenic causes include autonomic insufficiency and transient ischemic attacks (TIAs).

  1. Transient ischemic attacks (TIAs) are extremely rare causes of syncope. For syncope to occur, the vertebrobasilar circulation must be involved.

2. **Autonomic insufficiency** is common in elderly patients and patients with diabetes.

D. Cardiac causes

1. **Obstructive disorders.** Aortic, mitral, or pulmonic stenosis; idiopathic hypertrophic subaortic stenosis; atrial myxoma; and pulmonary embolism interfere with cardiac output and can precipitate a syncopal attack.

2. **Arrhythmias.** Disorders that lead to bradycardia (e.g., sick sinus syndrome, second- and third-degree atrioventricular (AV) block) or tachycardia (e.g., ventricular fibrillation, ventricular tachycardia, torsades de pointes, supraventricular tachycardia) also interfere with cardiac output.

3. **Other. Ischemic disorders** can precipitate an episode of syncope through low cardiac output or arrhythmias. **Aortic dissection** can lead to syncope through cardiac tamponade from hemopericardium or acute cerebrovascular insufficiency.

E. Orthostatic hypotension can cause syncope.

F. Psychogenic syncope is a diagnosis of exclusion.

G. Everything else

1. **Medications** (e.g., vasodilators, hypnotics, sedatives, nitrates, diuretics)

2. **Drugs** (e.g., cocaine, hypnotics, sedatives, alcohol)

III APPROACH TO THE PATIENT. The evaluation of a patient with syncope must be approached in a rigorous, stepwise fashion to avoid missing life-threatening disease.

A. History and physical examination. A thorough history and physical examination is a **very important** aspect of the evaluation and may establish the diagnosis in up to 45% of patients.

1. **Situational.** Was the episode preceded by urination, defecation, swallowing, coughing, exertion of arm muscles (subclavian steal), or manipulation of the neck (carotid sinus hypersensitivity)? Testing for carotid sinus hypersensitivity should be done carefully after excluding significant carotid artery stenosis and only while the patient is being monitored by ECG.

2. **Vasovagal.** Did a painful or emotional stimulus precede the event?

3. **Neurogenic.** Did anyone witness convulsions, bowel or bladder incontinence, or signs suggestive of a postictal state? A seizure is not syncope but could result in a loss of consciousness; therefore, it must be considered in the differential diagnosis.

4. **Cardiac.** A cardiac cause is more likely if the patient has any

history suggestive of cardiac disease. Has the patient complained of feeling lightheaded during exercise (suggestive of an obstructive cause)? Has the patient complained of "palpitations" (suggestive of an arrhythmic cause)? Patients may also complain of symptoms suggestive of cardiac ischemia.

5. **Orthostatic hypotension.** Does the patient report that he or she "got up too quickly?" Always check orthostatic vital signs in patients admitted with syncope.

6. **Psychogenic.** A psychogenic cause for the syncope (e.g., hyperventilation) should be considered after all other causes have been excluded.

7. **Everything else.** What prescription, over-the-counter, or illicit drugs might the patient have access to?

B. **Electrocardiogram (ECG).** All patients should have an ECG, although fewer than 10% of the causes of syncope can be identified by this test. Look for evidence of acute or remote myocardial infarction, preexcitation syndromes, arrhythmias, a long QT interval, and conduction system disease (i.e., bundle branch block).

C. **Risk assessment.** Patients should be **separated into two groups:** those without evidence of heart disease, and those who may have heart disease.

1. **No evidence of heart disease.** Patients who meet all the following criteria after a thorough history, physical examination, and ECG are at low risk for a cardiac cause, and additional cardiac testing may not be indicated. However, some patients may require additional evaluation and treatment. The criteria are:

   a. **Younger than 45 years of age**

   b. **No history or evidence of coronary artery disease or congestive heart failure**

   c. **Normal ECG**

2. **Evidence of heart disease.** Anyone who does not meet all the criteria in III C 1 is included in this group. If there is **suspicion of an ischemic or arrhythmic cause, admission and ECG monitoring** are indicated. Additional diagnostic tests to be considered include:

   a. **Ambulatory ECG monitoring.** This test is widely used but it establishes a diagnosis in only a small percentage of patients. Event or loop recorders may improve the diagnostic yield.

   b. **Exercise treadmill testing** can rule out exercise- or ischemia-induced syncope.

   c. **Echocardiography** allows assessment of valvular disease as well as left ventricular size and function.

   d. **Electrophysiologic studies (EPS)** are especially useful in patients at high risk for tachyarrhythmia (i.e., those with poor left ventricular function) when a diagnosis cannot be established using noninvasive methods. The yield of EPS is lower in patients without structural heart disease and in those with bradyarrhythmias.

   e. Tilt table test. This test can be useful in documenting vasovagal syncope but has poor specificity, especially when provocative agents such as isoproterenol are used.

IV TREATMENT is cause-specific.

A. The treatment of any **correctable cardiac abnormality** should be the first consideration (i.e., permanent pacemaker for patients with bradyarrhythmias, implantable cardiac defibrillators in patients with ventricular tachycardia, or valvular surgery for those with severe aortic stenosis).

B. Patients with **frequent vasovagal syncope** may benefit from a trial of β blockers, paroxetine, or disopyramide. In rare instances, patients with a significant cardioinhibitory component may benefit from permanent pacemaker placement.

C. **Orthostatic hypotension** is treated with volume resuscitation and discontinuation of culprit drugs. Rarely, support stockings, salt tablets, fludrocortisone, and midodrine may be added if autonomic insufficiency is present.

V PREVENTION

A. Medications and the use of alcohol or illicit drugs should be reviewed carefully.

B. Education about likely precipitants can help prevent recurrences.

References

Kapoor WN. Syncope. N Engl J Med 2000;343:1857–1862.

Martin TP, Hanusa BH, Kapoor WN. Risk stratification of patients with syncope. Ann Emerg Med 1997;29:459–466.

7. Arrhythmias

I INTRODUCTION

A. Bradyarrhythmias usually do not pose a diagnostic dilemma and have relatively few treatment options (e.g., atropine, pacemaker device).

B. Tachyarrhythmias may pose a significant challenge in diagnosis and often are treated very differently. All tachyarrhythmias can be classified according to whether they are regular (same distance between successive R waves) or irregular, and whether their QRS complex is narrow (< 0.12 second) or wide (> 0.12 second). Making these two determinations and consulting Table 7-1 can significantly narrow the diagnostic possibilities.

II NARROW, REGULAR TACHYARRHYTHMIAS

A. Differential diagnosis

   1. Sinus tachycardia

      a. Etiologies. Sinus tachycardia is usually a physiologic response to stress. Important etiologies include:

         (1) Low stroke volume states (e.g., from intravascular volume depletion or myocardial dysfunction)

         (2) Hypoxemia (e.g., from heart failure)

         (3) Hypercatecholamine states (e.g., from pheochromocytoma, pain, anxiety)

         (4) Drugs (e.g., inhaled β-agonists, theophylline, caffeine)

         (5) Systemic causes (e.g., fever, anemia, hyperthyroidism)

         (6) Myocarditis and pericarditis

      b. Electrocardiogram (ECG) appearance. Upright P waves in leads II, III, and aVF are always followed by a QRS complex.

HOT **KEY** The maximum predicted heart rate in sinus tachycardia = 220 minus the patient's age.

---

   2. Atrioventricular nodal reentrant tachycardia (AVNRT) accounts for more than 50% of all supraventricular tachyarrhythmias. [All narrow, regular tachyarrhythmias are supraventricular, but the term **supraventricular tachycardia**

TABLE 7-1. Classification of Tachyarrhythmias*

	Regular Rhythm	Irregular Rhythm

Narrow QRS	Sinus tachycardia
	AVNRT
	AT
	Atrial flutter
		Atrial fibrillation
		Atrial flutter with
		  variable block
		Multifocal atrial
		  tachycardia
		Frequent premature
		  atrial contractions

Wide QRS	Ventricular tachy-
	  cardia
	Supraventricular
	  tachycardia with
	  aberrancy
		Atrial fibrillation with
		  aberrancy*
		Ventricular tachycardia
		  (monomorphic or
		  polymorphic)

AT = atrial tachycardia; AVNRT = atrioventricular nodal reentrant tachycardia; AVRT = atrioventricular reentrant tachycardia.
*Because all arrhythmias characterized by an irregular rhythm and a narrow
QRS complex can become irregular with a wide QRS complex in the presence
of aberrant conduction, atrial flutter with variable block and multifocal atrial
tachycardia must also be considered here, although they are much less
common than atrial fibrillation.

is classically used for AVNRT, atrioventricular reentrant
tachycardia (AVRT), and atrial tachycardia (AT).]
  a. Characteristics include:
    (1) Heart rate of 160–200 beats/min
    (2) Isolated R waves, pseudo S waves, or inverted P waves
      on the ECG
  b. Mechanism. Many people have a dual atrioventricular
    (AV) node that contains a fast pathway with a long re-
    fractory period and a slow pathway with a short refractory
    period.
    (1) Sinus rhythm. During sinus rhythm, the impulse is
      conducted down the fast pathway to the ventricles.
      Conduction down the fast pathway is also able to tra-
      verse the AV node retrograde and block impulses on
      the slow pathway (Figure 7–1).
    (2) Excitation loop. The incidence of premature atrial
      contractions (PACs) increases with age. A PAC may
      be blocked at the fast pathway secondary to its long
      refractory period; the impulse is then conducted
      down the slow pathway, which has a short refractory

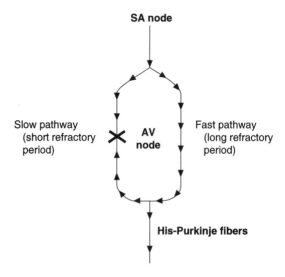

FIGURE 7-1. Dual atrioventricular node, sinus rhythm. *AV* = atrioventricular; *SA* = sinoatrial.

period (this is manifested as a long PR interval on the ECG immediately before the tachycardia's initiation. The impulse may then enter the fast pathway retrograde, which is no longer refractory, and activate the atria (slow-fast AVNRT or typical AVNRT) (Figure 7-2).

c. ECG appearance

   (1) In **typical AVNRT** (90% of cases), a PAC begins the loop of excitation. The P wave is inverted and occurs simultaneously with the QRS complex; **only R waves** are seen on the ECG.

   (2) In **atypical AVNRT** (10% of cases), a premature ventricular contraction (PVC) initiates the conduction of an impulse up the slow pathway and down the fast one (fast slow) (Figure 7-3). Because the retrograde P waves are formed from the slower pathway, they occur slightly later and can be seen as **pseudo S waves** in the inferior leads (II, III, avF) or as **inverted P waves** immediately following the QRS complex (usually with a short RP interval).

3. Atrioventricular reentrant tachycardia (AVRT) accounts for more than 30% of all supraventricular tachyarrhythmias.

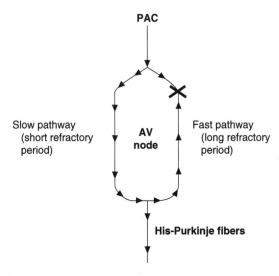

FIGURE 7-2. Atrioventricular nodal reentrant tachycardia (*AVNRT*) from premature atrial contractions (*PACs*). Following conduction down the slow pathway, the fast pathway is no longer refractory and may conduct retrograde, forming an excitation loop. *AV* = atrioventricular.

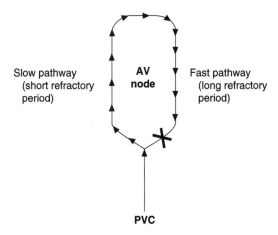

FIGURE 7-3. Atypical atrioventricular nodal reentrant tachycardia (AVNRT). *AV* = atrioventricular; *PVC* = premature ventricular contraction.

a. Characteristics. AVRT is characterized by a short RP interval on the ECG.

b. Mechanism. AVRT involves an **accessory pathway** (e.g., bundle of Kent in Wolff-Parkinson-White syndrome), an abnormal tract of fast conducting tissue between the atria and ventricles that bypasses the AV node. Accessory pathways often conduct in both an anterograde and retrograde direction.

c. ECG appearance

(1) Sinus rhythm

(a) During sinus rhythm, anterograde conduction results in ventricular preexcitation, manifested as a **short PR interval** and a **delta wave** on the ECG.

(b) If only retrograde conduction is possible (as is the case in approximately 25% of patients), no abnormality is seen during sinus rhythm (concealed bypass tract).

(2) Excitation loop

(a) Orthodromic conduction occurs when an impulse is conducted through the AV node and then up the accessory pathway in a retrograde direction (Figure 7–4). Because the loop is longer than that of AVNRT, the retrograde P wave is easily seen (i.e., it is not buried in the R wave). The interval from the R wave to the ensuing retrograde P wave will be less than that from the P wave to the next R wave (**short RP or RP < PR tachycardia**). This characteristic helps distinguish AVRT from AT and sinus tachycardia. The QRS complex remains narrow because the

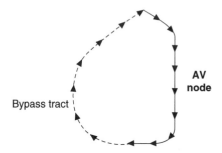

FIGURE 7–4. Orthodromic conduction leading to atrioventricular reentrant tachycardia (AVRT). *AV* = atrioventricular.

ventricle is depolarized normally (i.e., via the His-Purkinje system).

(b) **Antidromic conduction** occurs when the impulse is conducted antegrade down the bypass tract. Antidromic conduction produces a wide QRS complex because the tract terminates on ventricular muscle fibers. (Conduction from fiber to fiber is slow.)

4. **AT** accounts for 15% of all supraventricular tachycardias.
   a. **Characteristics**
      (1) The **atrial rate** (as reflected by the P waves on the ECG) is usually **less than 250 beats/min.** (In atrial flutter, the atrial rate is approximately 300 beats/min.)
      (2) A **long RP** interval is noted on the ECG.
   b. **Mechanism.** Enhanced automaticity of atrial tissue or atrial reentry with a focus usually located in the lower right atrium is thought to be the mechanism.
      (1) Patients often have **structural heart disease.**
      (2) Because digitalis increases atrial and ventricular automaticity and depresses conduction tissue, AT with variable degrees of AV nodal block is a common presentation of **digitalis toxicity.**
   c. **ECG appearance.** P wave has an unusual axis due to depolarization of the atria from a focus below the sinus node, and is followed by a narrow QRS complex (produced by conduction of the impulse down the AV node). The preceding P wave is linked to the R wave, and the PR interval is shorter than the RP interval (a long RP tachycardia).

HOT KEY

The supraventricular tachycardias can be classified according to the RP interval:
Short RP = AVRT and, occasionally, AVNRT
Long RP = AT and sinus tachycardia
No RP = AVNRT

---

5. **Atrial flutter**
   a. **Characteristics**
      (1) The atrial rate is often 300 beats/min, with the ventricular rate typically 150 beats/min. (In other words, a 2:1 AV block is commonly seen.) **Whenever the ventricular rate is approximately 150 beats/min, think of atrial flutter.**
      (2) Atrial flutter is typically transient, often degenerating to atrial fibrillation or returning to sinus rhythm. In general, the causes of atrial flutter are similar to those of atrial fibrillation (see chapter 8).

      b. Mechanism. Due to a macro-reentrant loop in the right atrium.

      c. ECG appearance. Because the waves often move in a superior-inferior direction (typical atrial flutter), flutter waves are best seen in the inferior leads (i.e., leads II, III, and avF).

B. Treatment

  1. Acute treatment depends on the patient's hemodynamic stability.

    a. Hemodynamically unstable (or ischemic) patient. Determine if the patient is in sinus rhythm.

      (1) If the patient is **not in sinus rhythm,** initiate **electrical cardioversion** immediately.

      (2) If the patient is **in sinus rhythm,** treatment is aimed at the underlying cause.

    b. Hemodynamically stable patient

      (1) Carotid sinus massage may increase vagal tone and block impulses at the level of the AV node. Carotid sinus massage is contraindicated in the presence of a carotid bruit and should be performed with continuous ECG monitoring and a crash cart available.

        (a) AVNRT and **AVRT,** tachycardias that involve reentrant loops through the AV node, may terminate.

        (b) AT is usually unaffected by carotid sinus massage but may terminate abruptly.

        (c) Sinus tachycardia. Carotid sinus massage may slow the atrial rate.

        (d) Atrial flutter usually becomes more obvious as the AV block increases and flutter waves appear; the tachycardia will not terminate.

      (2) Administer **adenosine** as a rapid intravenous (IV) push in incremental doses of 6 and 12 mg if carotid sinus massage is ineffective. (Halve the dose if administration is via a central line.) Adenosine is contraindicated in patients with acute bronchospasm and heart transplant patients; patients taking dipyridamole may have an increased sensitivity. The effects of adenosine occur within 15–30 seconds of administration and last for 10–20 seconds. Adenosine has effects similar to those of carotid sinus massage, but they are more pronounced as it results in transient complete AV nodal block.

        (a) AVNRT and **AVRT.** More than 90% of these tachycardias will be terminated with a 12 mg dose of adenosine.

        (b) AT rarely terminates. IV administration of verapamil or diltiazem is preferable for arresting atrial tachycardia and may decrease the ventricular response, even if the tachycardia persists.

c. **Sinus tachycardia** transiently slows. Additional treatment should be aimed at the underlying cause.

d. **Atrial flutter.** AV block increases and flutter waves are more evident. The heart rate returns to its previous accelerated rate as the effects of adenosine wane. Additional treatment may involve AV nodal blockade with digitalis, β blockers, or calcium channel blockers, followed by either chemical (e.g., procainamide, ibutilide) or electrical cardioversion. If the atrial flutter has been long-standing, cardioversion should only be considered after anticoagulation for 4 weeks or a transesophageal echocardiogram as with atrial fibrillation (see Chapter 8).

 HOT KEY In atrial flutter, type Ia agents should not be given before the administration of AV nodal blocking agents, because type Ia agents may slow atrial conduction sufficiently to permit 1:1 conduction through the AV node, thereby increasing the ventricular response.

---

(2) Electrical cardioversion starting at 25 J is a reasonable alternative to AV nodal blocking agents.

2. **Chronic treatment**

a. **AVNRT.** If the patient experiences sporadic episodes, control may be possible using vagal maneuvers. For patients who experience frequent or symptomatic episodes, antiarrhythmic drugs, AV nodal blocking agents, or radiofrequency ablation (RFA) may be used (>95% successful).

b. **AVRT.** Symptomatic patients with evidence of preexcitation on a baseline ECG should probably receive radiofrequency ablation. Patients with symptoms but no evidence of anterograde conduction (i.e., concealed bypass tract) can be treated with RFA or an initial trial of an AV nodal blocking agent.

c. **Atrial tachycardia.** Calcium channel blockers or β blockers are often the drugs of first choice. If pharmacologic therapy fails, ablation may be indicated.

d. **Atrial flutter.** RFA is 95% successful and should be considered in patients with recurrent symptoms. Antiarrhythmic drugs are typically less successful. Because of its high association with atrial fibrillation and independent association with stroke, anticoagulation also should be considered if there is evidence of advanced age, hypertension, or structural heart disease.

III NARROW, IRREGULAR TACHYARRHYTHMIAS

A. Differential diagnosis. In general, the members of this category can be differentiated easily on the basis of a 12-lead ECG. It is most difficult to distinguish atrial fibrillation from atrial flutter with variable block.

1. **Atrial fibrillation** is discussed in detail in Chapter 8. This arrhythmia is characterized by irregular atrial fibrillatory waves at a rate of 350–600 beats/min and a ventricular rate of usually 120–160 beats/min.

2. **Atrial flutter with variable block.** To help differentiate atrial flutter with variable block from atrial fibrillation:
   a. **Look at the inferior leads (II, III, avF).** With typical atrial flutter, flutter waves can often be "marched out" at a rate of approximately 300 beats/min. Variable block will produce a ventricular rate in proportion to the atrial rate (i.e., the ventricular response to 2:1, 3:1, and 4:1 AV block will be 150 beats/min, 100 beats/min, and 75 beats/min, respectively).
   b. **Increase AV block** by massaging the carotid sinus or administering adenosine. Flutter waves that may have been hidden will often become obvious.

3. **Multifocal atrial tachycardia**
   a. **Mechanism.** In approximately 60% of patients, multifocal atrial tachycardia is associated with pulmonary disease. For example, cor pulmonale causes right atrial stretch, producing different foci of atrial depolarization. Multifocal atrial tachycardia may also be caused by hypokalemia or hypomagnesemia.
   b. **ECG appearance.** Diagnosis requires the presence of three distinct P wave morphologies in the same lead and three separate PR intervals. As a result, the RR interval varies (i.e., **it is irregularly irregular**).

4. **Frequent PACs.** When frequent, PACs may give the appearance of an irregular rhythm.

B. Treatment

1. **Hemodynamically unstable (or ischemic) patients** with tachycardia and atrial fibrillation or atrial flutter with variable block should undergo immediate **electrical cardioversion.**

2. **Hemodynamically stable**
   a. **Atrial fibrillation.** Treatment is discussed in Chapter 8 VI.
   b. **Atrial flutter with variable block.** Treatment is the same as that for atrial flutter without variable block [see II B 1 b].
   c. **Multifocal atrial tachycardia.** Treat the underlying condition (usually related to bronchospasm, hypoxia, or metabolic derangements). Verapamil, magnesium, and β blockers are often tried, but this is a difficult arrhythmia to treat.

IV WIDE, REGULAR TACHYARRHYTHMIAS

A. Mechanism. Normally, the impulse is conducted from the sino-atrial (SA) node to the AV node, through the bundle of His, and through the left and right bundle branches (the Purkinje fibers). The bundles conduct rapidly and ventricular depolarization is efficient, producing a narrow QRS complex (< 100 msec in duration).

1. If one bundle is blocked, conduction will spread down the remaining bundle and then from muscle fiber to muscle fiber. This is a slow process that produces a wide QRS complex (> 120 msec in duration). A QRS complex between 100 and 120 msec in duration represents an incomplete bundle branch block and is often termed an interventricular conduction delay.

2. The QRS complex will be wide if the impulse starts in the ventricle and spreads fiber to fiber (as is the case with ventricular tachycardia) or if it starts above the ventricle but eventually spreads fiber to fiber (as is the case with supraventricular tachycardia with aberrancy). There are three mechanisms of aberrant conduction:

   a. **A preexisting underlying bundle branch block.**

   b. **A rate-related bundle branch block.** As the heart rate increases, one bundle (usually the right bundle) is unable to keep up with the other. The impulse is conducted down the faster bundle and then from fiber to fiber, producing a wide QRS.

   c. **An accessory pathway.** These tracts terminate on ventricular muscle, necessitating fiber-to-fiber conduction.

B. Differential diagnosis. The differential is **ventricular tachycardia versus supraventricular tachycardia with aberrancy.**

HOT **KEY** Patients with cardiac disease and a wide-complex tachyarrhythmia should be assumed to have ventricular tachycardia until proven otherwise.

The **Brugada criteria** can help distinguish between ventricular tachycardia and supraventricular tachycardia with aberrancy.[1] The precordial leads (V1–V6) are examined on a 12-lead ECG. Each criterion is extremely specific, but not particularly sensi-

[1]Brugada P, Brugada J, Mont L, Sweets J, Andreis EW. A new approach to the differential diagnosis of a regular tachycardia with a wide QRS complex. Circulation 1991;83(5):1649–1659.

tive, for ventricular tachycardia. Therefore, if a criterion is met, initiate treatment for ventricular tachycardia; if the criterion is not met, continue to the next.

1. **Absence of a true RS pattern in all the precordial leads.** An S wave is a discrete negative deflection. A broad negative deflection is an inverted T wave (as opposed to an S wave). If there is a monomorphic pattern (no RS) or "concordance," the arrhythmia is ventricular tachycardia.

2. **RS complex (from start of R to nadir of S) is greater than 100 msec.** Ventricular depolarization takes more time if it starts in the ventricle, rather than if it begins supraventricularly and is conducted aberrantly. If the RS complex is greater than 100 msec, then the arrhythmia is ventricular tachycardia.

3. **Evidence of AV dissociation** includes P waves marching through at different points of the wide complexes and fusion or capture beats. Although these clues are difficult to discern, they are diagnostic of ventricular tachycardia. If a diagnosis has still not been reached, morphologic criteria (given in several texts) can be used to arrive at a diagnosis.

C. **Treatment**

1. **Hemodynamically unstable (or ischemic) patients** should undergo cardioversion, starting with at least 200 J.

2. **Hemodynamically stable patients**

   a. **Ventricular tachycardia**

      (1) **Amiodarone.** Usual IV dosage is 150–300 mg bolus followed by 1 mg/min for 6 hours and then 0.5 mg/min.

      (2) **Lidocaine.** The initial bolus is 1–1.5 mg/kg administered intravenously, followed by an infusion of 1–4 mg/min.

      (3) **Procainamide** should be considered in patients who do not respond to amiodarone or lidocaine. Procainamide is effective at terminating ventricular tachycardia, but hypotension may occur.

   b. **Supraventricular arrhythmias with aberrancy. Carotid sinus massage** and **adenosine** should be employed as described in II B 1 b.

   c. **Undiagnosed**

      (1) **Amiodarone or Lidocaine.** The patient may be given a trial of either agent.

      (2) **Adenosine.** If there is no response, adenosine trials in 6- and 12-mg increments (half doses if administered via a central line) should be tried. If the patient has a history of cardiac disease, ventricular tachycardia is likely and needs to be treated immediately.

      (3) **Procainamide.** If the patient still fails to respond, a procainamide trial may be indicated.

V WIDE, IRREGULAR TACHYARRHYTHMIAS

A. Differential diagnosis. The differential diagnosis is atrial fibrillation with aberrancy versus ventricular tachycardia (monomorphic or polymorphic).

> **H O T**
>
> All members of the irregular, narrow category will appear irregular and wide with aberrant conduction.
> **K E Y**

1. **Atrial fibrillation** with aberrancy. There are three possible mechanisms of aberrant conduction.
   a. **Preexisting underlying bundle branch block.** If, upon comparing a previous 12-lead ECG with a current one, there is evidence of an old bundle branch block that has the same morphology as the present one, this diagnosis is extremely likely.
   b. **Rate-related bundle branch block** will usually have a right bundle branch block pattern on the ECG because the right bundle is usually slower than the left bundle.
   c. **Accessory pathway.** If there is evidence of preexcitation during sinus rhythm (i.e., a short PR interval, delta waves) on a prior 12-lead ECG, this diagnosis is extremely likely. Another clue to an accessory pathway is bizarre conduction (e.g., lead V1 suggests a left bundle but the nearby V2 lead suggests a right bundle). An accessory pathway is a dangerous situation because fibrillatory waves occur at rates of approximately 600 beats/min and the accessory pathway allows much faster conduction than does the AV node. Very fast ventricular rates (i.e., 200–300 beats/min) can be generated; this arrhythmia can quickly degenerate to ventricular fibrillation. AV nodal agents (e.g., verapamil) should be strictly avoided in all suspected cases.

> **H O T**
>
> Whenever you see a patient with a wide, irregular tachyarrhythmia with a rate greater than 200 beats/min, consider
> **K E Y** atrial fibrillation with an accessory pathway.

B. Treatment
   1. **Hemodynamically unstable (or ischemic) patients** should undergo **cardioversion** starting at 200 J.
   2. **Hemodynamically stable patients**

a. Procainamide is the drug of choice.
   (1) If the rhythm is atrial fibrillation with aberrancy, procainamide may convert the patient to sinus rhythm. If the cause of the patient's aberrant conduction is an accessory pathway, procainamide will slow conduction through the pathway, decreasing the ventricular rate, even though conversion may not occur.
   (2) Procainamide also treats ventricular tachycardia. However:
      (a) Procainamide is contraindicated in the setting of torsades de pointes. If a morphology consistent with torsades de pointes is present or there are strong epidemiologic factors suggestive of torsades de pointes (e.g., an increased baseline QT interval, use of quinidine or tricyclic antidepressants, or electrolyte disturbances such as hypokalemia or hypomagnesemia), procainamide is contraindicated because it will increase prolongation of the QT interval and promote further torsades. **Procainamide frequently leads to hypotension,** so patients with borderline blood pressures (i.e., 90–100 mm Hg) and fast heart rates may be better served with cardioversion.
b. AV nodal blocking agents (β blockers, calcium channel blockers, or digitalis) should only be considered when the patient shows strong evidence of atrial fibrillation with an underlying bundle branch block (i.e., a prior ECG shows the same bundle branch block during sinus rhythm). **Otherwise, AV nodal blocking agents should not be administered to patients with wide, irregular tachycardias** because if the patient has an accessory pathway, AV nodal blocking agents will promote conduction down the tract, thereby increasing heart rate.

VI VENTRICULAR TACHYCARDIA

A. Monomorphic ventricular tachycardia. In ventricular tachycardia, the rhythm may be irregular for the first 50 beats. A persistently irregular rhythm after 50 beats essentially rules out monomorphic ventricular tachycardia.
   1. Polymorphic ventricular tachycardia. Because the impulse is originating from different foci in the ventricle, the rhythm is irregular. Torsades de pointes is a type of polymorphic ventricular tachycardia that is associated with a prolonged QT interval and undulates around the isoelectric point.
   2. Acute treatment. Therapy for monomorphic ventricular tachycardia is as described earlier in IV C 2 a. For polymor-

phic ventricular tachycardia, emergently treat any reversible metabolic abnormalities and hold potentially dangerous drugs that may be prolonging the QT interval. Additional treatment typically involves IV magnesium or overdrive cardiac pacing with or without β blockers.

3. **Chronic treatment.** Patients with ventricular tachycardia, especially without a clear reversible cause, should be considered as candidates for **implantable cardiac defibrillators (ICD)**.

References

Cannom DS, Prystowsky EN. Management of ventricular arrhythmias: detection, drugs, and devices. JAMA 1999;281:172–179.

Ganz LI, Friedman PL. Supraventricular tachycardia. N Engl J Med 1995;332:162–173.

Mangrum JM, DiMarco JP. The evaluation and management of bradycardia. N Engl J Med 2000;342:703–709.

Morady F. Radiofrequency ablation as treatment for cardiac arrhythmias. N Engl J Med 1999;340:534–544.

8. Atrial Fibrillation

I INTRODUCTION

A. Epidemiology
1. Atrial fibrillation is the **most common chronic arrhythmia,** occurring in nearly 1% of the general population.
2. Its **incidence** varies with age: atrial fibrillation is rare in people younger than 50 years but occurs in 1 of 25 patients 60 years or older and in 1 of 10 patients 80 years or older.

B. Pathophysiology. Requires 1) an initial atrial ectopic event (typically from a focus in the pulmonary veins) and 2) a multiple wavelet reentrant circuit that is often sustained by structural disease in the left atrium (i.e., enlargement, scar).

C. Terminology. There are a number of terms used in association with atrial fibrillation.
1. **Valvular** refers to atrial fibrillation that is associated with valvular disease, most commonly rheumatic mitral valve disease. In the past, rheumatic heart disease accounted for the majority of cases of atrial fibrillation but currently accounts for less than one-third of cases. Atrial fibrillation associated with rheumatic heart disease carries a 5 times greater risk of stroke when compared to "nonvalvular" atrial fibrillation.
2. **Paroxysmal** refers to intermittent, brief episodes of atrial fibrillation unrelated to an acute illness.
3. **Persistent** refers to intermittent episodes lasting at least 7 days but responding to medical or electrical cardioversion to restore sinus rhythm.
4. **Chronic** refers to situations in which atrial fibrillation is the predominant rhythm and does not respond to cardioversion (or alternatively cardioversion is never attempted).
5. **Lone** refers to atrial fibrillation in the absence of structural heart disease [e.g., left ventricular hypertrophy, congestive heart failure (CHF), valve disease, cardiomyopathy] or hypertension. **In patients younger than 60 years of age, "lone" atrial fibrillation is associated with only a minimal risk of stroke or death.**
6. **Isolated** refers to atrial fibrillation that is secondary to another illness (e.g., hyperthyroidism, pneumonia, pulmonary embolism) and resolves when the illness is treated.

II CLINICAL MANIFESTATIONS OF ATRIAL FIBRILLATION

A. Symptoms are due to loss of the atrial kick and an increased heart rate, which results in decreased ventricular filling, de-

creased cardiac output, and an increase in cardiac demand. The most common symptoms reflect these processes.
1. **Dyspnea**
2. **Chest pain**
3. **Palpitations**
4. **Dizziness or syncope**
5. **Fatigue**

HOT KEY

Patients with atrial fibrillation may also be asymptomatic.

B. **Physical examination findings**
1. **Irregularly irregular pulse.** An irregularly irregular pulse is the **hallmark of atrial fibrillation.**
2. **Pulse of varying intensity** and **pulse deficit.** Because diastolic filling varies in length and is often reduced, pulses are of varying intensity and not all audible ventricular beats are palpable peripherally.
3. **Absent *a* waves** in the jugular venous pulse
4. **Variation in the intensity of the first heart sound (S₁)**

HOT KEY

Patients in atrial fibrillation never have an S_4.

C. **Electrocardiography**
1. The electrocardiogram (ECG) may show **f waves** (fine fibrillation of the atria at a rate of 350–600 beats/min) that are best visualized in lead V1. These f waves should be differentiated from more organized atrial activity (i.e., "sawtooths") in leads II, III, and aVF that might represent atrial flutter.
2. **P waves are absent.**
3. The **ventricular response** will be **irregularly irregular,** although this may be difficult to appreciate at higher heart rates.

III **CAUSES OF ATRIAL FIBRILLATION.** Because many of the causes of atrial fibrillation are correctable, an effort should be made to pinpoint the cause of the arrhythmia.

A. **Idiopathic.** In approximately 10% of patients, no etiology can be found; these patients are said to have "lone" atrial fibrillation if there is no structural heart disease and hypertension.

B. Cardiovascular disorders, including sick sinus syndrome, Wolff-Parkinson-White syndrome, coronary artery disease, congestive heart failure, cardiomyopathy (hypertrophic and dilated), myocarditis, hypertension, and congenital heart disease

C. Pulmonary disorders, including pulmonary embolism

D. Pericardial disease (e.g., pericarditis)

E. Metabolic disturbances, including hyperthyroidism

F. Infiltrative diseases, including amyloidosis, sarcoidosis, and hemochromatosis

G. Intoxication (e.g., alcohol, theophylline, β agonists)

H. Infection (e.g., endocarditis)

I. Stress-induced (e.g., post-surgery)

Causes of Atrial Fibrillation ("SWAMP CHILD")

Sick sinus syndrome, Stress
Wolff-Parkinson-White syndrome
Alcohol (intoxication, withdrawal, "holiday heart")
Myocarditis, Metabolic abnormality
Pericardial disease, Pulmonary disease
CHF, Coronary artery disease, Congenital heart disease
Hypertension, Hyperthyroidism, Hypertrophic cardiomyopathy
Infiltrative disease, Infection
Lone (idiopathic)
Dilated cardiomyopathy, Drugs

IV **APPROACH TO THE PATIENT.** Knowledge of the differential diagnosis will help direct diagnostic tests. All patients should undergo an ECG, a chest radiograph (to rule out pneumonia and other intrathoracic processes), a complete blood count (CBC), electrolyte studies, and thyroid function testing. An echocardiogram is usually obtained to examine cardiac function and atrial size as well as to rule out valve disease.

V **COMPLICATIONS.** The risk of **stroke** in all patients with "nonvalvular" atrial fibrillation is approximately 5% per year, 5 times the risk in those without atrial fibrillation. It is important to assess for five important factors that can allow you to further define your patient's risk for stroke:

Risk Factors for Stroke in Patients with "Nonvalvular" Atrial Fibrillation ("CHADS2" Index)

CHF (within 100 days or ejection fraction reduced)
Hypertension
Age 75 years or older
Diabetes mellitus
Stroke or transient ischemic attack in past

In calculating the CHADS2 risk score, each factor above is worth 1 point **except for stroke, which is worth 2 points.** For each 1-point increase in the CHADS2 risk score, the risk of stroke increases by 1.5 per 100 patient-years.

VI TREATMENT

A. **Acute treatment.** The goal of acute treatment of a patient with atrial fibrillation is **rate control.**
   1. **Pharmacologic therapy**
      a. **Atrioventricular (AV) node blocking agents.** There are several options for controlling heart rate:
         (1) **Diltiazem** [15–20 mg (0.25 mg/kg) intravenously over 2 minutes; repeat in 15 minutes if necessary; maintenance infusion is 5–20 mg/hr intravenously]
         (2) **Verapamil** (2.5–5.0 mg administered as an intravenous bolus over 1–2 minutes; if needed, repeat with a dose of 5 mg in 15–30 minutes; maximum dose is 15 mg)
         (3) **Esmolol** (250–500 μg/kg intravenously over 1 minute, followed by an intravenous maintenance infusion of 50–200 μg/kg/min)
         (4) **Digoxin** (0.5 mg intravenously followed by 0.25 mg intravenously every 6 hours to a total dose of 1 mg). Digoxin has weak AV nodal blocking properties but may be the only alternative in patients with borderline low blood pressures.
      b. AV node blocking agents are **contraindicated** in patients with irregular, wide complex tachycardia or extremely rapid ventricular rates (> 220) until atrial fibrillation with conduction down an accessory pathway (e.g., Wolff-Parkinson-White syndrome) has been excluded. If Wolff-Parkinson-White syndrome is present, these agents can precipitate fatal ventricular fibrillation.
   2. **Electrical Cardioversion**
      a. **Indications.** Cardioversion is indicated for any patient

with **rapid atrial fibrillation** and **life-threatening problems** (e.g., ischemia, severe hypotension, or severe pulmonary edema). You may begin with 100 J in the synchronized mode, but 360 J may be necessary.

  b. Contraindications. Unless there is an emergent indication, no patient with atrial fibrillation should be cardioverted until anticoagulation therapy has been initiated or until atrial thrombus has been excluded using transesophageal echocardiography. This usually includes patients who are thought to have "new onset" atrial fibrillation because it is difficult to estimate the length of time the patient has been in atrial fibrillation from the patient history. Patients who are cardioverted without undergoing anticoagulation therapy have a 3%-5% risk of stroke within 30 days.

B. Chronic treatment. The goals of the chronic treatment of atrial fibrillation are minimization of symptoms and reduction of the risk for stroke.

  1. Rate control. The goal is a resting heart rate lower than 90 beats/min. Treatment should be selected after considering the patient's other medical problems. For example:

  a. In patients with hypertension or coronary artery disease, a β blocker is a good choice because it addresses these problems as well as the atrial fibrillation. However, in patients with asthma or chronic obstructive pulmonary disease (COPD), a β blocker may not be a good choice because it induces bronchoconstriction.

  b. In patients with CHF, β blockers and digoxin can control the heart rate as well as improve symptoms of CHF. However, β blockers must be titrated up slowly, and in patients with chronic renal insufficiency, digoxin levels should be monitored very closely.

  c. AV node ablation with **pacemaker implantation** is used only under special circumstances when rate-control with drug therapy fails.

  2. Rhythm control. Theoretically, conversion to normal sinus rhythm returns the risk of stroke to baseline and relieves all rate-related symptoms. However, data from recent trials suggest that a strategy of rate-control and anticoagulation may be just as efficacious if patients are not significantly symptomatic.

  a. Electrical cardioversion should be undertaken only after atrial thrombus has been excluded or at least a 4-week course of anticoagulation, has been completed, unless there is an emergent indication.

  b. Pharmacologic therapy for cardioversion and to prevent recurrence. Rate must be controlled before the initiation of any antiarrhythmic medication.

(1) Procainamide and **quinidine** increase the time to relapse in treated patients, but both agents are proarrhythmic and have been associated with increased mortality rates. **Most patients should not be treated with these agents.**

(2) Amiodarone appears to be as effective as procainamide and quinidine for maintaining sinus rhythm without causing proarrhythmic effects. Amiodarone is likely to become the drug of choice, although there are significant side effects.

(3) Newer agents include ibutilide and dofetilide. Ibutilide, which cause torsades de pointes, should be avoided in patients with significant LV dysfunction or baseline QT prolongation.

   c. Radiofrequency ablation of pulmonary vein sources is a new option in select candidates with poorly controlled, paroxysmal atrial fibrillation.

3. Clot control. Stroke is the major cause of morbidity and mortality in patients with atrial fibrillation. Anticoagulation therapy is time-consuming and bothersome to patients, and the risks and benefits must be assessed on an individual basis.

   a. Warfarin treatment reduces the risk of stroke by 40%–90%. The target international normalized ratio should be 2.0–3.0. There is a small increase in the risk of major bleeding.

   b. Aspirin alone is a consideration for patients at low risk for stroke.

   c. Lower dose anticoagulation [i.e., a target international normalized ratio (INR) of 1.0–2.0] and combination therapy (e.g., aspirin plus warfarin) is considered ineffective.

References

Fuster V, Falk RH. Atrial fibrillation. N Engl J Med 2001;344:1067–1078.

Fuster V, Ryden LE, Asinger RW, et al. ACC/AHA/ESC guidelines for the management of patients with atrial fibrillation: executive summary. Circulation 2001;104:2118–2150.

Asinger RW, Gage BF, Waterman AD, Shannon W, et al. Validation of clinical classification schemes for predicting stroke: results from the National Registry of Atrial Fibrillation. JAMA 2001;285:2864–2870.

9. Chest Pain

I **INTRODUCTION.** Because chest pain (including "discomfort") is common and its etiologies range from a life-threatening myocardial infarction to benign musculoskeletal pain, a simple and reliable approach to the patient is necessary.

II **CAUSES OF CHEST PAIN.** One way to remember the causes of chest pain is to use an "outside-in" approach.

A. **Skin.** Varicella-zoster virus infection (shingles) often causes pain before vesicular lesions are noted. The pain usually occurs in a dermatomal distribution.

B. **Chest wall.** Musculoskeletal pain may result from shoulder arthritis or bursitis, intercostal injury, metastatic disease to the bones or chest wall, or costochondritis. Breast pathology (e.g., tumors, fibrocystic disease) and nerve root compression (from cervical disk herniation) may also lead to chest pain.

C. **Lungs.** Inflamed pleura from spontaneous pneumothoraces, pulmonary emboli, infections, malignancies, and connective tissue disorders can all cause chest pain, which is usually pleuritic (i.e., it worsens with inspiration or coughing).

D. **Heart and great vessels.** Pericarditis, myocardial ischemia and infarction, and aortic dissection can all cause chest pain.

E. **Gastrointestinal tract.** Esophageal disorders (including esophagitis, spasm, and rupture) are common causes of chest pain. Other gastrointestinal causes of chest pain include gastric and duodenal ulcers, pancreatitis, and biliary disease.

III **APPROACH TO THE PATIENT.** Although the outside-in approach is useful for remembering the differential diagnoses for chest pain, it fails to highlight the four acutely life-threatening causes:

HOT ▶ **KEY**

Four Killer Chest Pains

Myocardial infarction or ischemia
Pulmonary embolism
Aortic dissection
Spontaneous pneumothorax

Because chest pain may represent one of these emergencies, the usual order of evaluation (e.g., history, physical examination, diagnostic tests) may hinder critical early intervention. The first step should be a quick screen for the four killer chest pains, followed by a more in-depth evaluation if the etiology of the chest pain is still unclear.

A. Screen for the killer chest pains

1. **"Eyeball" the patient.** A patient who is clutching his chest, diaphoretic, and ashen can be presumptively diagnosed as suffering from myocardial infarction from across the room. Even if the presentation is not so classic, you can often decide who looks "sick" and may need a more rapid evaluation in a more monitored setting.

2. **Establish intravenous access and cardiac rhythm monitoring** immediately in patients who appear ill or who have cardiac risk factors.

3. **Evaluate the patient's vital signs**

HOT KEY

Any abnormality of the vital signs should alert you to the possibility that the chest pain has a potentially serious cause.

    a. **Check blood pressure in both arms.** Although a difference in pressure of 10 mm Hg or more may be seen in patients with aortic dissection, local atherosclerosis can also produce pressure differences. Therefore, the blood pressure reading is neither sensitive nor specific for aortic dissection.

    b. **Check respiratory rate and oxygen saturation.** Low oxygen saturation may accompany spontaneous pneumothorax, pulmonary embolism, and myocardial infarction (with pulmonary edema).

      (1) **Low oxygen saturation** (e.g., < 92%) is often an indication that an arterial blood gas should be ordered immediately.

      (2) **A normal oxygen saturation** may still be accompanied by a significant alveolar-to-arterial (A-a) oxygen gradient during hyperventilation. Therefore, arterial blood gas testing to evaluate the possibility of pulmonary embolism may still be necessary if the rest of the evaluation is unrevealing.

4. **Look at the electrocardiogram (ECG).** The ECG leads are often placed while the vital signs are being checked.

    a. ECG abnormalities that suggest **acute myocardial infarc-**

tion or **ischemia** (i.e., acute coronary syndromes) are always grounds for admission. Make sure the patient has intravenous access, a cardiac rhythm monitor, supplemental oxygen, and has been given an aspirin (usually 325 mg) orally. (The emergent treatment of acute coronary syndromes is discussed in more detail in Chapter 11.)

    b. Normal ECG. A normal ECG does not rule out myocardial infarction or ischemia. **Nitroglycerin** (0.3–0.6 mg sublingually or via aerosol) may be administered and the dose repeated every 3–5 minutes as both a diagnostic challenge and as potential therapy in patients with persistent chest pain.

5. Take a preliminary history

HOT KEY In patients with a history of coronary artery disease or cardiac risk factors and no alternative explanation for the chest pain after careful evaluation, an admission to rule out myocardial infarction (ROMI) is usually appropriate.

---

    a. Cardiac history and risk factors. First, ask about any prior cardiovascular problems.

        (1) If there is a history of coronary artery disease, the patient has ischemia until proven otherwise.

        (2) With a negative cardiac history, you can quickly establish the pretest probability of myocardial infarction by assessing cardiac risk factors (i.e., age, male gender, smoking, diabetes, hypertension, high cholesterol, and positive family history).

    b. Other risk factors. The preliminary history can also help elucidate any predisposing factors to the other killer chest pains. For example, a history of cancer or inactivity may contribute to pulmonary embolism, and uncontrolled hypertension may increase the likelihood of aortic dissection (or myocardial infarction).

6. Perform a preliminary physical examination. Frequently, you will have a few brief moments between tests during which you can look at the neck veins, listen to the heart and lungs, palpate the upper abdomen for tenderness, and evaluate the pulses in the arms and legs.

7. Evaluate the chest radiographs. Always compare the new films to old films, if they are available.

    a. Spontaneous pneumothorax can be subtle and you need to look carefully, especially in the apices.

    b. Esophageal rupture may lead to air in the mediastinum (pneumomediastinum).

    c. Myocardial infarction or aortic dissection may be accompanied by enlargement of the heart or mediastinum, respectively; however, these structures are often exaggerated on anteroposterior films. The presence of pulmonary edema may also be suggestive of myocardial infarction.

  8. Order an arterial blood gas analysis. If not performed earlier, an arterial blood gas analysis with the patient breathing room air is usually necessary.

B. Further define the cause of the chest pain

  1. Take a more detailed patient history

    a. Type of chest pain. Pulmonary embolism frequently presents with pleuritic chest pain; myocardial infarction may present with "crushing" chest pain or only a mild "discomfort"; and aortic dissection is often characterized by a ripping pain that radiates to the back.

    b. Radiation of chest pain. Pain that radiates to the neck or left arm should be considered cardiac until proven otherwise.

      (1) Atypical patterns may still indicate ischemia and include pain, tingling, or numbness in the left fingertips unaccompanied by arm pain and pain in the outer left shoulder.

      (2) It is wise to consider any neck, upper abdominal, or upper back pain as cardiac in origin until proven otherwise.

    c. Onset of chest pain. Spontaneous pneumothorax, aortic dissection, and pulmonary embolism usually present with abrupt pain, whereas pain from myocardial infarction or ischemia may build more gradually. Spontaneous pneumothorax and pulmonary embolism often occur while the patient is at rest, whereas aortic dissection and myocardial infarction may occur with rest or exertion.

    d. Duration of chest pain. Pain that only lasts seconds or that has been constant for more than 24 hours is usually not caused by one of the four killer chest pains. A myocardial infarction is almost always associated with more than 20 minutes of chest pain.

    e. Associated symptoms. Dyspnea, diaphoresis, or lightheadedness should alert you to a probable serious cause of chest pain.

    f. Aggravating and mitigating factors

      (1) Deep inspiration often aggravates pain from the pleura or pericardium (e.g., pleurisy from a pulmonary embolism or pericarditis).

(2) Exertion may worsen the pain from myocardial infarction or aortic dissection. Rest may ease the pain from cardiac ischemia, usually gradually.

(3) Position. Patients with pericarditis often feel worse when supine and better when sitting up. Patients with musculoskeletal pain may feel worse in certain positions. The pain of myocardial infarction is usually unaffected by changes in position, but this is not always the case.

(4) Food intake. Pain on swallowing localizes the problem to the gastrointestinal tract. Chest pain after a meal may indicate gastrointestinal pathology, but it also may occur with myocardial infarction.

(5) Nitroglycerin. If chest pain decreases with nitrates (e.g., sublingual nitroglycerin), a cardiac etiology should be presumed; however, esophageal spasm may also respond to this therapy.

2. Perform a complete physical examination. Pay extra attention to the following parts of the exam.

a. Jugular venous pressure. An elevated jugular venous pressure should alert you to the possibility of a serious disorder (e.g., myocardial infarction, pulmonary embolism, or tension pneumothorax), but a normal jugular venous pressure does not exclude these disorders.

b. Cardiac examination

(1) Heart sounds. Listen carefully for a third heart sound (S_3) or fourth heart sound (S_4) gallop, which may indicate impaired ventricular contractility or ventricular relaxation, respectively. Both impaired ventricular contractility and impaired relaxation can accompany cardiac ischemia.

(2) Murmurs may also increase the likelihood of a cardiac etiology of chest pain. A mitral regurgitant murmur may accompany a myocardial infarction with papillary muscle dysfunction, whereas an ejection murmur may indicate aortic stenosis or hypertrophic cardiomyopathy (both of these conditions may predispose the patient to ischemia).

c. Lung examination. Listen carefully for rales (e.g., from myocardial infarction with pulmonary edema) and pleural friction rubs (e.g., from pulmonary embolism, infection, or other pleural processes).

d. Chest wall examination. Minimal tenderness to palpation is nonspecific, but if the chest pain is *exactly* and *reliably* reproduced (especially in a well-localized area), a musculoskeletal etiology is likely. Briefly inspect the skin for lesions.

    e. Abdominal examination. Palpate for any upper abdominal tenderness that may indicate a gastrointestinal cause of the chest pain.

    f. Pulses. Check pulses in the arms and legs bilaterally.

3. Pearls

    a. Myocardial infarction

      (1) Because coronary artery disease is such a common disease, it is always better to admit patients for ROMI if there is any doubt as to the diagnosis, even in young patients.

      (2) More than 20 minutes of unexplained chest pain may represent a myocardial infarction, whereas chest pain that lasts less than 20 minutes but increases in frequency, duration, or occurs with minimal exertion often represents unstable angina; both patterns are indications for admission.

      (3) Frequently, patients with chest pain are given an antacid and lidocaine swish and swallow ("GI cocktail") to evaluate possible reflux esophagitis. **Many patients who "benefit" from this "diagnostic test" may actually have ischemic pain that is improving spontaneously or from bed rest and oxygen therapy.**

    b. Pulmonary embolism. Clinical suspicion is critical. There is often no evidence of deep vein thrombosis, and subtle symptoms and signs may be inappropriately rationalized away. If you have a high clinical index of suspicion, administer heparin before sending the patient for diagnostic tests.

    c. Aortic dissection

      (1) Most dissections occur either within several centimeters of the aortic valve (Type A or ascending aortic dissection) or just distal to the left subclavian artery takeoff (Type B or descending aortic dissection). If the patient has abrupt onset of symptoms, pain that radiates to the back, unequal blood pressures, or other suspicious findings, aortic dissection should be ruled out emergently.

      (2) Both computed tomography (CT) and transesophageal echocardiography are equally effective in diagnosing aortic dissection. The choice of test to use depends on the patient (e.g., poor renal function may weigh against a CT scan) and institutional preferences. If clinical suspicion is high, a surgeon should be consulted immediately for his or her input regarding subsequent evaluation, because the mortality rate may be as high as 1% per hour during the first 48 hours. Transthoracic echocardiography is not sensitive enough to rule out dissection, especially in the descending aorta.

(3) If dissection is strongly suspected, blood pressure control and strict avoidance of anticoagulants becomes essential.

(4) Increasingly, patients with symptoms of dissection are identified as having "intramural" aortic hematoma due to rupture of vasa vasorum within the thoracic aorta. Although data are limited, prognosis and therapy appear to be similar to those with true aortic dissection.

References

Bennett J. ABC of the upper gastrointestinal tract. Oesophagus: Atypical chest pain and motility disorders [Review]. BMJ 2001;323(7316):791–794.

Goldman L, Cook EF, Johnson PA, Brand DA, Rouan GW, Lee TH. Prediction of the need for intensive care in patients who come to the emergency departments with acute chest pain. N Engl J Med 1996;334(23):1498–1504.

Lee TH, Goldman L. Evaluation of the patient with acute chest pain. N Engl J Med 2000;342:1187–1195.

Panju AA, Hemmelgarn BR, Guyatt GH, Simel DL. The rational clinical examination. Is this patient having a myocardial infarction? JAMA 1998;280(14):1256–1263.

Schwartz L, Bourassa MG. Evaluation of patients with chest pain and normal coronary angiograms. Arch Intern Med 2001;161(15):1825–1833.

10. Angina

I | INTRODUCTION

A. Definition. Myocardial ischemia results when the oxygen supply is inadequate to meet the oxygen demands of the cardiac muscle. Although other diseases may reduce the oxygen supply (e.g., coronary artery spasm, hypoxemia, anemia) or increase the oxygen demand (e.g., tachycardia as a result of infection, thyrotoxicosis), the most common cause of myocardial ischemia is **underlying coronary artery disease** due to atherosclerosis.

B. Risk factors for atherosclerosis include:
1. **Age and gender:** Men older than 45 years and women older than 55 years
2. **Hypertension**
3. **Diabetes mellitus**
4. **Smoking**
5. **Dyslipidemia:** Elevated low-density lipoprotein (LDL) cholesterol and low high-density lipoprotein (HDL) cholesterol
6. **Family history** (first-degree male or female relative with premature atherosclerosis)

II | CLINICAL MANIFESTATIONS OF CORONARY ARTERY DISEASE

A. Symptoms
1. **Angina** is the typical symptom associated with myocardial ischemia. It is described as a chest pain beneath or left of midsternum that increases with physical exertion or stress, often lasts from a few minutes up to 20 minutes, and subsides gradually with rest or nitroglycerin.
   a. Additional features. If chest pain radiates to the neck or left arm or is accompanied by dyspnea, diaphoresis, or lightheadedness, the likelihood of myocardial ischemia is increased, but these features need not be present.
   b. Classification. Angina may be **stable** or **unstable:**
      (1) Stable angina usually results from a fixed atherosclerotic plaque that limits oxygen delivery to the cardiac tissue. The oxygen mismatch that results causes a predictable and stable pattern of chest pain during exertion.
      (2) Unstable angina usually results when an atherosclerotic plaque ruptures with the development of superimposed thrombus. As a result, oxygen supply

becomes acutely inadequate at lower activity levels
or event at rest (discussed more in Chapter 11).

   c. **"Anginal equivalents."** Other symptoms unaccompanied
   by chest pain (e.g., dyspnea) may actually represent "anginal equivalents." **Importantly, some patients with myocardial ischemia may not have any symptoms at all.**

B. **Physical examination findings.** A normal physical examination
   does not rule out the possibility of chronic ischemic heart disease. Transient signs may occur during ischemic episodes including hypertension or, less commonly, hypotension; ventricular or supraventricular arrhythmias; a third or fourth heart
   sound (S_3 or S_4); or a holosystolic murmur over the apex (rep-
   resentative of mitral regurgitation as a result of papillary muscle ischemia). The presence of elevated jugular venous pressure, pulmonary edema, a gallop rhythm, pathologic murmurs,
   or signs of cardiac risk factors (e.g., peripheral vascular disease
   from diabetes) should all increase suspicion of coronary artery
   disease.

III APPROACH TO THE PATIENT. Angina and ischemic heart
   disease need to be differentiated from the many other causes
   of chest pain (see Chapter 9).

A. **Patient history.** In patients with classic symptoms, the diagnosis
   of stable or unstable angina can be made on the basis of history
   alone. An assessment of a patient's atherosclerotic risk profile
   is critical for determining your overall suspicion for ischemic
   heart disease.

B. **Resting electrocardiography.** Chronic ischemic heart disease
   can be diagnosed in asymptomatic patients by finding evidence
   of old myocardial infarctions or active ischemia on a resting
   electrocardiogram (ECG) [e.g., ST segment depressions and T
   wave inversions].

C. **Patients with episodes of prolonged chest pain or rapidly accel-
   erating angina should have cardiac biomarkers [i.e., creatine kinase (CK) or troponin] evaluated to rule out recent myocardial
   infarction.**

D. **Stress tests** may be helpful both diagnostically in patients with
   atypical chest pain and prognostically in patients with typical
   angina.

   1. **Types**

      a. **Exercise electrocardiography (ECG).** The presence of 1
         mm of downsloping or horizontal ST-segment depression
         on ECG with exercise is considered a positive test for isch-
         emia. Although this test gives excellent prognostic infor-
         mation, it is limited to patients who can exercise with rea-

sonably normal baseline ECGs (i.e., without left bundle branch block or left ventricular hypertrophy with strain). Unfortunately, interpretation is often limited by baseline abnormalities.

b. Myocardial perfusion scintigraphy is often performed in conjunction with exercise electrocardiography and involves the injection of thallium 201 (^{201}Tl) or Technetium 99 (^{99}Tc) based agents (sestamibi) into the peripheral venous blood. Cardiac muscle cells that are ischemic or infarcted do not take up these tracers well in comparison to normally perfused, living cells.

(1) Reversible defects, areas that lack thallium on exercise images but "fill in" on rest images (i.e., after 3–4 hours), indicate non-infarcted, ischemic tissue. **Fixed defects** are present on both exercise and rest imaging and denote prior infarction.

(2) In patients who are unable to exercise vigorously, vasodilators, such as **dipyridamole, adenosine,** or **dobutamine** that produce vasodilatation in normal coronary arteries out of proportion to that produced in atherosclerotic vessels, can be used to shunt thallium away from cardiac regions served by diseased vessels. Dipyridamole and adenosine are contraindicated in patients with significant reversible airway disease because they may facilitate bronchospasm.

c. Exercise or dobutamine stress echocardiography. If exercise results in a decrease in ejection fraction or segmental wall motion abnormalities, cardiac ischemia is presumed. Intravenous **dobutamine** increases oxygen demand by increasing heart rate and contractility and may be used as an alternative to exercise.

d. Other studies such as electron-beam computed tomography (EBCT) and magnetic resonance imaging (MRI) are still under investigation.

2. Choosing a test. Although one stress test cannot be universally recommended over the others, certain caveats apply:

a. Patients with ECG abnormalities may not be evaluated appropriately with standard exercise electrocardiography alone. Scintigraphy is frequently added to increase sensitivity and specificity.

b. Echocardiography is more likely to be inadequate in obese patients and patients with chronic obstructive pulmonary disease because of poor images.

c. Patients with significant baseline wall motion abnormalities on their echocardiogram may have difficult images to interpret using stress echocardiography.

E. Cardiac catheterization with coronary angiography is the gold standard for diagnosing obstructive coronary artery disease. If catheterization demonstrates severe coronary artery disease, revascularization with coronary artery bypass surgery or percutaneous coronary intervention (PCI) may be indicated.

IV TREATMENT

A. General measures. Because angina is a symptom of atherosclerosis and coronary artery disease, an indispensable part of the treatment is aimed at identifying and treating cardiac risk factors.

1. **Smoking cessation**
2. **Control of dyslipidemia** [target LDL goal < 100 mg/dl]; HMG-CoA reductase inhibitors (or "statins") are the drugs of choice
3. **Control of hypertension** (at least systolic < 140 mm Hg and diastolic < 90 mm Hg)
4. **Control of diabetes mellitus**
5. **Regular exercise** (e.g., brisk walking for 30 minutes 4 times weekly)
6. **Weight loss**
7. **Treatment of other factors that may aggravate angina** (e.g., anemia, hypoxemia, thyrotoxicosis)

B. Specific measures for the relief of angina

1. **Pharmacologic therapy** is generally aimed at increasing myocardial oxygen supply (by coronary vasodilation), decreasing oxygen demand (by decreasing heart rate, contractility, preload, or afterload), and preventing acute thrombotic events. Most patients are initially given an aspirin, β blocker, and short-acting nitrates, unless there are contraindications.

   a. **Aspirin** (usually 81–325 mg/day) inhibits platelet aggregation and coronary thrombosis and therefore prevents acute coronary syndromes.

   b. **Nitrates** lower oxygen demand by decreasing preload and afterload and may increase oxygen supply by vasodilating coronary arteries (less important mechanism).

   (1) **Short-acting nitrates.** Nitroglycerin 0.3–0.6 mg sublingually or by aerosol may be used for **angina prophylaxis** (the dose is taken 5 minutes before an activity known to result in angina) or **immediate therapy** (the dose is administered every 3–5 minutes until the pain is relieved; if pain is not relieved in 20 minutes, the patient should get to a hospital immediately).

   (2) **Long-acting nitrates** (e.g., isosorbide dinitrate, isosorbide mononitrate, transdermal nitroglycerin patches).

An interval of approximately 8–10 hours per day without nitrate therapy is needed to prevent tachyphylaxis, so the last dose is often given after dinner and patches are removed overnight. Headaches may occur with the initiation of nitrate therapy; if they can be managed conservatively, they frequently resolve after 1–2 weeks.

c. β **blockers** decrease heart rate and myocardial contractility, resulting in symptomatic control of angina by lowering oxygen demands. In addition, unlike other anti-anginal agents, they have been shown to have a mortality benefit in patients with coronary artery disease who have already experienced myocardial infarction.

   (1) Frequently used β blockers include **metoprolol** (50–100 mg orally 2 times daily) and **atenolol** (50–100 mg orally once daily).

   (2) Gradually, the dose of the β blocker may be increased until the symptoms are controlled, side effects develop (e.g., postural lightheadedness), blood pressure falls below approximately 100/60 mm Hg, resting heart rate falls below approximately 55 beats/min, or the maximal dose is reached. If symptoms are still not controlled, long-acting nitrates may be added and increased as needed with attention to the patient's symptoms, side effects, and blood pressure.

   (3) β blockers are contraindicated in patients with significant bradyarrhythmias. In patients with chronic obstructive pulmonary disease (COPD), a β_1-selective agent (e.g., metoprolol or atenolol) should be used; β blockers may need to be avoided in patients with severe COPD. Patients with impaired left ventricular function benefit from β blockers; however, candidates must be started with a low dose (e.g., 2.5–5 mg metoprolol) and titrated up gradually with frequent patient monitoring.

d. **Calcium channel blockers** lower oxygen demand (by decreasing heart rate, contractility, and afterload) and may increase oxygen supply (by inducing vasodilation of the coronary arteries).

   (1) Agents include **verapamil, diltiazem,** and **dihydropyridines (nifedipine, felodipine, amlodipine),** in order of increased effect on lowering systemic vascular resistance and decreased effect on myocardial inotropy and chronotropy. Verapamil and diltiazem are usually preferred for angina but should be used carefully with β blockers.

(2) Calcium channel blockers have not been associated with improved survival after myocardial infarction and may lead to a worse outcome; therefore, they are **not the initial drugs of choice for most patients with coronary artery disease,** particularly if LV dysfunction is present. **Amlodipine alone has been shown to be safe in those with ejection fractions less than 40%.**

HOT **KEY** Angiotensin-converting enzyme (ACE) inhibitors do not acutely improve angina symptoms. However, tissue-based ACE inhibitors (i.e., ramipril) reduce mortality rates in patients with ischemic heart disease, likely due to coronary plaque stabilization.

---

2. **Revascularization.** The indications for **coronary artery bypass surgery** or **PCI** are controversial. Studies are underway to address the relative advantages and disadvantages of each strategy.
   a. **Coronary artery bypass surgery** is generally considered superior in the treatment of patients with left main coronary artery disease (greater than 50% diameter occlusion) or three-vessel disease (greater than 70% diameter occlusion) associated with decreased left ventricular function (less than 50%). Diabetics also seem to benefit more from bypass surgery when compared with PCI.
   b. Bypass surgery may also benefit patients with three-vessel disease and severe angina (class III or IV) and patients with proximal left anterior descending occlusion associated with two-vessel disease; nevertheless, there is less of a consensus on whether bypass surgery, angioplasty, or medical therapy is appropriate in these instances.
   c. Patients with angina refractory to medical therapy and patients with a recent myocardial infarction or unstable angina and continuing symptoms or signs of ischemia are also candidates for revascularization.
   d. Often the final choice between bypass or PCI depends on the **coronary anatomy's suitability** for revascularization (i.e., good "targets" for bypass surgery, approachable lesions for PCI, etc.)

References

Ades PA. Cardiac rehabilitation and secondary prevention of coronary heart disease. N Engl J Med 2001;345(12):892–902.

Channer K, Morris F. ABC of clinical electrocardiography: myocardial ischaemia. BMJ 2002;324(7344):1023–1026.

Lee TH, Boucher CA. Clinical practice. Noninvasive tests in patients with stable coronary artery disease. N Engl J Med 2001;344(24):1840–1845.

Pretre R, Turina MI. Choice of revascularization strategy for patients with coronary artery disease. JAMA 2001;285(8):992–994.

11. Myocardial Infarction

I **INTRODUCTION.** Unstable angina, non-ST segment elevation myocardial infarction (NSTEMI), and ST segment elevation myocardial infarction (STEMI) make up the **acute coronary syndromes (ACS).** The term encompasses the entire range of presentations associated with acute ischemic heart disease and, importantly, reflects the diagnostic uncertainty present on initial evaluation. ACS are a leading cause of death in the United States. The failure to recognize ACS in the emergency room has led to inappropriate patient discharges, resulting in an abundance of malpractice claims. Many therapies have a proved mortality benefit in the treatment of ACS; however, studies show that patients frequently receive suboptimal therapy.

II **PATHOPHYSIOLOGY OF ACS.** ACS usually results from the rupture of unstable atherosclerotic plaques with subsequent thrombosis of a coronary artery. This leads to inadequate blood flow and oxygen delivery, which in turn results in myocardial cell death. Less common causes of ACS include coronary vasospasm (usually associated with coronary artery disease), severe hypotension, emboli (e.g., from mitral valve disease), aortic dissection (usually with right coronary artery involvement), vasculitis, and cocaine use (atherosclerosis, vasospasm, and platelet aggregation are presumed etiologies).

III **CLINICAL MANIFESTATIONS OF MI.** Typical symptoms and signs associated with cardiac ischemia are discussed in Chapters 9 and 10. The **chest pain** associated with ACS differs from that of stable angina in that it frequently begins while the patient is at rest or has minimal exertion, lasts more than 20 minutes, is more severe, and is unrelieved with sublingual nitroglycerin; however, these findings are variable. **Pain that lasts for more than 20 minutes should be considered due to MI** (either NSTEMI or STEMI) until proved otherwise.

IV **DIAGNOSIS.** Because unstable angina and MI share similar pathophysiology, it is not surprising that they frequently cannot be distinguished by clinical criteria alone. Patients are often admitted for "unstable angina/rule out MI (ROMI)"; serial electrocardiograms (ECGs) and cardiac biomarker studies are required for a definitive diagnosis. If ECGs show evidence of injury (i.e., ST elevation) or if cardiac biomarkers show evidence of cell death, then myocardial infarction is diagnosed.

 HOT KEY The diagnosis of MI is made by the presence of cardiac biomarker elevation in the setting of 1) typical symptoms and signs of MI or 2) ECG changes consistent with an MI.

A. **Patient history and physical examination.** Chest pain is the most common symptom of MI, but other signs and symptoms may also signal MI (e.g., flash pulmonary edema, hypotension, dyspnea).
B. **Electrocardiography. An initial ECG is the key to triaging patients with ACS and should be performed as soon as possible in the emergency room.** Following admission of the patient, serial ECGs are usually obtained on a frequent basis until resolution of symptoms occurs and the ECG changes stabilize; a daily ECG and an ECG following reports of any symptoms are usually obtained thereafter. Specific ECG findings for MI or ischemia include hyperacute (peaked) T waves, ST elevations, ST depressions, Q waves, or inverted T waves.

 HOT KEY In up to 10% of cases of documented MI, the ECG is normal.

---

1. **ST segment depressions and elevations may reflect both myocardial ischemia and injury.**
   a. The subendocardial region is the most susceptible to ischemia because it is perfused "last" (i.e., the coronary arteries course from the outer epicardial surface inward), and this is typically manifested by ST segment depression. Because the subendocardium is on the inner surface of the heart away from the ECG leads on the chest wall, **subendocardial injury** may be seen as **ST segment depression.** Epicardial injury, in contrast, is near the ECG leads and typically occurs with transmural ischemia; it most often results in a larger amount of myocardial damage and is evident as ST segment elevation on ECG. ST segment ele-

vations also may occur with transient ischemia (e.g., from vasospasm).

   b. Traditional terminology that identifies ST segment depressions as **"ischemia"** and ST segment elevations as **"infarct"** is oversimplified. ST depressions may occur with infarction, and ST segment elevations may occur with transient epicardial ischemia (e.g., from coronary vasospasm). ST segment changes in ACS are more accurately thought of as representing myocardial **"injury."**

  2. **Q waves** signify electrical activity moving away from the area of the heart where they are seen; they therefore indicate dead muscle (previous MI) in that region. Q wave MIs may occasionally disappear on ECG over years.

  3. A **right-sided ECG** (leads V1 and V2 reversed, with the other leads placed in corresponding positions on the right side of the chest) should be obtained in all patients with an acute inferior wall MI. Right ventricular infarction may complicate the clinical course of a myocardial infarction and is associated with a higher in-hospital mortality rate. ST segment elevation in leads RV4 or RV3 on a right-sided ECG indicates right ventricular infarction.

C. Cardiac biomarker studies

  1. MI is usually associated with an elevation in serum creatine kinase (CK) levels. Detection of the CK-MB isoenzyme has increased specificity for cardiac muscle and maintains a high sensitivity. **CK with isoenzyme studies** are usually ordered every 8 hours for 24 hours or until a peak level is reached (usually 16–18 hours).

  2. More recently, **cardiac troponin levels** have been introduced as a more useful means of diagnosing acute MI. Cardiac troponin levels are more sensitive and specific than CK for the detection of myocardial infarction. These biomarkers usually rise within 4–6 hours of cell death, peak at 18–24 hours, and may remain elevated for up to 7–10 days.

  3. **Myoglobin levels** rise quickly (within 2 hours), but are nonspecific to cardiac injury.

V **APPROACH TO THE PATIENT.** The treatment of ACS requires both precision and speed. The following stepwise approach allows you to make critical treatment decisions immediately, followed by those that are less urgent. Whenever a patient is admitted with an ACS, it is helpful to answer three questions: 1) What is the patient's hemodynamic status? 2) Is reperfusion [i.e., thrombolysis or primary percutaneous coronary intervention (PCI)] indicated? 3) What other treatments may benefit the patient?

A. What is the patient's hemodynamic status?
1. **Assessment.** Hemodynamic status can be approximated by examination of the volume status (i.e., jugular venous pressure [JVP] and lungs) and peripheral perfusion (i.e., extremities examination).
   a. **Low-risk patients** have normal JVP, clear lungs, and warm extremities associated with normal peripheral pulses. The presence of clear lungs usually indicates normal left ventricular filling pressures [i.e., a normal pulmonary capillary wedge pressure (PCWP)], and normal findings on examination of the extremities imply adequate cardiac output.
   b. **Intermediate-risk patients** have a normal extremity exam, but elevated JVP and pulmonary rales are found on exam. In these patients, elevated right and left-sided filling pressures (i.e., right atrial pressure [RAP] > 10 mm Hg and PCWP > 18 mm Hg) are suspected.
   c. **High-risk patients** have rales and cool extremities with diminished peripheral pulses. These patients are in **cardiogenic shock.** The presence of pulmonary edema suggests that the PCWP, an estimate of end-diastolic volume, is elevated. Normally, according to the Starling curve, a high end-diastolic volume ensures that the stroke volume will be maximized. If the heart is unable to adequately perfuse the end organs despite adequate filling (i.e., a high PCWP), cardiogenic shock is diagnosed.
2. **Management**
   a. **Low-risk patients** are hemodynamically stable and have a low mortality rate. Management of these patients entails deciding whether reperfusion therapy (i.e., thrombolysis or primary PCI) is indicated, and what other forms of therapy might benefit the patient (see V B C).
   b. **Intermediate-risk patients** have evidence of pulmonary edema, which may decrease oxygenation while increasing oxygen demand (increased sympathetic tone increases the heart rate and myocardial contractility).
      (1) **Agents frequently used in the treatment of MI** (e.g., **nitrates, morphine**) may also treat pulmonary edema by decreasing preload.
      (2) **Intravenous diuretics** should be given as needed.
   c. **High-risk patients** have **cardiogenic shock.**
      (1) **Pulmonary artery (PA) line placement** is indicated for monitoring cardiac output, systemic vascular resistance, and PCWP. In patients with ACS, only those with evidence of cardiogenic shock generally require hemodynamic monitoring with a PA line.
      (2) Pharmacologic therapy is dictated by the **patient's**

blood pressure. Although cardiogenic shock is often accompanied by **hypotension,** blood pressure may still be normal with low flow states due to a significant increase in systemic resistance.

HOT

> Do not assume that normal blood pressure indicates adequate end-organ flow.

KEY

(a) **Systolic blood pressure > 90–100 mm Hg**
  (i) **Dobutamine** is often started intravenously at a dose of 2.5 μg/kg/min. The dose may be increased gradually (up to 15–20 μg/kg/min) until the cardiac output rises and the PCWP falls. Dobutamine raises cardiac output by increasing myocardial contractility and by decreasing systemic vascular resistance. Because blood pressure is the product of cardiac output and systemic vascular resistance, it may remain stable, increase, or decrease depending on how much the cardiac output increases in comparison with the decrease in systemic vascular resistance. A decrease in blood pressure commonly occurs with dobutamine therapy, so the systolic blood pressure should be greater than 90 mm Hg (and preferably greater than 100 mm Hg) before the initiation of therapy.
  (ii) **Sodium nitroprusside** is an alternative to dobutamine, but often requires a higher starting blood pressure or the concomitant administration of an inotrope.
(b) **Systolic blood pressure < 90 mm Hg**
  (i) Intravenous **dopamine** is usually given. Dopamine usually causes **renal artery dilatation** at doses of 1–2 μg/kg/min ("renal dose" dopamine), **increased inotropy** from β_1-receptor stimulation at doses of 5–10 μg/kg/min, and vasoconstriction from α-receptor stimulation at higher doses; **however, significant overlap and variability exist.** Once the systolic blood pressure is greater than 90–100 mm Hg, dobutamine is often added and the dopamine is titrated down (preferably to "renal doses") as tolerated by the blood pres-

sure. Because arrhythmias may complicate dobutamine or dopamine therapy, patients require careful rhythm monitoring, and electrolytes should be maintained in the normal range (especially potassium and magnesium levels).

   (ii) Placement of an **intra-aortic balloon pump (IABP)** increases cardiac output, reduces systemic resistance, and improves coronary blood flow by improving perfusion pressure during diastole. When available, it should be considered in all hypotensive patients with acute ischemia.

  3. **Emergent PCI** is the only therapy that has been shown to decrease mortality rates in patients with cardiogenic shock from ACS and is clearly the **treatment of choice.**

B. **Is reperfusion therapy with thrombolysis or primary PCI indicated?** The initial triage ECG is critical in determining whether patients are appropriate candidates for immediate reperfusion therapy. In patients with chest pain of 6 hours or less duration (and possibly up to 12 hours or longer) and ST elevations of at least 1 mm in two consecutive ECG leads (i.e., STEMI) or evidence of a new left bundle branch block, there is a mortality benefit from immediate coronary reperfusion. Unless contraindicated, all such patients should therefore undergo thrombolysis or primary PCI. Importantly, studies in patients with unstable angina and NSTEMI have not shown any benefit with immediate reperfusion strategies and, in the case of thrombolytics, potential harm.

  1. **Primary PCI** is the treatment of choice in centers that can perform the procedure quickly and with expertise. It also may be favored when there are contraindications to thrombolytic therapy, and select patients should be transferred to a specialized center if necessary.

  2. **Thrombolysis**
     a. **Contraindications**
        (1) **Absolute contraindications** generally include the presence of:
            (a) **Central nervous system (CNS) disease.** Recent trauma or surgery, aneurysms, arteriovenous malformations, tumors, or a history of hemorrhagic stroke at any time or nonhemorrhagic stroke within 3 months are usually considered contraindications.
            (b) **Active gastrointestinal** or **genitourinary bleeding**
            (c) **Pregnancy**
        (2) **Relative contraindications** generally include:

    (a) **Traumatic** or **prolonged cardiopulmonary resuscitation**
    (b) **Recent trauma** or **surgery** (within 2 weeks)
    (c) **Diabetic retinopathy**
    (d) **Sustained hypertension** (e.g., blood pressure > 180/130 mm Hg after appropriate treatment)
    (e) **Coagulopathy, thrombocytopenia,** or **current oral anticoagulation therapy**
    (f) **Recent trauma to noncompressible arterial or venous puncture sites during intravenous access attempts**

  b. Other considerations. Patients who have had **prior coronary artery bypass grafting** do not benefit as much from either thrombolysis or PCI but should still be considered candidates for reperfusion with appropriate.

  c. Agents. The two most commonly used thrombolytic agents are **streptokinase** (usually 1.5 million units over 1 hour) and **tissue plasminogen activator (t-PA),** usually 100 mg. If t-PA is used, **heparin** must be given during or following therapy to decrease the high early reocclusion rate; no benefit of additional heparin has been shown with streptokinase. There may be slight advantages to one or the other agent, depending on the clinical situation.

    (1) t-PA. Young patients with anterior MIs who present within 4 hours of the onset of symptoms may benefit the most from t-PA. t-PA is also preferred for patients who have had a recent streptococcal infection or received streptokinase within the past 6 months, and for patients with borderline low blood pressure (because t-PA causes less hypotension than streptokinase).

    (2) Streptokinase. Overall, t-PA is associated with a slightly higher risk of hemorrhagic stroke than streptokinase (approximately 0.7–0.8% versus 0.5%). Patients who are older than 70 years and those with high blood pressure (i.e., systolic blood pressure > 160 mm Hg) have a higher risk of hemorrhagic stroke; therefore, streptokinase may be the preferred agent in these patients.

  d. General recommendations. The mortality benefit decreases drastically with delay in therapy, so speed is of the essence. Make sure a large-bore peripheral intravenous catheter (usually 16-gauge) is in place before therapy and limit venous and arterial blood draws. It is clear that the type of agent used is less important than ensuring that all patients who meet appropriate criteria and do not have contraindications receive thrombolytic therapy as rapidly as possible.

HOT KEY

Time elapsed = myocardium lost

    e. Signs of successful reperfusion include a prompt decrease in chest pain, normalization of the ST segment, an accelerated idioventricular rhythm, or an early peak of the CK enzymes (within 12 hours).

    f. If thrombolytic agents do not appear to result in thrombolysis, then **salvage PCI** should be considered in high-risk patients with ongoing signs of ischemia/infarction.

C. What other treatments may benefit the patient with ACS? Specific forms of therapy with nitrates, β blockers, and calcium channel blockers as well as potential contraindications are outlined in Chapter 10. The **coronary care unit (CCU) or specialized telemetry units** are the best place to manage patients with ACS, given the need for frequent vital checks and continuous rhythm monitoring.

    1. General measures

        a. Bed rest and a **stool softener** are usually prescribed.

        b. Subcutaneous heparin (5000 units twice daily) is usually administered to prevent deep venous thrombosis in patients who are otherwise not receiving systemic anticoagulation.

        c. Analgesia. Initially, **nitrates** are usually given to relieve pain, but **morphine sulfate** (2–4 mg intravenously) may be used for persistent pain (careful titration of dose may be needed in patients who have borderline low blood pressure).

    2. Aspirin and other oral antiplatelet agents. Aspirin (usually 325 mg orally) has been shown to have a mortality benefit in all patients with ACS, even in patients with STEMI who receive thrombolytics. **Therefore, aspirin should be given as soon as possible in all patients with suspected ACS. Clopidogrel,** a thienopyridine that inhibits ADP-induced platelet aggregation, has recently been shown in clinical trials to reduce recurrent ischemic events in unstable angina and NSTEMI when used concomitantly with aspirin. **In addition, clopidogrel should be used in all patients undergoing PCI with intracoronary stent placement for at least 4 weeks** (and up to 9 months). Active bleeding is a contraindication to both these agents.

    3. Oxygen (e.g., 2–4 L/min) is often administered, although the benefit in patients with normal oxygen saturation is questionable.

4. **Nitrates** are usually given unless the patient is hypotensive or has evidence of a low cardiac output. Nitrates should be used cautiously (if at all) in patients with right ventricular infarction given their dependence on preload.

5. **β blockers** have been shown to decrease mortality rates in patients with MI and are especially useful in patients with tachycardia, hypertension, or both. Use these cautiously, however, in patients with borderline low blood pressures or heart rates.

6. **Calcium channel blockers** have not been shown to have a mortality benefit in patients with MI and, in some studies, have been associated with increased mortality rates. In general, these agents **should be avoided** in the acute management of MI.

7. **Angiotensin-converting enzyme (ACE) inhibitors** are useful in the chronic management of patients with ischemic heart disease, but are associated with an increased mortality rate when given intravenously in the acute setting (see VII B 1 a).

8. **Heparin** is useful in the treatment of patients with NSTEMI and high-risk patients with unstable angina. Low-molecular weight heparin (such as enoxaparin) appears to decrease recurrent ischemic events better than unfractionated heparin and has the benefit of being easier to dose. Patients with STEMI benefit from heparin only when: 1) it is used with t-PA thrombolysis, 2) there is an anterior wall myocardial infarction associated with significant LV dysfunction, or 3) there is a documented LV thrombus.

9. **Glycoprotein IIb/IIIa (GIIb/IIIa) inhibitors.** GIIb/IIIa inhibitors block platelet glycoprotein IIb/IIIa receptors, the final common pathway for all platelet aggregation. Three intravenous agents are currently available: abciximab, eptifibatide, and tirofiban. Any of the three agents may be used in **high-risk unstable angina cases** (i.e., dynamic ECG changes) and **NSTEMI. Contraindications include** severe renal insufficiency and bleeding diathesis (thrombocytopenia). Abciximab might be better if early PCI is planned, whereas tirofiban has been shown to be beneficial even without PCI. Recent studies have failed to demonstrate mortality benefits from a combined use of GIIb/IIIa inhibitors and half-dose thrombolytics.

10. **Early coronary angiography and PCI.** In high-risk patients with unstable angina (dynamic ECG changes) and NSTEMI, there is accumulating evidence that a strategy of early coronary angiography and revascularization (either PCI or coronary bypass surgery) improves outcomes when compared with conservative management (i.e., risk stratification with exercise stress testing). In low-risk patients with NSTEMI or those with

STEMI who have received thrombolytic therapy, a conservative strategy is more reasonable. Typically, this involves a noninvasive assessment of both LV function and ischemic burden. Patients with a decreased LV function (ejection fraction < 40%) and/or significant ischemia on their stress test should undergo coronary angiography with possible revascularization as needed. Low-risk patients with unstable angina (no dynamic ECG changes with negative cardiac biomarkers) should also undergo noninvasive exercise stress testing before coronary angiography.

VI ACS COMPLICATIONS

A. **Arrhythmias** are most common during the initial 12–24 hours.
  1. **Tachyarrhythmias** are evaluated and treated as discussed in Chapter 7. Of note, **prophylactic lidocaine and magnesium are no longer recommended.** Lidocaine is reserved for patients with sustained or nonsustained ventricular tachycardia. Patients with tachyarrhythmias (ventricular tachycardia/fibrillation or nonsustained ventricular tachycardia [NSVT]) 24–48 hours after presentation are considered at high long-term risk for sudden cardiac death. These patients should be evaluated for the placement of **implantable cardiac defibrillators (ICDs)**, especially if they have LV dysfunction (see VII C 1).
  2. **Bradyarrhythmias** are more common with inferior wall MI because the sinoatrial (SA) and atrioventricular (AV) nodes are more dependent on blood flow from the right coronary artery.
     a. **Intravenous atropine** (0.5–1 mg every 3–5 minutes, up to 3 mg) is usually effective for sinus bradycardia and symptomatic Wenckebach (Mobitz type 1) second-degree AV block.
     b. Temporary pacing is generally indicated for patients with acute MI and:
        (1) Symptomatic sinus bradycardia and Wenckebach block that is unresponsive to atropine
        (2) Mobitz type 2 second-degree AV block or third-degree AV block
        (3) New bifascicular block, including alternating left and right bundle branch block, right bundle branch block with left anterior or posterior fascicular block, and left bundle branch block with first-degree AV block
B. **Recurrent ischemia or chest pain** following MI that is not responsive to medical management is usually a urgent indication for **coronary angiography** and **revascularization.**
C. **Pump dysfunction.** Severe left ventricular failure is managed as

outlined for cardiogenic shock. In severe cases, IABP and **left ventricular assist devices** may also be used until more definitive therapy (i.e., **cardiac transplantation**) can be performed.

D. Right ventricular infarction should always be suspected when hypotension accompanies an inferior MI. Treatment involves **large fluid boluses** to increase right-sided cardiac output and left ventricular filling. **Inotropic agents** (i.e., dobutamine) with hemodynamic monitoring may also be required. Nitrates should be avoided because these patients are preload-dependent.

E. Mechanical complications usually occur 2–7 days after infarction.

1. **Cardiac tamponade** from free wall rupture usually leads to abrupt hypotension and death.

2. **Ventricular septal defect** or **papillary muscle rupture leading to acute mitral regurgitation**
   a. **Clinical signs and symptoms**
      (1) These disorders are often heralded by hypotension, pulmonary edema, or both. Any abrupt change in hemodynamics should increase clinical suspicion of one of these mechanical complications.
      (2) A holosystolic murmur may be present in both conditions, but the location is usually at the left sternal border in ventricular septal defect and at the apex in papillary muscle rupture.
   b. **Diagnosis.** An **emergent surface echocardiogram** is the quick and easy way to make the diagnosis. Hemodynamic monitoring with a PA line is usually necessary for treatment and may also be used diagnostically—an increased oxygen saturation between the right atrium and pulmonary artery is seen with ventricular septal defect, and both disorders may display prominent v waves.
   c. **Treatment.** Nitroprusside or IABP may be used temporarily to decrease afterload and improve forward cardiac output. **Emergent surgical repair** is indicated for definitive therapy.

3. **Left ventricular aneurysm** or **pseudoaneurysm**
   a. **LV aneurysm** most often occurs after large anterior wall MIs. **Warfarin therapy** for 3–6 months is often administered to patients with large anterior wall MIs even in the absence of a LV thrombus. LV aneurysms may also be associated with refractory heart failure or arrhythmias and require surgical correction.
   b. **Pseudoaneurysms** are contained LV free-wall ruptures distinguished by a relatively narrow neck and a predisposition for an inferior-posterior location; **surgical correction** is generally performed to prevent delayed rupture.

VII RISK REDUCTION

A. **General measures** include **aspirin therapy** (usually 81–325 mg/day), which has a mortality benefit, and **aggressive risk factor reduction** (see Chapter 10 I B). Patients intolerant of aspirin should be given clopidogrel or ticlopidine.

B. **Additional diagnostic testing and preventive therapy.** Because the major complications of MI are heart failure, recurrent ischemia, and arrhythmias, diagnostic testing is aimed at identifying and treating these disorders (risk stratification).

1. **LV function assessment.** The post-MI **left ventricular ejection fraction** is the single best predictor of survival. For this reason, patients usually receive echocardiograms or another noninvasive assessment of their ejection fraction before discharge from the hospital.

   a. **ACE inhibitors** have been shown to decrease mortality rates in patients who have a **left ventricular ejection fraction** of **less than 40%** post-MI. Recent data suggest that ACE inhibitors may also be beneficial in patients with ischemic heart disease and normal ejection fractions.

   b. β **blockers** decrease post-MI mortality rates. Patients with the lowest left ventricular ejection fractions who can tolerate β blockers have the greatest survival advantage. β blockers may decrease the likelihood of arrhythmias and progressive heart failure in these high-risk patients.

2. **Stress testing** (see Chapter 10)

   a. In low-risk patients with unstable angina and patients with uncomplicated STEMI who have received thrombolysis, stress testing can be considered before discharge for further risk stratification. Patients usually undergo a **submaximal** stress test before discharge. Maximal or symptom-limited stress tests at 2–4 weeks can be considered in select patients at low risk who are ambulating without any difficulties. Patients with evidence of significant ischemia should undergo coronary angiography.

   b. **Early coronary angiography with revascularization** is usually indicated for patients with 1) unstable angina and high-risk features (i.e., dynamic ECG changes), 2) NSTEMI, 3) completed STEMI and high-risk features (recurrent ischemia, inadequate reperfusion therapy, stress tests that show significant ischemia, and baseline LV dysfunction).

C. **Arrhythmia monitoring**

1. Patients with **sustained ventricular tachycardia** or **symptomatic nonsustained ventricular tachycardia** (three or more consecutive ventricular premature beats lasting less than 30 seconds) require treatment, generally with ICD placement.

HOT **KEY** Ventricular arrhythmias that occur within 24 hours of MI generally do not worsen the patient's long-term prognosis; however, subsequent episodes are associated with a higher mortality rate and often necessitate chronic therapy.

2. Patients with **asymptomatic nonsustained ventricular tachycardia** may also be treated, although the benefit of therapy is less clear. Electrophysiologic testing in these patients may be valuable.

3. Recent data suggest that all patients with ejection fractions less than 30% derive a mortality benefit from ICD placement.

4. No antiarrhythmic agents, including amiodarone, have been shown to consistently reduce mortality rates in this setting.

References

Boden WE, McKay RG. Optimal treatment of acute coronary syndromes—an evolving strategy. N Engl J Med 2001;344:1939–1942.

Braunwald E, Antman EM, Beasley JW, et al. ACC/AHA guidelines for the management of patients with unstable angina and non-ST elevation myocardial infarction: executive summary and recommendations. Circulation 2000;102:1193–1209.

Hamm CW, Bertrand M, Braunwald E. Acute coronary syndrome without ST elevation: implementation of new guidelines. Lancet 2001;358(9292):1533–1538.

Morris F, Brady WJ. ABC of clinical electrocardiography: acute myocardial infarction: Part I. BMJ 2002;324(7341):831–834.

12. Congestive Heart Failure

I   INTRODUCTION

A. Definition. Congestive heart failure (CHF) is a **syndrome** that is the final common pathway for several different disease processes. It occurs when the heart is unable to supply sufficient amounts of blood at normal filling pressures to match the metabolic demands of the body.

B. Clinical manifestations classically include fatigue, lethargy, dyspnea on exertion or at rest, paroxysmal nocturnal dyspnea (PND), orthopnea, weight gain, and leg swelling.

C. Incidence. CHF is a common disorder, primarily affecting older individuals (10% of the U.S. population older than 75 years of age have this diagnosis). There are approximately 500,000 new cases diagnosed each year.

D. Mortality rates. The 1- and 5-year mortality rates for all patients with CHF are 25% and 65%, respectively. For those with pure diastolic dysfunction, the annual mortality rate is less (9%).

II   CLASSIFICATION.
There are many different classification schemes. The most useful include the following:

A. New York Heart Association (NYHA) functional classification
1. **Class I:** Symptomatic only with extraordinary activity
2. **Class II:** Symptomatic during ordinary activity
3. **Class III:** Symptomatic with less than ordinary activity
4. **Class IV:** Symptomatic at rest

B. American College of Cardiology/American Heart Association (ACC/AHA) Staging System
1. **Stage A:** Patients at high-risk for developing CHF but with no structural heart disease
2. **Stage B:** Patients with structural heart disease that are **asymptomatic**
3. **Stage C:** Patients with structural heart disease and past or current symptoms
4. **Stage D:** Patients with end-stage disease requiring specialized therapy (i.e., mechanical support devices, intravenous inotropic agents)
5. This new classification was established 1) to complement the NYHA functional class system, which primarily assesses the symptom severity of patients in Stage C and D, and 2) to target therapy.

C. Forward versus backward failure. Forward failure is primarily

characterized by low cardiac output and its associated symptoms of fatigue and weakness. Backward failure results in "congestive" symptoms of pulmonary and peripheral edema.
  D. **Left-sided versus right-sided failure.** It is important to decide if patients have evidence of left-sided failure, because these patients can present with significant hypoxemia and therefore may need to be treated urgently (see IV D). The distinction between left-sided and right-sided failure is based primarily on signs found during physical examination—but all these findings can be insensitive and nonspecific especially in patients with chronic heart failure.
     1. **Left-sided failure.** Signs of left-sided failure include **a left-sided third heart sound (S_3), rales, wheezes** ("cardiac asthma," a manifestation of interstitial edema), and **tachypnea.**
     2. **Right-sided failure.** Signs of right-sided failure include a **right-sided S_3** (i.e., one that increases with inspiration), **an elevated jugular venous pressure, abnormal hepatojugular reflux, ascites, peripheral edema,** and an **enlarged liver.**
        a. Most of the time, evidence of biventricular failure is found during physical examination because **the most common cause of right-sided failure is left-sided failure.**
        b. Other causes of right-sided failure include:
           (1) Pulmonary hypertension [most commonly caused by chronic obstructive pulmonary disease (COPD)]
           (2) Right ventricular infarction (usually occurring in the setting of left-sided inferior wall infarction)
           (3) Right-sided endocarditis
  E. **Systolic versus diastolic dysfunction.** Left ventricular failure can be either systolic or diastolic. This is the most important distinction to make because it affects treatment.
     1. **Systolic dysfunction** means that the heart's contractility is compromised. The most useful clinical measure of contractility is the **ejection fraction,** which is **considered significantly abnormal below 40%.** Causes of systolic dysfunction include:
        a. **Myocardial infarction** and **ischemic heart disease**
        b. **"Burned out" hypertensive** or **valvular heart disease.** Initially, these disorders lead to diastolic dysfunction, but with time, the heart dilates and the ejection fraction decreases.
        c. **Dilated cardiomyopathies** (a cardiomyopathy is a disorder of the myocardium not caused by coronary artery disease, hypertension, valvular disease, or congenital heart disease).

Common Causes of Dilated Cardiomyopathy ("PIPED")

Postmyocarditis
Idiopathic
Peripartum
Ethanol
Drugs (cocaine and heroin)

d. Myocarditis
2. **Diastolic dysfunction** means that the heart has normal contractility, but its ability to relax and allow adequate filling during diastole is compromised. These patients have a **normal or supranormal ejection fraction.** Causes of diastolic dysfunction include:
   a. Ischemia
   b. Disorders that lead to left ventricular hypertrophy, such as:
   (1) Hypertension
   (2) Aortic stenosis
   (3) Hypertrophic cardiomyopathy
   c. Restrictive cardiomyopathy. This disorder is usually caused by infiltrative diseases (e.g., hemochromatosis, amyloidosis, sarcoidosis, or scleroderma) or injury such as postradiation fibrosis.
3. In most patients, evidence of both diastolic and systolic dysfunction coexist; however, 20%–40% of patients have predominantly diastolic dysfunction. Both types of dysfunction have similar clinical manifestations.

HOT **KEY** CHF with a low ejection fraction = systolic dysfunction
CHF with a normal or high ejection fraction = diastolic dysfunction

---

III APPROACH TO THE PATIENT

A. Determine if the patient's symptoms are truly due to CHF. Given substantial limitations of the physical exam, this can be particularly difficult. Importantly, accumulating data suggest that B-type natriuretic peptide (BNP) may aid in separating breathlessness from CHF from noncardiac causes, especially in the emergency department setting. Once CHF is suspected, assess how symptomatic the patient is.
B. On the basis of the patient's history, physical examination findings, and chest radiographs, categorize the failure as predominantly left-sided, right-sided, or biventricular.
C. If the patient has left-sided CHF, determine whether the dysfunction is predominantly systolic or diastolic, using the ejection fraction as a basis for the determination. Ejection fraction can be assessed using echocardiography, multiple gated acquisition (MUGA) scans or gated single-photon emission computed tomography (SPECT), or cardiac catheterization. **Re-**

member, if a patient with a normal ejection fraction has cardio-genic pulmonary edema or additional evidence for elevated fill-ing pressures or low cardiac output, then the dysfunction is di-astolic.

D. Determine the underlying cause of CHF (e.g., coronary artery disease, valvular disease, hypertension, cardiomyopathy).

E. If the patient's symptoms have worsened acutely (this is usually the scenario in patients evaluated in the emergency depart-ment), you must decide what precipitated the CHF exacerba-tion:

Factors That Can Exacerbate CHF ("FAILURE")

Forgot meds
Arrhythmia or **A**nemia
Infections, Ischemia, or Infarction
Lifestyle (e.g., increased sodium intake, stress)
Upregulators (e.g., thyroid disease, pregnancy)
Rheumatic valve or worsening of other valvular diseases
Embolism (pulmonary)

IV TREATMENT

A. **Goals** of treatment of CHF (and most other diseases) are two-fold:
  1. **Reduce symptoms**
  2. **Reduce mortality**

B. **Chronic systolic dysfunction.** Treatment primarily involves the following:
  1. **Vasodilators.** Peripheral arterial vasodilators [e.g., an-giotensin-converting enzyme (ACE) inhibitors, angiotensin-receptor blockers, hydralazine, isosorbide dinitrate] are drugs that have been shown to reduce both symptoms and mortality rates in both asymptomatic and symptomatic pa-tients (ACC/AHA Stages B and C). The ACE inhibitors are considered first-line therapy for systolic dysfunction. If ACE inhibitors are unable to be tolerated because of cough, an-giotensin-receptor blockers are reasonable second-line agents.
  2. **β blockers.** These agents should be used in all potential pa-tients with CHF. The key is to start treatment when the pa-tient is stable (i.e., not after a recent exacerbation) and at low doses with slow titration.
  3. **Digoxin.** This age-old treatment for CHF has been shown to reduce symptoms but has never been shown to decrease

mortality rates. Digoxin should be used in patients who are symptomatic despite other therapy.

4. **Diuretics** are effective for treating symptoms of fluid overload (e.g., rales, peripheral edema). Aldactone, a potassium-sparing diuretic, has been shown to improve mortality rates in patients with NYHA Class III and IV.

5. **Diet.** A low-salt diet is also primarily used for control of fluid overload. The number of patients admitted to the hospital for CHF exacerbations significantly increases the day after Thanksgiving, undoubtedly as a result of increased salt consumption.

6. **Arrhythmias.** Sudden cardiac death remains the leading cause of death in patients with CHF. Patients with significant symptoms (i.e., syncope) and/or ventricular tachyarrhythmias should be considered candidates for implantable cardiac defibrillators (ICD). Biventricular pacemakers may also be beneficial in patients with severe systolic dysfunction and intraventricular conduction delays.

C. **Chronic diastolic dysfunction.** Digoxin and vasodilators do not play a major role in the treatment of patients with predominantly diastolic dysfunction. Treatment focuses on controlling blood pressure and heart rate, maintaining fluid balance, and minimizing ischemia if present. Some agents, such as β blockers and centrally acting calcium channel blockers (e.g., diltiazem, verapamil), are thought to improve left ventricular relaxation directly. None of these drugs have been shown to reduce mortality rates.

D. **Acute pulmonary edema.** If a patient experiencing acute pulmonary edema is not treated correctly and promptly, he or she may die. Both systolic and diastolic dysfunction can lead to acute pulmonary edema; however, in the beginning, initiating prompt therapy is more important than determining the exact cause of the patient's rapid decompensation. Reducing preload is the primary goal of therapy in patients with acute pulmonary edema. Some patients may require the addition of intravenous inotropes (e.g., dobutamine, milrinone) to aid with diuresis. It is easy to remember how to treat "wet" patients:

Treatment of Acute Pulmonary Edema ("MOIST 'N DAMP")

Morphine (2–4 mg intravenously as long as the blood pressure is adequate)

Oxygen (as much as necessary to raise the oxygen saturation over 90%)

Intubation, if necessary (pulmonary edema is rapidly reversible, but if the patient is tiring, intubation can be life-saving)

Sit 'em up (to reduce preload)

Tourniquet (rotating tourniquets to decrease preload were once used)

Nitrates (acutely decrease preload)

Diuretics (20–40 mg furosemide intravenously to first decrease preload and then induce a diuresis)

Albuterol (may help bronchospastic patients)

More morphine, more nitrates, and more diuretics as needed

Phlebotomy (was once used to reduce preload)

References

Cowie MR, Mendez GF. BNP and congestive heart failure. Prog Cardiovasc Dis 2002; 44(4):293–321.

Hunt SA, Baker DW, Chin MH, et al. ACC/AHA guidelines for the evaluation and management of chronic heart failure in the adult: executive summary. Circulation 2001;104:2996–3007.

Nohria A, Lewis E, Stevenson LW. Medical management of advanced heart failure. JAMA 2002;287(5):628–640.

Schrier RW, Abraham WT. Hormones and hemodynamics in heart failure. N Engl J Med 1999;341:577–585.

Zile MR, Brutsaert DL. New concepts in diastolic dysfunction and diastolic heart failure: part I: diagnosis, prognosis, and measurements of diastolic function. Circulation 2002;105(11):1387–1393.

Zile MR, Brutsaert DL. New concepts in diastolic dysfunction and diastolic heart failure: part II: causal mechanisms and treatment. Circulation 2002;105(12):1503–1508.

13. Shock

I INTRODUCTION

A. **Definition.** Shock occurs when the arterial circulation is unable to keep up with the metabolic demands of the body.
B. **Clinical manifestations** of shock—regardless of etiology—usually include:
   1. **Hypotension**
   2. **Tachycardia**
   3. **Altered mental status**
   4. **Decreased urine output**
   5. **Cool skin**

II CAUSES OF SHOCK.
The many causes of shock must be remembered because treatment must address both the manifestations of shock as well as its underlying cause.

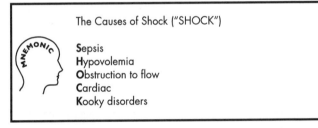

The Causes of Shock ("SHOCK")

Sepsis
Hypovolemia
Obstruction to flow
Cardiac
Kooky disorders

A. **Sepsis** is a common cause of shock. Bacteremia caused by **gram-negative rods** (e.g., *Escherichia coli, Klebsiella, Proteus, Pseudomonas*) or **gram-positive cocci** (e.g., *Staphylococcus, Streptococcus*) is the usual cause of septic shock.
B. **Hypovolemia.** Any process that causes a significant reduction in intravascular volume (e.g., trauma, gastrointestinal bleeding, hematoma, burns, pancreatitis, hyperosmolar states, vomiting, diarrhea) can lead to hypovolemic shock.
C. **Obstruction to flow.** Disorders such as cardiac tamponade, pulmonary embolism, tension pneumothorax, and severe aortic or mitral valve stenosis can lead to shock. Tamponade and tension pneumothorax should always be considered promptly because early treatment can save the patient's life.
D. **Cardiac causes.** Cardiogenic shock is most commonly the result of "pump failure," caused by a myocardial infarction (of either

97

the left or right ventricle) or dilated cardiomyopathy. Other cardiac causes include tachyarrhythmias or bradyarrhythmias, acute valvular regurgitation (mitral or aortic), and rupture of the septum or ventricular wall.

E. "Kooky" disorders. This category includes diseases only a medical school "DEAN" could remember:

"Kooky" Disorders Leading to Shock ("DEAN")

Drug toxicity (primarily vasodilating drugs)
Endocrine disorders (adrenal insufficiency or myxedema)
Anaphylaxis
Neurogenic (especially after spinal cord injury)

III APPROACH TO THE PATIENT

A. Physical examination. The ABCs (**airway, breathing,** and **circulation**) should be assessed first.

1. **Blood pressure** should be verified with a manual cuff. Hypotension is usually defined as a systolic pressure that is less than 90 mm Hg but can vary across individuals. Pulsus paradoxus (a greater than 10 mm Hg drop in systolic pressure with inspiration) suggests tamponade.

2. **Temperature.** If the patient is febrile or hypothermic, septic shock is likely.

3. **Oxygen saturation** should be obtained during the initial assessment.

4. **Neck vein assessment.** Elevated neck veins in a hypotensive patient are usually indicative of:
   a. Tamponade
   b. Tension pneumothorax
   c. Pulmonary embolism (with right ventricular failure)
   d. Right ventricular infarct (typically associated with an inferior wall myocardial infarction)
   e. Biventricular dysfunction (the only entity on this list that will also cause rales)

5. **Lung sounds**
   a. **Rales** usually indicates a cardiac cause.
   b. **Wheezing** should increase suspicion of anaphylaxis.
   c. **Asymmetric breath sounds** may represent pneumothorax.

6. **Cardiac auscultation.** Important findings include an abnormal rate or rhythm, distant heart sounds, a third heart sound (S_3), or new murmurs.

7. **Abdominal palpation** is helpful in evaluating whether pan-

creatitis, a perforated viscus, or an infected hepatobiliary source is the cause of shock.

    8. Rectal examination is important, especially if gastrointestinal bleeding is likely.

    9. Skin inspection. A **scarlatiniform rash** may be indicative of toxic shock syndrome, whereas **urticaria** can be a sign of anaphylaxis.

    10. Neurologic examination is useful to assess mental status and to ensure that the patient does not have spinal cord compression.

B. Laboratory tests. Useful tests include:

    1. A **complete blood count (CBC)**

    2. A **chemistry panel,** including blood urea nitrogen (BUN) and creatinine levels

    3. Liver function tests

    4. Urinalysis

    5. Blood cultures

    6. Arterial blood gases

C. A **chest radiograph** and **electrocardiogram (ECG)** are **mandatory.**

D. Other diagnostic modalities [e.g., computed tomography (CT), echocardiography, endoscopy, ventilation-perfusion ($\dot{V}/\dot{Q}$) scan, cardiac biomarkers, or evaluation of thyroid-stimulating hormone (TSH) level or serum cortisol] should be enlisted promptly if warranted by clinical suspicion.

E. Occasionally, patients are hypotensive but the cause is not clear. In these situations, **pulmonary artery (PA) catheterization** can be useful, especially in patients who are both hypotensive and hypoxemic (Table 13-1).

HOT

KEY

    Hypotension + Hypoxemia = PA line

IV   TREATMENT. The goal is to maintain the mean arterial pressure above 60 mm Hg (calculated by adding 2/3 of the diastolic pressure to 1/3 of the systolic pressure) while treating the underlying disorder causing the shock. Treatment is usually instituted even before a definitive cause of shock has been determined.

A. Place the patient in the **Trendelenburg position** (head down).

B. Provide **supplemental oxygen.** Intubation may be necessary.

C. Administer **fluids** rapidly through two large-bore intravenous lines, unless the patient clearly has biventricular failure.

D. Insert a **Foley catheter** to monitor urine output.

TABLE 13-1. Pulmonary Artery (PA) Catheterization Findings in Specific Disease States

Disease	RAP	PCWP	SVR	CO	Comments
Sepsis	↓	↓	↓	↑	Few other disorders have a low SVR
Hypovolemia	↓	↓	↑	↓	Source of fluid loss must be identified
Tamponade	↑	Normal to ↓	↑	↓	PCWP = CVP = PADP
Pulmonary embolism	Normal to ↑	Normal	↑	↓	PADP is often 5 mm Hg > PCWP
Biventricular failure	↑	↑	↑	↓	Diagnosis is usually apparent on physical examination and chest x-ray
Right ventricular infarct	↑	↓	↑	↓	If the patient is hypoxemic and the chest x-ray is normal, consider a right-to-left shunt
Neurogenic shock	↓	↓	↓	Normal to ↓	Hemodynamics can be similar in adrenal insufficiency

RAP = right atrial pressure (equivalent to central venous pressure); normal: 0–8 mm Hg
PCWP = pulmonary capillary wedge pressure; normal: 5–12 mm Hg
SVR = systemic vascular resistance; normal: 900–1300 dyne/sec/cm^{-5}
CO = cardiac output; normal: 3.5–7 L/min
PASP = pulmonary artery systolic pressure; normal: 15–30 mm Hg
PADP = pulmonary artery diastolic pressure; normal: 5–12 mm Hg
CVP = central venous pressure
↑ = increased; ↓ = decreased

E. Place an **intra-arterial catheter** (either in the radial or femoral artery) for closer hemodynamic monitoring, especially if manual blood pressure measurements are unreliable.

F. Consider **vasopressor medications.** The decision to use "pressors" is often difficult; usually, they are used if the patient has not responded to a trial of aggressive fluid resuscitation. The choice of which pressor to use depends on the clinical situation and should be guided by hemodynamic monitoring.

1. **Mechanism of action.** Vasopressors act on the **autonomic nervous system.** Once you understand what each receptor does (Table 13-2), it is easy to remember the actions of each pressor.

2. **Agents.** Table 13-3 contains the most commonly used vasopressors, in order from α_1-adrenergic agents to β_2-adrenergic agents. Get used to remembering the drugs in this order. [If you need a mnemonic to help you, you can think of the following scenario: A patient, Edward, who has severe congestive heart failure (CHF), calls himself "Eddie." Unfortunately, he is a poor speller, so he spells his name "Edi." Every time you see him, you inquire whether he has paroxysmal nocturnal dyspnea (PND). You ask, "PND EDI?"]

Vasopressors ("PND EDI?")

Phenylephrine
Norepinephrine
Dopamine
Epinephrine
Dobutamine
Isoproterenol

TABLE 13-2. Review of Autonomic Nervous System

Receptor	Major Location	Action
α_1	Peripheral vascular and coronary smooth muscle	Constricts
β_1	Myocardium	Increases heart rate and contractility
β_2	Bronchial, peripheral vascular, and coronary smooth muscle	Dilates
Dopamine	Vascular smooth muscle (renal, gastrointestinal)	Dilates

TABLE 13-3. Vasopressors

Drug	Action	Dose	Indications
Phenylephrine	α_1-Adrenergic	10–200 µg/min	Sepsis
Norepinephrine	α_1-Adrenergic, β_1-adrenergic	2–64 µg/min	Sepsis
Dopamine*	Dopaminergic	1–2 µg/kg/min	Sepsis, hypotensive cardiogenic shock
	β_1-Adrenergic	2–10 µg/kg/min	
	α_1-Adrenergic	10–20 µg/kg/min	
Epinephrine	α_1-Adrenergic, β_1-adrenergic, β_2-adrenergic	1–4 µg/min	Pulseless arrest, sepsis
Dobutamine	β_1-Adrenergic, β_2-adrenergic	1–20 µg/kg/min	Cardiogenic shock (but not by itself if patient is hypotensive), congestive heart failure
Isoproterenol	β_1, β_2	1–4 µg/min	Bradycardia

*Action depends on the dose.

3. Vasopressin. Vasopressin, a hormone typically responsible for osmotic control in the renal collecting ducts, recently has been shown to have significant vasopressor effects through direct constriction of vascular wall smooth muscle cells. Its effect may be seen even when high doses of other agents fail.

References

Abraham E, Matthay MA, Dinarello CA, et al. Consensus conference definitions for sepsis, septic shock, acute lung injury, and acute respiratory distress syndrome: time for a reevaluation. Crit Care Med 2000;28(1):232–235.

Hollenberg SM, Kavinsky CJ, Parrillo JE. Cardiogenic shock. Ann Intern Med 1999; 131(1):47–59.

Landry DW, Oliver JA. Pathogenesis of vasodilatory shock. N Engl J Med 2001; 345:588–595.

PART III

PULMONARY AND CRITICAL CARE

14. Acute Dyspnea

I **INTRODUCTION.** Acute dyspnea is a common cause of emergency room visits, hospital admissions, and decompensation among hospitalized patients.

II **CAUSES OF ACUTE DYSPNEA.** Dyspnea is often the chief complaint of patients with a variety of disorders, many of which can be immediately life-threatening (Table 14-1).

A. **Pulmonary**
   1. **Pneumothorax** is a sudden event that is often accompanied by very acute dyspnea and pleuritic chest pain. This diagnosis should be considered carefully in a patient with significant bullous lung disease, recent chest wall trauma, or on a ventilator.
   2. **Pulmonary embolism** is a difficult diagnosis to make because of the poor sensitivity and specificity of the history and physical examination. Consider the diagnosis early, as specialized diagnostic testing is often required.
   3. **Airflow limitation** should be suspected in patients with known obstructive lung disease, such as chronic obstructive pulmonary disease (COPD) or asthma. Wheezing is the hallmark physical finding.
   4. **Aspiration** should be suspected in patients with swallowing dysfunction, alcohol abuse, seizure disorder, or a diminished level of consciousness. Always ask family members or nurses about witnessed aspiration. Importantly, aspiration events are often not witnessed.
   5. **Pneumonia.** Patients will usually have other symptoms of infection, including fever or hypothermia, chills, or a productive cough.
   6. **Upper airway obstruction.** A very acute onset of symptoms with inspiratory stridor should prompt consideration of this diagnosis.

TABLE 14-1. Common Causes of Acute Dyspnea		
Pulmonary	**Cardiac**	**Other**
Pneumothorax	Myocardial ischemia or infarction	Sepsis
Pulmonary embolism	Congestive heart failure	Metabolic acidosis
Airflow limitation	Arrhythmias	Anemia
Aspiration	Pericardial tamponade	Anxiety
Pneumonia		
Upper airway obstruction		
Acute respiratory distress syndrome		

7. **Acute respiratory distress syndrome (ARDS).** ARDS is a clinically defined entity encountered most commonly in patients with sepsis, trauma, massive blood transfusion, or pancreatitis.

B. Cardiac

1. **Myocardial ischemia** or **infarction.** Dyspnea may occur in the absence of chest pain and thus may represent an anginal equivalent.

2. **CHF.** In hospitalized patients with CHF, acute dyspnea is often precipitated by fluid administration or myocardial ischemia.

3. **Arrhythmias.** Patients may have a history of palpitations. Specific etiologies cannot be reliably diagnosed on physical examination; a 12-lead electrocardiogram (ECG) or a rhythm strip is required.

4. **Pericardial tamponade** is rare but should always be considered in patients with breast and lung cancer, renal failure, recent myocardial infarction, or blunt trauma to the chest.

C. Metabolic

1. **Sepsis.** Dyspnea and an acute respiratory alkalosis may be the earliest findings in sepsis.

2. **Metabolic acidosis.** Dyspnea is common as patients hyperventilate to compensate for their acidosis.

D. Hematologic. Acute anemia (from hemorrhage or hemolysis) can cause acute dyspnea due to the decreased oxygen carrying capacity of blood. Anemia can easily be missed on history and physical examination.

E. Psychiatric. Anxiety can be a primary cause of acute dyspnea; however, a diagnosis of primary anxiety should be considered only after ruling out the more serious possibilities.

III **APPROACH TO THE PATIENT.** The key to evaluating a patient with acute dyspnea is to focus on recognizing the most serious disorders.

A. Patient history. There are four key areas of inquiry:
   1. What was the **speed of onset** of the dyspnea?
   2. Are there any **associated symptoms** (e.g., chest pain, cough, chills)?
   3. **What happened immediately before** the onset of the dyspnea? What medications or fluids was the patient receiving?
   4. What are the patient's **other medical problems**? If already hospitalized, what is the admission diagnosis?
B. Physical examination. Focus on five key areas:
   1. Vital signs. Significantly abnormal vital signs in an acutely dyspneic patient may signify impending respiratory failure. An oxygen saturation should be obtained.

> **HOT**
> Remember, a normal oxygen saturation does not exclude the possibility of a serious disorder!
> **KEY**

   2. Chest. Pay particular attention to the symmetry of breath sounds and the presence of wheezing or rales. Look for tracheal deviation (toward a pneumothorax or collapsed lung, away from an effusion).
   3. Heart. A complete examination should be performed, focusing on the findings of right-sided and left-sided heart failure. Also note the heart rate (too fast? too slow?).
   4. Extremities. Look for edema (unilateral versus bilateral) and cyanosis.
   5. Mental status. Evaluating the patient's mental status is crucial for two reasons:
       a. A significantly depressed level of consciousness may necessitate intubation for airway protection.
       b. The finding of altered mental status as a result of the dyspnea suggests a significant homeostatic insult.
C. Diagnostic studies. Four studies should routinely be performed when the patient is acutely dyspneic.
   1. 12-Lead ECG
   2. Arterial blood gas analysis
   3. Chest radiograph
   4. Complete blood count (CBC)

IV **TREATMENT.** Treatment should be aimed at the underlying cause. The following are a few general principles:

A. Supplemental oxygen. All patients with acute dyspnea should be administered supplemental oxygen, with the goal of normalizing oxygen saturation($> 90\%$) and partial pressure of oxygen ($PaO_2 \geq 60$ mm Hg). A history of COPD or carbon dioxide retention should not prevent oxygen therapy for hypoxemic patients; however, patients at risk for carbon dioxide retention should be monitored closely. Approximately 35% oxygen can be delivered by standard nasal cannula, with close to 100% oxygen available with a non-rebreather face mask.

B. Diuretics. Cardiogenic pulmonary edema should respond rapidly to diuretic therapy. Other processes associated with excess lung water (e.g., ARDS, aspiration, pneumonia) may also improve with diuresis.

C. β agonists. Regardless of the cause, wheezing will likely improve somewhat with nebulized β agonist therapy. Albuterol can be given continuously if indicated but may cause undesired tachycardia. Ipratropium (an anticholinergic agent) may be used in conjunction with albuterol but is given only every 4 hours.

D. Mechanical ventilation (see Chapter 26). The need for mechanical ventilation (either invasive endotracheal intubation or noninvasive face mask) should be assessed. Indications for mechanical ventilation include:

1. Refractory hypoxemia ($PaO_2 < 60$ mm Hg despite maximal oxygen therapy)

2. Hypercapnea (generally manifested by an increasing $PaCO_2$ despite therapy)

3. Inability to protect the airway

4. Impending upper airway obstruction

HOT KEY

Hypoxemic or hypercapneic respiratory failure may respond to noninvasive positive pressure ventilation (NIPPV) in patients who are alert and able to tolerate the pressurized mask. Inability to protect the airway demands immediate endotracheal intubation. Impending upper airway obstruction should be approached cautiously, with immediate percutaneous tracheostomy available should endotracheal intubation prove impossible.

References

Dyspnea. Mechanisms, assessment, and management: a consensus statement. American Thoracic Society. Am J Respir Crit Care Med 1999;159(1):321–340.

Mahler DA, Harver A. Do you speak the language of dyspnea? Chest 2000;117(4): 928–929.

15. Massive Hemoptysis

I **INTRODUCTION.** Hemoptysis, defined as the expectoration of blood, can be an insignificant symptom of a benign illness, a first manifestation of serious malignancy, or a fatal process in and of itself. Hemoptysis is usually classified as either **massive** or **nonmassive**.

A. Massive hemoptysis, variably defined as expectorating > 200–500 ml of blood in a 24-hour period, requires immediate evaluation; it is the focus of this chapter.

B. Nonmassive hemoptysis, usually defined as expectorating < 200–500 ml of blood in a 24-hour period, accounts for more than 90% of cases. Patients with nonmassive hemoptysis warrant close attention, because they may develop massive hemoptysis in an unpredictable fashion. However, many can be managed effectively as outpatients.

HOT ▶ **KEY** While the precise volume of expectorated blood is usually difficult to ascertain, if a patient says he has coughed up about one cup or more of blood in the last 24 hours, consider this "massive" hemoptysis.

II **CAUSES OF HEMOPTYSIS.** The list of differential diagnoses is long. The following mnemonic can help you to remember the many causes of hemoptysis—think of soldiers in a "BATTLE CAMP" coughing up blood.

Causes of Hemoptysis ("BATTLE CAMP")

Bronchiectasis* or **B**ronchitis
Aspergillosis*
Tumor*
Tuberculosis*
Lung abscess*
Emboli
Coagulopathy
Arteriovenous malformation, **A**rteritis, or **A**lveolar hemorrhage
Mitral stenosis
Pneumonia

*Most common causes of **massive** hemoptysis

A. Bronchitis is the most common cause of hemoptysis but rarely causes massive bleeding.

B. Bronchiectasis is relatively rare in the United States because the number of cases of tuberculosis and untreated pneumonia has declined. Massive hemoptysis can occur from arteriovenous shunts that develop in areas of bronchiectatic lung.

C. Aspergillosis. Any fungal pneumonia can cause hemoptysis, but infection with the angioinvasive *Aspergillus fumigatus* is the most common cause. This usually occurs in immunocompromised patients and can cause massive hemoptysis.

D. Tuberculosis. Massive hemoptysis in patients with tuberculosis is often caused by the rupture of dilated pulmonary arteries that traverse the tuberculous cavities (so-called Rasmussen's aneurysms).

E. Emboli. Pulmonary embolism can cause lung infarction, which can bleed as it necroses.

F. Coagulopathy. Anticoagulation is often associated with hemoptysis but is generally not causative in and of itself. An underlying lesion should be sought. Rarely, anticoagulation can cause alveolar hemorrhage (see below).

G. Arteriovenous malformation is usually congenital and is often associated with hereditary hemorrhagic telangiectasia (Osler-Weber-Rendu syndrome).

H. Arteritis. Many vasculitides can involve the lungs (e.g., Churg-Strauss syndrome, Wegener's granulomatosis).

I. Alveolar hemorrhage is usually caused by autoimmune processes that lead to alveolar capillary damage ("capillaritis"). Some of these conditions may also involve the kidneys [e.g., Goodpasture's syndrome, systemic lupus erythematosus (SLE)], causing hematuria and a cellular ("active") urinary sediment.

J. Mitral stenosis causing pulmonary hypertension can lead to hemoptysis.

K. Pneumonia associated with hemoptysis is often necrotizing (e.g., that caused by *Staphylococcus aureus* or *Pseudomonas aeruginosa*).

III APPROACH TO THE PATIENT

A. Maintain airway patency and oxygenation. Arterial blood gas analysis and chest radiographs should be performed immediately to assess oxygenation and determine the extent of blood retained in the lung. Because death from massive hemoptysis usually results from alveolar flooding and hypoxemia, ensuring adequate oxygenation is the most important first step.

HOT KEY

To prevent aspiration of blood into the unaffected lung in a patient with massive hemoptysis, have the patient lie in the lateral decubitus position with the bleeding side down. How do you know which lung is bleeding? Ask the patient; he or she may know (clues: known cancer, recent procedure or surgery).

1. If emergent intubation is indicated (see Chapter 14) a large-bore endotracheal tube should be used to enable adequate suctioning and allow for urgent bronchoscopy.

2. In cases of unilateral hemorrhage, selective right or left mainstem intubation with specialized endotracheal tubes protects against spread of blood to the unaffected lung.

B. Identify the bleeding lesion

1. **Ensure a bronchopulmonary source.** It is necessary to ensure that the patient truly has bronchopulmonary bleeding; gastrointestinal and nasopharyngeal bleeding commonly masquerade as hemoptysis. If the source of the bleeding is not obvious, helpful techniques include the following:

   a. **Evaluation of the pH of the expectorated substance** can provide clues—gastrointestinal contents are usually acidic, whereas pulmonary expectorations are usually alkaline.

   b. **Examination of the pharynx** and **larynx** may reveal the cause of the bleeding to be epistaxis.

2. **Lung auscultation** and **chest radiographs** can help to localize the bleeding but may not be helpful if the bleeding is diffuse or if blood has been aspirated from one lung into the other. A chest radiograph may show a mass lesion or cavity.

3. **Urinalysis** and **assessment of renal function** may show proteinuria, dysmorphic red cells or red cell casts, suggesting a vasculitis or pulmonary-renal syndrome.

4. **Computed tomography (CT)** may reveal a space-occupying lesion (e.g., lung cancer or abscess).

5. **Early bronchoscopy** is indicated for most patients for both therapeutic and diagnostic purposes.

6. **Arteriography** is useful for actively bleeding patients for purposes of localization of the bleeding lesion and therapy.

C. Control the hemorrhage

1. General measures indicated for all patients with massive hemoptysis include bed rest, cough suppressants, sedatives, and stool softeners or laxatives, which help prevent sudden increases in intrathoracic pressure, thereby minimizing intravascular pressure.

2. Coagulopathies should be corrected if present.

3. Bronchoscopic maneuvers such as ice-saline irrigation, topi-

cal application of epinephrine or thrombin, or balloon tamponade may be useful in selected patients.

4. External radiation therapy may be effective for reducing bleeding from tumors.

5. Definitive therapy for massive hemoptysis often requires angiographic arterial embolization or surgical lung resection.

H O T

 Consult a pulmonologist immediately if the patient presents with massive hemoptysis.

K E Y

References

Dweik RA, Stoller JK. Role of bronchoscopy in massive hemoptysis. Clin Chest Med 1999;20(1):89–105.

Jean-Baptiste E. Clinical assessment and management of massive hemoptysis. Crit Care Med 2000;28(5):1642–1647.

Tasker AD, Flower CD. Imaging the airways. Hemoptysis, bronchiectasis, and small airways disease. Clin Chest Med 1999;20(4):761–773.

16. Approach to the Chest Radiograph

I **INTRODUCTION.** It is often necessary to rely on your own interpretation of a chest radiograph pending a formal reading. This chapter provides a consistent, easy-to-use approach to the evaluation of a chest radiograph.

II **PRELIMINARY CONSIDERATIONS**

A. What kind of radiograph should I order?
1. A **posterior-anterior (PA) view** is always preferable to an anterior-posterior (AP) view because the latter exaggerates the size of the heart and other mediastinal structures. However, in an emergency situation, an AP view is often the only option.
2. A **lateral view** should also be obtained to provide supplemental information and to confirm findings on the PA view.

B. Is it a good film? Assessing the quality of the radiograph may help avoid common misinterpretations.
1. **Inspiration.** Count the number of ribs; a good inspiration will reveal 10 posterior ribs. A poor inspiration may result in the false appearance of an interstitial process, leading to a misdiagnosis of pulmonary edema or atypical pneumonia.
2. **Rotation.** Look at the clavicles and see if they are asymmetrical (an indication of rotation). Rotation often leads to erroneous estimates of cardiac, pulmonary artery, aortic, and mediastinal dimensions.
3. **Penetration.** You should be able to see individual vertebrae in a film that is appropriately penetrated. Decreased penetration will make the lungs seem denser. Mild pulmonary edema or a small infiltrate will appear to be significant pulmonary edema or a large infiltrate, and even normal interstitial markings may appear abnormal.

C. Is there an old film available for comparison? There is no substitute for comparison with prior films. A new subtle area of consolidation may be found in a patient with suspected pneumonia, a nodule may be unchanged for 10 years and therefore presumed to be benign, or the mediastinum may be wider in a patient with suspected aortic dissection. In all cases, you need to make sure the view was the same (i.e., AP versus PA). In addition, you must "mentally adjust" for variations in technique (i.e., inspiration, rotation, and penetration).

III THE OUTSIDE—IN APPROACH. The structures visible
on a chest radiograph can be evaluated in any order, but you
should be consistent every time you read a film. The outside-
in approach is frequently used and ensures that commonly
overlooked structures (e.g., bones) are not forgotten.

A. **Bones and soft tissues.** Look for lytic or blastic lesions that may
signal a metastatic malignancy. Evidence of osteoporosis or
compression fractures may also be found. Look for subcutaneous air to suggest pneumothorax or pneumomediastinum. Soft
tissue masses may also be apparent.

B. **Pleura.** Follow the pleural border of each lung, looking for evidence of focal thickening suggesting scarring or mass, blunting
of the costophrenic angle suggesting effusion, or calcifications
suggesting old pleural inflammation from empyema or asbestos
exposure.

C. **Lungs.** Look at both lung fields in an orderly fashion. Pay special attention to the diaphragms, the cardiac borders, and the
apices. Although symmetrical abnormalities may occur (e.g.,
with pulmonary edema or bilateral pneumonia), asymmetrical
findings are particularly suspicious. Infiltrates are generally
described as "alveolar" or "intersitial." Alveolar infiltrates
are generally fluffy, confluent, poorly demarcated opacities.
There may be air-bronchograms (lucent airways surrounded
by opaque consolidated lung) visible within them. An alveolar
infiltrate may be blood, pus, water, or cells; commonly, hemorrhage, pneumonia, cardiogenic pulmonary edema, and
ARDS are all considerations. Interstitial infiltrates are generally linear, well-defined, reticular (lattice-like), occasionally
nodular opacities. Interstitial infiltrates suggest atypical pneumonia, interstitial lung disease, and lymphatic congestion
(seen in heart failure and malignancy).

1. **Diaphragms**

   a. If one of the diaphragms is obscured, either an infiltrate is
   present in the respective lower lobe or there is a pleural
   effusion.

   b. The retrocardiac area is a common place for abnormalities to be overlooked. The left hemidiaphragm should be
   visible behind the heart. An obscured left hemidiaphragm
   suggests atelectasis or an infiltrate. The presence of air
   bronchograms favors consolidation.

   c. Flattened diaphragms are often found in chronic obstructive pulmonary disease (COPD).

   d. An elevated hemidiaphragm suggests diaphragmatic paralysis, a subpulmonic pleural effusion, or a subdiaphrag-
   matic process.

   e. Air under the diaphragm on an upright chest radiograph

in patients presenting with abdominal pain suggests visceral perforation and is a surgical emergency.

   f. A depressed lateral hemidiaphragm with a poorly visible costophrenic angle and surrounding hyperlucency ("deep sulcus sign") suggests a pneumothorax.

2. **Cardiac borders**

   a. A **lingular infiltrate** (lower portion of the left upper lobe) is suggested if the left cardiac border is obscured.

   b. A **right middle lobe infiltrate** is suggested if the right cardiac border is obscured.

3. **Apices**

   a. **Apical pneumothoraces** are easy to miss; always look carefully for these in patients with chest pain or shortness of breath. Follow the interstitial markings to the chest wall to ensure that no pneumothorax is present.

   b. **Congestive heart failure (CHF): Pulmonary venous congestion** is characterized by **cephalization** (redistribution of blood flow toward the apices). Other common findings with CHF include cardiomegaly, pleural effusions, prominent pulmonary arteries, Kerley B lines (horizontal lines in the periphery), and alveolar infiltrates due to pulmonary edema.

   c. **Tuberculosis:** Reactivation disease often presents with apical cavitary infiltration. A **lordotic view** may be ordered if the apex is not well visualized.

D. Heart

1. **Increased cardiac silhouette.** The cardiac silhouette should be less than one half of the thoracic diameter on a PA film; anything larger suggests cardiomegaly or pericardial effusion.

2. **Chamber enlargement**

   a. The left side of the cardiac silhouette represents the left ventricle, whereas the right side represents the right atrium. Prominence in either location may represent enlargement of the respective chamber.

   b. Left atrial enlargement may be signified by:

   (1) The loss of the normal concavity on the left side of the heart

   (2) An elevated left mainstem bronchus

   (3) The **"double-density" sign,** which is seen as two parallel lines on the right side of the heart representing the right atrial and the enlarged left atrial borders

   c. Right ventricular enlargement is not visible on PA or AP films, but can be seen on a lateral film as filling of the retrosternal space.

3. **Pulmonary hypertension.** The diameter of the pulmonary artery should generally not exceed that of a dime; promi-

nent pulmonary arteries may signify pulmonary hypertension.

E. Mediastinum

1. Aortic dissection. Mediastinal widening may signify aortic dissection, but the sensitivity and specificity of this finding are suboptimal.

2. Lymphadenopathy. A widened paratracheal stripe (normally a narrow opaque stripe along the right side of the trachea) and fullness of the aortic-pulmonary window (a triangular space on the left side of the mediastinum below the aortic arch) often signify mediastinal lymphadenopathy.

References

Dixon AK. Evidence-based diagnostic radiology. Lancet 1997;350(9076):509–512.

Hansell DM. Thoracic imaging—then and now. Br J Radiol 1997;70(Spec No: S153–61).

Ravin CE, Chotas HG. Chest radiography. Radiology 1997;204(3):593–600.

17. Hypoxemia

I INTRODUCTION

A. Hypoxemia is not a diagnosis; it is a manifestation of an underlying disease.
B. Hypoxemia is common in hospitalized patients.
C. Patients with hypoxemia should always be evaluated promptly.

II CLINICAL VALUES

A. Arterial oxygen tension (Pao₂). In strictest terms, one needs to obtain an arterial blood gas report to confirm the presence of hypoxemia. A **normal** Pa_{O_2} at sea level is **80–100 mm Hg.**
B. Oxygen (O₂) saturation. The arterial O_2 saturation is the percentage of oxyhemoglobin in arterial blood. It can be measured by pulse oxymetry (indirect) or arterial blood gas analysis (direct).

HOT

KEY

The pulse oximetry has a variability of at least ±4%. Thus, when in doubt, check an arterial blood gas.

C. Alveolar-to-arterial (A-a) gradient. The A-a gradient helps determine the cause of hypoxemia and provides a rough estimate of how ill a patient is.
1. A **normal A-a gradient** is **less than the patient's age divided by 4 plus 4.** For example, a 24-year-old patient should have an A-a gradient less than 10.
2. Calculating the A-a gradient is easy using the alveolar gas equation and values from the arterial blood gas report.
   a. First, the alveolar oxygen tension (PA_{O_2}) is calculated using the **alveolar gas equation:**

$$PA_{O_2} = (P_{barometric} - P_{water})\, FI_{O_2} - Pa_{CO_2}/0.8,$$

   where
   $P_{barometric}$ = the barometric pressure (760 mm Hg at sea level)
   P_{water} = the vapor pressure of water at body temperature (47 mm Hg)
   FI_{O_2} = the fraction of oxygen in the inspired gas (0.21 on room air)

117

HOT KEY

Remember, for the simplified equation to work, the patient must be breathing room air.

$Paco_2$ = the arterial carbon dioxide tension

Thus, at sea level, the equation simplifies to:

$$\mathbf{PAO_2 = 150 - Paco_2/0.8}$$

The value for $Paco_2$ is obtained from the arterial blood gas report.

  b. To calculate the A-a gradient, subtract the Pao_2 (obtained from the arterial blood gas report) from the PAo_2 (obtained from the alveolar gas equation):

$$\mathbf{A\text{-}a \ gradient = PAO_2 - Pao_2}$$

III MECHANISMS OF HYPOXEMIA. There are five pathophysiologic mechanisms that cause hypoxemia (Table 17-1).

TABLE 17-1. Causes of Hypoxemia	
Pathophysiologic Mechanism	**Clinical Examples**
Ventilation-perfusion ($\dot{V}/\dot{Q}$) mismatch	Pneumonia, CHF, ARDS, atelectasis, tumor-filled alveoli
Right-to-left shunting	Any of the causes of $\dot{V}/\dot{Q}$ mismatch if $\dot{V}/\dot{Q}$ = 0, congenital cardiac abnormalities, pulmonary arteriovenous malformation
Diffusion defects	Interstitial lung disease, *Pneumocystis carinii* pneumonia
Hypoventilation	COPD, CNS disorder (damage to respiratory neurons), mechanical impairment of the breathing apparatus (poliomyelitis, Guillain-Barré syndrome, myasthenia gravis, kyphoscoliosis, Pickwickian syndrome)
Low inspired O_2 tension	High altitude

ARDS = acute respiratory distress syndrome; *CHF* = congestive heart failure; *CNS* = central nervous system; *COPD* = chronic obstructive pulmonary disease; O_2 = oxygen.

A. Ventilation-perfusion ($\dot{V}/\dot{Q}$) mismatch accounts for more than 95% of cases of hypoxemia. $\dot{V}/\dot{Q}$ mismatch occurs when ventilation in a part of the lung is decreased in comparison to perfusion.

B. Right-to-left shunting occurs when systemic venous blood (PvO_2 = 40 mm Hg) enters the left side of the heart without coming in contact with oxygen-rich alveolar air.

1. Right-to-left shunting may result from cardiac abnormalities (e.g., patent foramen ovale, atrial septal defect) or pulmonary abnormalities (e.g., arteriovenous malformations, hepatopulmonary syndrome).

2. A shunt exists whenever ventilation equals zero but perfusion continues.

C. Diffusion defects leading to hypoxemia are uncommon. The causes include interstitial lung diseases (e.g., idiopathic pulmonary fibrosis), environmental lung disease, and *Pneumocystis carinii* pneumonia.

D. Hypoventilation is defined by an elevated $PaCO_2$ and a normal A-a gradient. There are many causes of this abnormality; to find the cause, a systematic approach, starting at the head and working to the lungs, is best.

E. Low inspired oxygen tension. Unless the patient is at a high altitude, this cause can be ruled out.

References

Henig NR, Pierson DJ. Mechanisms of hypoxemia. Respir Care Clin North Am 2000; 6(4):501–521.

Tierney LM Jr., Whooley MA, Saint S. Oxygen saturation: a fifth vital sign? Western J Med 1997;166(4):285–286.

White AC. The evaluation and management of hypoxemia in the chronic critically ill patient. Clin Chest Med 2001;22(1):123–134.

18. Pulmonary Function Tests

I | INTRODUCTION

A. **Uses.** Pulmonary function tests can be used to:
   1. Differentiate obstructive lung disease from restrictive lung disease
   2. Assess the severity of lung disease
   3. Evaluate response to therapy
B. **Types of information assessed.** Pulmonary function tests allow assessment of three types of information:
   1. **Lung volumes**
      a. The **total lung capacity (TLC)** is the volume of air in the lungs after a maximal inspiratory effort.
      b. The **vital capacity (VC)** is the maximal volume of air that can be expelled from the lungs following a maximal inspiration.
      c. The **residual volume (RV)** is the volume of air remaining in the lungs after a maximal expiratory effort.
   2. **Expiratory flow rate.** The **forced expiratory volume in 1 second (FEV_1)** is the most commonly used screening test for airway disease. FEV_1 represents the volume of air expired during the first second of expiration.
   3. **Diffusion capacity.** Evaluation of the diffusing capacity for carbon monoxide ($DLCO$) indicates the adequacy of alveolar—capillary gas exchange. Common causes of a decreased $DLCO$ are emphysema, interstitial lung disease, and pulmonary vascular disease.
C. **Interpretation.** An organized and systematic approach to interpretation is required. When interpreting the results of pulmonary function testing, it is important to note both the observed values and the percent predicted. The range of normal for all values will vary slightly depending on the pulmonary function testing laboratory.

II | OBSTRUCTIVE VERSUS RESTRICTIVE LUNG DISEASE

A. The **relationship between flow rate, lung volume, resistance, and compliance** is as follows: **Flow Rate = Lung Volume/ (Airway resistance)(Compliance)** Therefore, the flow rate (as measured by FEV_1) will decrease if the lung volume decreases (as seen in restrictive disorders), airway resistance increases (as seen in asthma or chronic bronchitis), or compliance increases (as seen in emphysema).

B. Obstructive disorders cannot be distinguished from restrictive disorders on the basis of FEV_1 alone. To distinguish between obstructive and restrictive lung disorders, the lung volume must be eliminated from the equation; dividing by the FVC will accomplish this goal: **$FEV_1(\%) = FEV_1/FVC.$** The $FEV_1(\%)$ is the percent of the forced vital capacity expelled in 1 second.

   1. If the **$FEV_1(\%)$** is **decreased** ($< 80\%$), then the patient has **airflow limitation,** suggestive of obstructive disease.

   2. If the **$FEV_1(\%)$** is **normal** or **increased** in the setting of a low FEV_1, then the patient may have **restrictive disease.**

III APPROACH TO THE INTERPRETATION OF PULMONARY FUNCTION TESTS

A. Look at the FEV_1 first.

   1. If the patient has a normal FEV_1, TLC, and DLCO, the patient is unlikely to have significant pulmonary disease.

   2. If the FEV_1 is low, look at the $FEV_1(\%)$ to document airflow limitation (obstructive disease) or to suggest restrictive disease.

   a. If the $FEV_1(\%)$ is normal or high, the patient may have restrictive disease (which will be confirmed by a low TLC).

   b. If the $FEV_1(\%)$ is less than 80%, the patient has airflow limitation, suggesting obstructive disease.

   (1) If the patient has airflow limitation, then determine if it is reversible.

   (a) If the FEV_1 improves by more than approximately 12% after bronchodilator administration, reversible airflow limitation is present. Such patients will probably benefit from treatment with inhaled corticosteroids. If there is no improvement following the administration of bronchodilators, the patient has fixed airway obstruction [possibly due to chronic obstructive pulmonary disease (COPD)].

B. Now look at the lung volumes.

   1. Increased TLC, RV: This suggests hyperinflation and gas trapping, consistent with obstructive lung disease.

   2. Decreased TLC, RV: This suggests restriction and is diagnostic of restrictive lung disease.

C. Finally, look at the DLCO.

   1. DLCO values should always be corrected for hemoglobin (DLCO-C) and alveolar volume (DLCO/VA).

   2. If the patient has restrictive disease, a low DLCO/VA implies that interstitial lung disease is the cause. If the DLCO is low but the DLCO/VA is normal, the patient's restrictive disease is likely due to low lung volumes (e.g., obesity, skeletal deformities).

3. If the patient has obstructive disease, a low DLCO-C suggests the presence of emphysema.

References

Celli BR. The importance of spirometry in COPD and asthma: effect on approach to management. Chest 2000;117(Suppl 2):15S-19S.

Crapo RO. Pulmonary-function testing. N Engl J Med 1994;7;331(1):25–30.

Ferguson GT, Enright PL, Buist AS, Higgins MW. Office spirometry for lung health assessment in adults: a consensus statement from the National Lung Health Education Program. Chest 2000;117(4):1146–1161.

19. Obstructive Lung Disease

I INTRODUCTION

A. **Disorders.** There are four major obstructive lung diseases:
1. **Asthma**
2. **Chronic obstructive pulmonary disease (COPD)**
3. **Bronchiectasis**
4. **Cystic fibrosis**

B. **Definitions.** Asthma and COPD are by far the most common obstructive lung diseases; therefore, these two disorders are the focus of this chapter. All obstructive diseases are marked by **airflow limitation,** characterized by a **low forced expiratory volume in 1 second (FEV_1)** and a **low $FEV_1(\%)$.** [$FEV_1(\%)$ = percent of the forced vital capacity expelled in 1 second.]
1. **Asthma** is characterized by reversible narrowing of the distal airways as a result of chronic inflammation and airways hyperreactivity. Pathologic changes include smooth muscle hypertrophy, mucosal edema, hypermucus secretion, and mucus plugging. The airflow limitation is **usually reversible** with bronchodilators.
2. **COPD.** The airflow limitation in COPD is usually **not reversible.** There are two types of COPD:
   a. **Chronic bronchitis,** defined clinically as a productive cough lasting for at least 3 months over 2 consecutive years, results from chronic airway inflammation and hyperproduction of mucus.
   b. **Emphysema** is defined pathologically as permanent enlargement of the airspaces distal to the terminal bronchioles with parenchymal destruction. This is also the result of chronic airway inflammation.

II CLINICAL MANIFESTATIONS OF ASTHMA AND COPD

A. **Asthma** is usually seen in children and young adults. Clinical manifestations may include:
1. Episodic wheezing, chest tightness, and dyspnea
2. Chronic cough
3. Tachypnea, reliance on the accessory muscles, and intercostal retraction
4. A prolonged expiration phase and hyperresonance
5. Pulsus paradoxus

B. COPD usually presents in the fifth or sixth decade of life. Most patients have components of both chronic bronchitis and emphysema.

1. **Chronic bronchitis ("blue bloaters")**
   a. Stocky build
   b. Prominent, productive cough
   c. Mild dyspnea
   d. Early hypoxemia and hypercarbia
   e. Wheezes and rhonchi

2. **Emphysema ("pink puffers")**
   a. Barrel-chested with a thin build
   b. Mild cough with severe dyspnea
   c. Hypoxemia and hypercarbia only in end-stage disease
   d. Diminished breath sounds on examination

III DIAGNOSIS OF ASTHMA AND COPD. These disorders are diagnosed on the basis of the patient's history, physical examination findings, and abnormal pulmonary function test results.

A. Asthma. Patients with asthma are usually diagnosed based on history, pulmonary function testing, and responsiveness to therapy. When the diagnosis is in question, specialized testing can be performed (e.g., methacholine provocation, exercise spirometry) to aid in the diagnosis. Remember, **not all that wheezes is asthma.** A physician who "CARES" will always rule out other causes of wheezing:

Other Causes of Wheezing ("CARES")

Cardiac asthma (i.e., CHF), **C**hurg-Strauss syndrome, or vocal **C**ord dysfunction
Allergic bronchopulmonary aspergillosis
Reflux esophagitis
Exposures (irritants, medications), **E**mbolism (pulmonary)
Sinusitis, *Strongyloides* infection

B. COPD. Patients with COPD often have a history of chronic cough, sputum production, and dyspnea that may have been present for many years. The etiology is almost always prolonged cigarette smoking; however, α_1-antitrypsin deficiency should be suspected in patients who are younger than 40 years of age, especially if they have predominantly basilar emphysema.

IV TREATMENT. The treatment of acute exacerbations of both asthma and COPD is very similar.

A. **Albuterol** and **ipratropium** are first-line agents and have similar efficacy. Ipratropium may be more effective in COPD. β agonists appear to have a more rapid onset of action and should be nebulized if patients are too distressed to use metered dose inhalers effectively.

B. **Steroids** are critical in asthma exacerbations and have been shown to benefit hospitalized patients with COPD flares, also called acute exacerbation of chronic bronchitis (AECB). Steroids improve symptoms after 4–6 hours and should be used for at least 5–10 days in patients with severe exacerbations. Oral therapy is generally as efficacious as parenteral, if patients are tolerating feeds.

C. **Theophylline** is cautiously used because of concerns regarding toxicity and proven efficacy of other agents. If used, levels should be checked carefully and dosage modified accordingly.

D. **Humidified oxygen** should be used in all patients who are hypoxemic, but caution is needed in rare patients susceptible to carbon dioxide retention.

Agents Used To Treat Exacerbations of Asthma or COPD ("ASTHMA")

Albuterol or ipratropium (**A**trovent)
Steroids (oral or intravenous)
Theophylline
Humidified oxygen, **H**eliox
Magnesium
Antibiotics

E. **Heliox,** a mixture of oxygen and helium (instead of nitrogen) has improved laminar flow and may be beneficial in patients with airflow limitation. There are data to support its use in asthma, although its efficacy is debated.

F. **Intravenous magnesium,** although controversial, may be beneficial in patients with severe asthma.

G. **Antibiotics** are likely to benefit patients with AECB who have dyspnea and a change in sputum production or color, even in the absence of fevers and a clear radiographic infiltrate. Asthmatic patients should be treated only if a bacterial infection is suspected.

References
Barnes PJ. Chronic obstructive pulmonary disease. N Engl J Med 2000;343(4):269–280.
Georgitis JW. The 1997 Asthma Management Guidelines and therapeutic issues re-
    lating to the treatment of asthma. National Heart, Lung, and Blood Institute.
    Chest 1999;115(1):210–217.
Ryu JH, Scanlon PD. Obstructive lung diseases: COPD, asthma, and many imitators.
    Mayo Clin Proc 2001;76(11):1144–1153.

20. Restrictive Lung Disease

I **INTRODUCTION.** Restrictive lung disease is an uncommon but important group of disorders that is often diagnosed by pulmonary function testing to evaluate dyspnea or by an abnormal chest radiograph. There are more than 100 causes of restrictive lung disease, and distinguishing among them is of critical importance to prognosis and treatment.

A. Definition. The **sine qua non** of restrictive lung disease is a **reduction in lung volumes [total lung capacity (TLC), vital capacity (VC), residual volume (RV)]**. The $FEV_1(\%)$ [i.e., the forced expiratory volume in 1 second (FEV_1) divided by the forced vital capacity (FVC)] may be increased, but this finding is not necessary to make the diagnosis.

B. Etiology. Although interstitial lung disease is the focus of this chapter because it is perhaps the most important cause of restrictive lung disease, there are many other causes of restrictive lung disease. Diseases of the pleura, chest wall, and nervous system can also cause restriction. Use the following mnemonic to "PAINT" a mental picture of the causes of restrictive lung disease.

Causes of Restrictive Lung Disease ("PAINT")

Pleural (scarring, effusions, pneumothorax)
Alveolar (edema, hemorrhage, inflammation)
Interstitial lung disease
Neuromuscular (myasthenia, phrenic nerve dysfunction, myopathy)
Thoracic or extrathoracic (kyphoscoliosis, obesity, ascites, pregnancy)

II **CAUSES OF INTERSTITIAL LUNG DISEASE (ILD)**

A. Interstitial processes can be remembered using the mnemonic "HITS FACED." (For some, the mnemonic may be easier to remember if the "S" is placed before the "H.")

Causes of Interstitial Lung Disease ("HITS FACED")

Histiocytosis X or **H**ypersensitivity pneumonitis
Idiopathic interstitial pneumonia
Tuberculosis or **T**umor
Sarcoidosis

Fungal infection
Alveolar proteinosis
Collagen vascular disease
Environmental or **E**osinophilia-associated
Drugs

1. **Pulmonary histiocytosis X (eosinophilic granuloma)** is an idiopathic disorder that may progress to fibrosis.
   a. **Diagnosis.** The typical patient is a 30- to 40-year-old smoker. The upper lung zones are most frequently involved. Bierberbach granules (X bodies) are seen within mononuclear cells on biopsy.
   b. **Treatment** involves smoking cessation and often requires high-dose steroids.
2. **Hypersensitivity pneumonitis** is an immune-mediated inflammatory process that results from repeated inhalation of organic dusts (e.g., mold, grain, bird droppings). The disease can be acute, subacute, or chronic; unrecognized disease can progress to fibrosis.
   a. **Diagnosis** is usually made by history and characteristic radiographic findings. Occasionally lung biopsy is required.
   b. **Treatment.** The source of the antigen should be avoided; this may involve moving or changing jobs. High-dose steroids may be necessary as well.
3. **Idiopathic interstitial pneumonia (IIP)** is the most common diagnosis for patients presenting with ILD. The disease presents in the sixth to seventh decade of life with the insidious onset of dyspnea and a cough. It has several subtypes, defined by their pathologic appearance. The most common of these is idiopathic pulmonary fibrosis (IPF), which has a distinctly worse prognosis and response to treatment.
   a. **Diagnosis.** A careful history must be taken to exclude other causes of ILD. The chest radiograph generally shows interstitial abnormalities with a lower lobe predominance, and high-resolution computed tomography scanning can be helpful in identifying subtypes [e.g., IPF, desquamative interstitial pneumonia (DIP), nonspecific interstitial pneumonia (NSIP), respiratory bronchiolitis

interstitial lung disease (RBILD)]. Lung biopsy is generally required for definitive subclassification.

b. Treatment. Most subtypes of IIP respond well to steroids. IPF does not, and newer therapies aimed at stopping fibroproliferation are under investigation (e.g., gamma interferon). Lung transplantation should be considered in appropriate patients.

4. **Tuberculosis.** Diffuse micronodular infiltrates can occur with tuberculosis if the infection is disseminated (i.e., miliary tuberculosis). Diffuse parenchymal infiltration can occur during reactivation of disease, usually in immunocompromised hosts.

    a. Diagnosis requires the identification of acid-fast organisms on sputum or tissue stain, and culture or PCR should be obtained to confirm it is Mycobacterium tuberculosis.

    b. Treatment entails combination antibiotic therapy for tuberculosis.

5. **Tumor.** ILD due to malignancy is usually due to lymphangitic spread. The most common etiologies are lung and breast cancer.

    a. Diagnosis is suggested by diffuse reticular abnormalities on chest radiograph with Kerley B lines. Lung biopsy is often required.

    b. Treatment depends on the malignancy and previous radiation and chemotherapy received.

6. **Sarcoidosis** is an idiopathic systemic granulomatous disease usually presenting in the third to fourth decade of life; there is lung involvement in 90% of cases. The incidence is higher in African-Americans and in women.

    a. Diagnosis is suggested by lymphadenopathy (characteristically bilateral hilar involvement), rash, erythema nodosum, and hepatosplenomegaly. There may be an elevated angiotensin-converting enzyme (ACE) level; however, this finding is neither sensitive nor specific.

    b. Treatment. Many patients with mild disease improve without therapy. Steroids may be appropriate for some patients.

7. **Fungal infections**

    a. Histoplasmosis is found in the central and eastern United States and presents as diffuse ILD, often in a miliary pattern, during reactivation in immunocompromised hosts. **Coccidioidomycosis** is endemic in the southwestern United States. Rarely, diffuse involvement occurs during primary infection; it is more common during reactivation in immunocompromised hosts.

    b. Diagnosis. A history of travel to endemic areas and typical radiography are often diagnostic. Serologic tests may be helpful to confirm exposure. Lung biopsy can confirm the diagnosis.

   c. **Treatment.** Active disease is most commonly treated with amphotericin B.

8. **Alveolar proteinosis** is a rare disorder resulting from deposition of phospholipid material in alveolar spaces. The disease can be primary (idiopathic) or secondary (postviral or post-tuberculous). Diagnosis can be made by high-resolution computed tomography scanning and bronchoscopic lavage. Treatment entails periodic whole lung lavage by bronchoscopy.

9. **Collagen vascular diseases.** ILD is only one manifestation of pulmonary involvement in these disorders. Rheumatoid arthritis and scleroderma are the two diseases most commonly associated with ILD that ultimately leads to fibrosis. These diseases are often histopathologically indistinguishable from idiopathic interstitial pneumonia. Diagnosis often requires lung biopsy, although empiric therapy with steroids is often prescribed.

10. **Environmental exposures** can include organic dusts (leading to hypersensitivity pneumonitis) or inorganic dusts (e.g., asbestos, silica, beryllium) leading to pneumoconioses. Particle deposition leads to inflammation, which can progress to fibrosis. There are dozens of known pneumoconioses, and a careful occupational and environmental history is critical in identifying an agent. Diagnosis is usually made by history and chest radiography. Lung biopsy is occasionally performed. Treatment entails removal from the source of exposure, and steroids are occasionally helpful.

11. **Eosinophilia-associated lung diseases** are generally characterized by pulmonary infiltrates, eosinophilic bronchoalveolar lavage fluid, and in many cases, peripheral eosinophilia. Figure 20–1 shows an easy way to remember the major diseases that cause pulmonary infiltrates with eosinophilia (PIE). These diseases are often diagnosed by history, chest radiograph, and bronchoalveolar lavage. Occasionally, lung biopsy is required. Most of these conditions are exquisitely steroid responsive, although prolonged steroid therapy is sometimes required. Relapses are common.

12. **Drugs.** The most common drugs to cause ILD are antineoplastic drugs, antibiotics (sulfa drugs, penicillins), sulfonylureas, gold, phenytoin, penicillamine, and amiodarone. The diagnosis is made by history. Removal of the offending agent is critical. If continued, progressive fibrosis can occur.

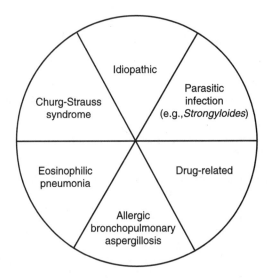

FIGURE 20-1. Major diseases that cause pulmonary infiltrates with eosinophilia. Just think of six pieces of PIE!

III APPROACH TO THE PATIENT

A. Patient history and physical examination. Although the symptoms of cough and dyspnea are of foremost concern to the patient, they are almost universal and do not distinguish one disease from another. The history should focus on exposures to environmental agents and drugs. The review of systems should be comprehensive; look for symptoms of infection or evidence of collagen vascular disease (e.g., history of rash, arthralgias, photosensitivity, ulcers).

B. Chest radiograph. A chest radiograph is helpful. It will usually reveal bilateral interstitial (reticular) abnormalities. However it can be diagnostic in other ways:

1. Pleural thickening or effusions in the absence of parenchymal disease will reveal the pleura as the cause of the restrictive physiology. Pleural plaques suggest asbestosis.

2. A normal chest radiograph with evidence of restriction on pulmonary function testing suggests the possibility of a neuromuscular disorder.

3. A chest radiograph may be diagnostic if normal parenchyma is seen in combination with spinal pathology (e.g., kyphoscoliosis) or small lung volumes (e.g., ascites, obesity).

C. Other tests. The most common dilemma occurs when ILD is seen on the chest radiograph and the patient history and physical examination findings are unrevealing. Many tests are available, each with its own sensitivities and specificities. Tests should be selected according to the patient's situation and the list of likely diagnostic possibilities.

1. **High-resolution computed tomography (HRCT)** is a logical next step after the history, physical, and chest radiograph. HRCT has been reported to have high specificities for the diagnosis of idiopathic pulmonary fibrosis, sarcoidosis, asbestosis, silicosis, and many other forms of ILD.

2. **Bronchoscopy.** Bronchoalveolar lavage can be diagnostic by revealing infectious organisms or malignant cells. Cell count and differential analysis of lavage fluid is rarely helpful, except when looking for eosinophilic lung disease, alveolar hemorrhage, or pulmonary alveolar proteinosis.

3. **Transbronchial biopsy** increases the risk of pneumothorax and hemorrhage but enables diagnosis of diseases not identified on lavage, particularly sarcoidosis and histiocytosis X. Although it cannot reliably diagnose many forms of ILD, transbronchial biopsy may be beneficial in patients who are too ill to tolerate surgical lung biopsy.

4. **Surgical lung biopsy** is the diagnostic gold standard. It may be performed by open thoracotomy or thoracoscopically. **Video-assisted thoracoscopic surgery (VATS)** involves the insertion of a rigid thoracoscope into the pleural cavity to biopsy the lung. It appears to have a similar yield to open thoracotomy but decreased morbidity.

HOT **KEY** If the diagnosis is unclear, repeating the history and physical examination (i.e., "the basics") will often lead to the diagnosis as quickly as ordering a battery of invasive and expensive tests.

References

Gross TJ, Hunninghake GW. Idiopathic pulmonary fibrosis. N Engl J Med 2001; 345(7):517–525.

Michaelson JE, Aguayo SM, Roman J. Idiopathic pulmonary fibrosis: a practical approach for diagnosis and management. Chest 2000;118(3):788–794.

Raghu G. Interstitial lung disease: a diagnostic approach. Are CT scan and lung biopsy indicated in every patient? Am J Respir Crit Care Med 1995;151(3 Pt 1):909–914.

21. Community-Acquired Pneumonia

I INTRODUCTION

A. Epidemiology. Community-acquired pneumonia is a leading cause of death and the number one cause of infectious disease-related mortality in the United States. Hospitalized patients with community-acquired pneumonia have an in-hospital mortality rate of up to 25%.

B. Classification. Attempting to classify community-acquired pneumonia as "typical" or "atypical" using clinical information is not very useful for predicting the underlying pathogen.

II CLINICAL MANIFESTATIONS OF COMMUNITY-ACQUIRED PNEUMONIA

A. Symptoms commonly include subjective fever, cough, sputum production, pleuritic chest pain, and dyspnea.

B. Signs commonly include fever, tachypnea (> 20 respirations/min), and signs of lobar consolidation (bronchial breath sounds, egophony, dullness to percussion, crackles).

III CAUSES OF COMMUNITY-ACQUIRED PNEUMONIA

A. Organisms

1. *Streptococcus pneumoniae* is the most common organism and can be quite virulent.

2. *Haemophilus influenzae* is an especially common cause of community-acquired pneumonia in patients with chronic obstructive pulmonary disease (COPD).

3. *Legionella* **species** can cause severe pneumonia. Gram staining usually reveals numerous polymorphonuclear neutrophils (PMNs) but no organisms.

4. **Aerobic gram-negative rods.** For example, *Klebsiella* infection is seen in alcoholics (in whom it can present as a "bulging fissure" on a chest radiograph).

5. *Staphylococcus aureus* infection is usually seen in patients who have influenza or who are immunocompromised.

6. **Other.** This category includes **respiratory viruses** [e.g., influenza virus, respiratory syncytial virus (RSV)], *Mycoplasma pneumoniae, Moraxella catarrhalis, Chlamydia*

pneumoniae, Mycobacterium tuberculosis, Pneumocystis carinii, and **fungi.**

B. **Polymicrobial aspiration** must be considered in patients with altered mental status, a history of seizures or alcohol abuse, swallowing difficulties, or patients transferred from a nursing home.

1. If aspiration occurs in the upright position, the lower lobes are affected (the right side more often than the left). The distribution follows the law of gravity.
2. It is more of a "PUSL" to remember which lobes are involved if aspiration occurs during recumbency—the posterior segment of the upper lobe and the superior segment of the lower lobe.

IV APPROACH TO THE PATIENT

A. **Diagnostic tests**
  1. **Complete blood count (CBC)**
  2. **Electrolytes, blood urea nitrogen (BUN),** and **creatinine**
  3. **Peripheral blood cultures** on samples drawn from two separate sites should usually be performed.
  4. **Arterial blood gas**
  5. **Chest radiograph** [posterior-anterior (PA) and lateral views]
  6. **Sputum analysis**
     a. Gram staining and culture of even a properly expectorated sputum sample may not be the best way to detect or identify the responsible organism (it has a high sensitivity, low specificity); therefore, this test is not routinely recommended by some experts.
     b. If there is concern that *M. tuberculosis* or *P. carinii* is the cause of the pneumonia, sputum analysis using special stains should always be done.
  7. **Thoracentesis.** If a pleural effusion is present, pleural fluid may be sent for a cell count and differential, Gram staining and culture, total protein, lactate dehydrogenase (LDH), pH, and glucose to further evaluate presence of an empyema (see Chapter 24)

B. **Criteria for hospital admission.** There are no absolute criteria for hospital admission, but there are specific risk factors associated with a complicated clinical course, increased mortality, or both. The following mnemonic can help you remember some of the most important criteria for admitting a patient: "ADMIT NOW." However, sometimes the most important criterion is the "eyeball" test (i.e., how sick a person looks to an experienced physician).

Criteria for Hospital Admission of Patients with Community-Acquired Pneumonia ("ADMIT NOW")

Age > 65 years
Decreased immunity (e.g., cancer, diabetes, AIDS, splenectomy)
Mental status changes
Increased A-a gradient
Two or more lobes involved

No home (i.e., homeless patients)
Organ system failure (increased creatinine, bone marrow suppression, severe hypotension, liver failure)
WBC count greater than 30,000/mm³ or less than 4000/mm³

Ⅴ TREATMENT

A. Empiric therapy. There are several guidelines that exist for the management of patients with community-acquired pneumonia. The American Thoracic Society recommends stratifying patients by place of therapy (outpatient or inpatient) and the presence of significant risk factors (e.g., nursing home residence, cardiopulmonary disease, alcoholism, immunosuppression). Inpatients should be treated empirically until a pathogen is identified by sputum or blood culture (if a pathogen is identified, appropriate specific therapy for the organism should be used). In general, antimicrobial therapy should be given for 10–14 days.

1. Group 1: Inpatients, not in intensive care, without risk factors. These patients can be treated with a newer intravenous macrolide or fluoroquinolone.

2. Group 2: Inpatients, not in intensive care, with risk factors. These patients should be treated with intravenous β-lactam plus macrolide or intravenous fluoroquinolone alone.

3. Group 3: Inpatients in intensive care, without risk factors for Pseudomonas infection (bronchiectasis, immunosuppression, recent antibiotics, or malnourished). These patients can be treated with intravenous β-lactam plus macrolide or plus intravenous fluoroquinolone.

4. Group 4: Inpatients in intensive care, with risk factors for Pseudomonas infection. These patients can be treated with an antipseudomonal β-lactam plus an antipseudomonal fluoroquinolone (or an intravenous aminoglycoside).

B. Response to therapy. Most patients will have some improvement by 3 days. However, cough and crackles usually take longer to respond (1 week and 3 weeks, respectively). The chest radiograph can take even longer to return to normal (4–12 weeks depending on patient age and if there is underlying lung disease). In patients not responding to therapy consider the following:
   1. Bacterial resistance to antimicrobial agent(s) chosen
   2. Unusual pathogen (e.g., *Mycobacterium tuberculosis, Pneumocystis carinii,* viral infection)
   3. Complication of the infection (e.g., empyema, lung abscess)
   4. Underlying malignancy leading to postobstructive pneumonia
   5. Additional noninfectious causes (e.g., congestive heart failure, Churg-Strauss syndrome)
C. In patients failing to respond to what appears to be appropriate therapy, consider obtaining a pulmonary consultation (and bronchoscopy) and further imaging (e.g., chest computed tomography).

References

Bartlett JG, Dowell SF, Mandell LA, et al. Practice guidelines for the management of community-acquired pneumonia in adults. Infectious Diseases Society of America. Clin Infect Dis 2000;31(2):347–382.

Metlay JP, Kapoor WN, Fine MJ. Does this patient have community-acquired pneumonia? Diagnosing pneumonia by history and physical examination. JAMA 1997; 278(17):1440–1445.

Niederman MS. Guidelines for the management of community-acquired pneumonia. Current recommendations and antibiotic selection issues. Med Clin North Am 2001;85(6):1493–1509.

Niederman MS, Mandell LA, Anzueto A, et al. American Thoracic Society. Guidelines for the management of adults with community-acquired pneumonia. Diagnosis, assessment of severity, antimicrobial therapy, and prevention. Am J Respir Crit Care Med 2001;163(7):1730–1754.

22. Pulmonary Hypertension

I INTRODUCTION

A. Pulmonary hypertension is diagnosed when pulmonary artery pressures exceed 25/8 mm Hg (normal). This can be directly measured by pulmonary arterial catheterization, indirectly measured by echocardiography, or suggested by physical examination.

B. Untreated pulmonary hypertension carries a high mortality rate, but identification and treatment of reversible causes can significantly benefit the patient.

II CLINICAL MANIFESTATIONS OF PULMONARY HYPERTENSION

A. Symptoms include:
1. Progressive dyspnea
2. Chest pain (partially as a result of right ventricular ischemia)
3. Fatigue
4. Syncope or near syncope
5. Peripheral edema (from right ventricular failure)

B. Signs. Pulmonary hypertension often presents with physical examination findings that **reflect right ventricular failure.**

HOT **KEY**

Evidence of right ventricular failure almost always indicates pulmonary hypertension.

The following findings are typical:
1. Increased jugular venous pressure
2. A right-sided third or fourth heart sound (S_3 or S_4)
3. A right ventricular lift
4. Pulmonic component of the second heart sound (P_2) louder than the aortic component of the second heart sound (A_2)
5. Murmurs of tricuspid and pulmonary regurgitation
6. Peripheral cyanosis and edema

III CAUSES OF PULMONARY HYPERTENSION

A. Primary causes. Primary pulmonary hypertension (plexogenic pulmonary arteriopathy) is seen most commonly in young women who present with dyspnea and, occasionally, right-sided heart failure. Most patients have rapid deterioration; the average survival time from diagnosis is 2–3 years.

B. Secondary causes must be ruled out before diagnosing primary pulmonary hypertension. To remember the many secondary causes of pulmonary hypertension, think "backward" from the left ventricle to the lungs. Pulmonary hypertension is often divided into two anatomic categories: **postcapillary pulmonary hypertension** (caused by processes distal to the pulmonary capillary bed) and **capillary/precapillary pulmonary hypertension** (caused by problems at or proximal to the capillary bed).

1. Postcapillary pulmonary hypertension
  a. Left ventricular dysfunction. Disorders include:
    (1) Systolic or diastolic dysfunction
    (2) Constrictive pericarditis
  b. Increased left atrial pressure with normal left ventricular pressures. Disorders include:
    (1) Mitral valve disease
    (2) Left atrial myxoma (rare)
    (3) Cor triatriatum (rare)
  c. Pulmonary veno-occlusive disease. Fibrotic narrowing and destruction of the pulmonary veins and venules. It may be idiopathic or associated with:
    (1) Malignancy
    (2) Chemotherapy
    (3) Bone marrow transplantation

2. Capillary/precapillary causes
  a. Obstructive lung disease
  b. Restrictive lung disease
  c. Pulmonary vascular disease
    (1) Vasculitis/collagen-vascular disease
    (2) Pulmonary embolism
    (3) Cirrhosis
    (4) Schistosomiasis
  d. Miscellaneous causes
    (1) Hypoxemia causes pulmonary vasoconstriction which, over time, leads to pulmonary hypertension.
    (2) Intracardiac left-to-right shunt (Eisenmenger's syndrome) causes increased flow through the pulmonary circulation, thereby raising pressures.
    (3) Congenital absence or abnormality of the right or left

pulmonary artery leads to increased flow through the normal artery and increased pressures.

HOT KEY

Sleep apnea is increasingly being recognized as a cause of hypoxemia and secondary pulmonary hypertension.

IV APPROACH TO THE PATIENT

A. Preliminary evaluation
  1. **Physical examination findings**
     a. Carefully compare the components of the second heart sound at the upper sternal border. A P_2 (pulmonic component) that is louder than the A_2 (aortic component) suggests pulmonary hypertension.
     b. Listen carefully for a left-sided S_3 or S_4, which may indicate left ventricular dysfunction. Also listen for diastolic murmurs indicating mitral stenosis and a variable S_1 and intermittent "plop" that may indicate a left atrial myxoma.
     c. Look for elevated jugular venous pressure (JVP), prominent V waves, hepatojugular reflux, and lower extremity edema suggesting right-sided heart failure.
  2. **Laboratory findings.** Polycythemia is often present with chronic hypoxemia.
  3. **Radiographic findings**
     a. Pulmonary hypertension from all etiologies will usually result in enlarged central pulmonary arteries visible on the chest radiograph. Right ventricular and atrial enlargement may also be seen in severe, chronic cases.
     b. Evidence of the underlying cause may also be visible radiographically. For example:
        (1) In emphysema, there may be apical blebs, "pruning" of distal vessels, hyperinflation, or flat diaphragms.
        (2) In left ventricular dysfunction, there may be left ventricular or atrial enlargement or evidence of pulmonary edema.
  4. **Electrocardiographic findings.** The ECG typically shows right axis deviation. Right ventricular hypertrophy and right atrial enlargement are also common findings (see Chapter 5 IV; VI B and D).
B. Confirmation. There are many invasive and noninvasive diagnostic tests that may be used to further define the nature of the patient's pulmonary hypertension. Obtaining tests in the fol-

lowing order is a reasonable way to approach patients with pulmonary hypertension.

1. **Echocardiography**
   a. **Doppler echocardiography.** Measurement of pulmonary pressures can confirm or dispute the initial clinical diagnosis.
      (1) Right ventricular hypertrophy or enlargement, paradoxical motion of the interventricular septum, and right atrial enlargement may also accompany pulmonary hypertension.
      (2) The presence of left ventricular dysfunction, mitral stenosis, or left atrial myxoma confirms a diagnosis of postcapillary pulmonary hypertension; no additional workup is necessary and appropriate treatment can be instituted.
   b. **Bubble study.** A bubble study allows detection of a right-to-left intracardiac shunt.
2. **Pulmonary function tests with arterial blood gases**
   a. Hypoxemia, a decreased diffusing capacity for carbon monoxide ($DLCO$), and a mild restrictive defect are common findings regardless of the cause of pulmonary hypertension.
3. **Sleep studies** are usually indicated in patients with risk factors for sleep apnea (i.e., male gender, obesity, and a history of snoring). However, sleep studies do not correlate well with the degree of pulmonary hypertension.
4. **Ventilation—perfusion ($\dot{V}/\dot{Q}$) lung scanning.** If no cause of postcapillary hypertension has been found and chronic obstructive pulmonary disease (COPD) has been excluded, evaluation for chronic thromboembolic disease is usually necessary (see Chapter 23 IV F).
5. **Pulmonary angiography** and **right-heart catheterization.** If the diagnosis is still elusive, invasive studies become necessary. Although there is concern about the safety of right-heart catheterization in the presence of pulmonary hypertension, most studies have not shown major morbidity or mortality, and the consequence of not diagnosing a treatable condition is severe. These tests can often be done one right after the other.
   a. A positive pulmonary angiogram obviates the need for right-heart catheterization.
   b. Right-heart catheterization may be necessary to rule out postcapillary pulmonary hypertension (i.e., from diastolic dysfunction that may have been missed on echocardiography) and an intracardiac shunt as etiologies. In addition, this procedure may serve to guide vasodilator therapy.

V TREATMENT

A. **Primary pulmonary hypertension**
   1. **Oxygen therapy** decreases pulmonary vasoconstriction in hypoxic patients, slowing the progression of pulmonary hypertension.
   2. **Pharmacologic therapy.** Some authorities recommend chronic anticoagulation and vasodilator therapy (guided by pulmonary artery catheterization). Calcium channel blockers or continuous prostacyclin infusion may offer the best medical treatment. Newer agents, such as endothelin receptor antagonists, show significant promise.
   3. Heart—lung transplantation is being used with increasing frequency for patients with end-stage disease.

B. **Secondary pulmonary hypertension**
   1. **General measures**
      a. **Oxygen therapy** should be initiated to counteract hypoxia, regardless of the etiology. More than 15 hours per day has a long-term mortality benefit in hypoxic patients with COPD.
      b. **Phlebotomy.** Patients showing polycythemia with a hematocrit that exceeds 60% may undergo phlebotomy to reduce blood viscosity.
      c. **Salt restriction, diuretics,** and sometimes, **digitalis** (controversial) are used to treat cor pulmonale.
   2. **Specific measures.** Treatment is always aimed at the underlying disease.
      a. **Postcapillary pulmonary hypertension** is generally easier to treat than precapillary/capillary pulmonary hypertension.
      b. **Capillary/precapillary pulmonary hypertension**
         (1) **COPD** can be treated with smoking cessation, bronchodilators, and oxygen therapy when appropriate.
         (2) **Thromboembolic disease** is treated with chronic anticoagulation therapy. Thromboendarterectomy may benefit certain patients who develop pulmonary hypertension as a result of major pulmonary thromboembolism.
         (3) **Sleep apnea** can be treated with weight reduction, avoidance of alcohol and sedatives, and nighttime oxygen with or without continuous positive airway pressure (CPAP).

References
Krowka MJ. Pulmonary hypertension: diagnostics and therapeutics. Mayo Clin Proc 2000;75(6):625–630.
Nauser TD, Stites SW. Diagnosis and treatment of pulmonary hypertension. Am Fam Physician 2001;63(9):1789–1798.

23. Pulmonary Embolism

I **INTRODUCTION.** Pulmonary embolism causes more than 50,000 deaths per year; however, prompt treatment may significantly reduce the mortality rate.

II **CAUSES OF PULMONARY EMBOLISM**

A. Most pulmonary emboli (95%) arise from **deep venous thrombosis of the lower extremities.** The highest risk for pulmonary embolism occurs with proximal deep venous thrombosis (i.e., thrombosis of the popliteal, superficial femoral, or common femoral vein).

B. Pulmonary embolism can also originate from **upper extremity** or **pelvic venous thrombosis** and **right atrial thrombi.**

C. Rare causes of nonthrombotic pulmonary embolism include fat embolism, amniotic fluid embolism, septic embolism, and tumor embolism.

III **CLINICAL MANIFESTATIONS OF PULMONARY EMBOLISM.** The symptoms and signs of pulmonary embolism are nonspecific, occurring in many disorders.

A. **Symptoms.** The presence of **chest pain,** especially the pleuritic variety, is the most common symptom, followed closely by **dyspnea.** A feeling of **apprehension** or impending doom is frequently described.

B. **Signs. Tachypnea** is present in most patients with pulmonary

---

Risk factors for pulmonary embolism include:

HOT
▶
KEY

Age older than 40 years
History of venous thromboembolism
Malignancy
Prolonged immobility
Congestive heart failure
Myocardial infarction
Stroke
Fracture of the lower extremity (including hip)
Obesity
Major surgery (especially orthopedic)
Congenital or acquired abnormalities in hemostasis

---

embolism. **Tachycardia, low-grade fever,** and evidence **of lower extremity swelling** or **tenderness** are other important signs.

IV **APPROACH TO THE PATIENT.** Pulmonary embolism can pose a substantial diagnostic challenge. The differential diagnosis includes other cardiac and pulmonary disorders that cause dyspnea, chest pain, and hypoxemia. Common competing diagnoses are pneumonia, congestive heart failure (CHF), asthma, chronic obstructive pulmonary disease (COPD), pneumothorax, myocardial infarction, and aortic dissection.

A. **Patient history** and **physical examination** are essential to the diagnosis. A sudden onset of chest pain and dyspnea is typical. The physical examination may reveal an edematous, erythematous and tender extremity suggesting deep venous thrombosis.

B. **Chest radiograph.** The chest radiograph provides valuable information in a patient with dyspnea, chest pain, or hypoxemia.
   1. A common misconception is that most patients with pulmonary embolism have a normal chest radiograph. **In fact, most patients with pulmonary embolism have an abnormal chest radiograph.** Atelectasis and parenchymal opacities are the most common findings.
   2. There are several classic roentgenographic signs of pulmonary embolism:
      a. **Westermark's sign** is a region of oligemia (decreased vascularity) visible as a focal radiolucent area.
      b. **Hampton's hump** is a peripheral wedge-shaped density that may reflect pulmonary infarction.
      c. **Subsegmental atelectasis,** a **small pleural effusion,** an **enlarged central pulmonary artery,** and an **elevated hemidiaphragm** are other common signs.
   3. These classic radiographic signs of pulmonary embolism are nonspecific and cannot definitively establish the diagnosis. Therefore, the main utility of a chest radiograph is in identifying alternative diagnoses (e.g., pneumonia, pneumothorax, pulmonary edema).

C. **Electrocardiogram (ECG).** Most patients with pulmonary embolism will have an abnormal ECG. The findings, however, are nonspecific.
   1. The most common finding is **sinus tachycardia;** other arrhythmias are rare.
   2. The classic **findings of acute right-sided heart strain** are seen in only approximately 25% of patients. These include:
      a. **Right bundle branch block**
      b. **P pulmonale**
      c. **Right axis deviation**

    d. $S_1Q_3T_3$ (a large S wave in lead I, a large Q wave in lead III, and an inverted T wave in lead III)—remember, these patients are **SiQ** from **Thrombus!**

D. Arterial blood gases. Patients with pulmonary embolism may have alveolar hyperventilation (low $Paco_2$), hypoxemia (low Pao_2), a **widened alveolar-to-arterial (A-a)** gradient, or any combination of the three. Although most patients with pulmonary embolism have a widened A-a gradient, up to 15% may be normal.

E. D-dimer assay. The use of D-dimers in the diagnostic evaluation of suspected pulmonary embolism has been evaluated in several studies. Unfortunately, the poor specificity of an elevated level prevents one from ruling in pulmonary embolism if the test is positive without conducting further testing. Some facilities use a quantitative D-dimer assay (using ELISA) that has been shown to have a very high sensitivity for pulmonary embolism or deep venous thrombosis. At present, the variability of the types of assays available in different hospitals prevents the routine use of this test in patients with suspected pulmonary embolism.

F. Ventilation—perfusion ($\dot{V}/\dot{Q}$) scanning. If the $\dot{V}/\dot{Q}$ scan shows perfusion defects in areas of normal ventilation, a pulmonary embolism occluding blood flow is probable. $\dot{V}/\dot{Q}$ scans are interpreted as normal or showing low, intermediate, or high probability of pulmonary embolism based on standardized criteria.

    1. The likelihood ratio for pulmonary embolism can be calculated for each category of $\dot{V}/\dot{Q}$ scan result (Table 23-1).

    2. Using the $\dot{V}/\dot{Q}$ scan result, the probability of pulmonary embolism in a given patient can be calculated.

      a. Generate the pretest probability of pulmonary embolism, using the patient history, physical examination findings, and data provided by the chest radiograph, ECG, and arterial blood gas report.

TABLE 23-1. Correlation of Ventilation-Perfusion ($\dot{V}/\dot{Q}$) Scans and Likelihood Ratios

$\dot{V}/\dot{Q}$ Scan Result	Likelihood Ratio
High probability	13
Intermediate probability	1.1
Low probability	0.4
Normal	0.1

Based on data from PIOPED investigators: Value of the ventilation/perfusion scan in acute pulmonary embolism. JAMA 1990;263:2753–2759.

b. Convert the pretest probability to posttest probability using the method described in Chapter 2 III C 1. In general, a very low posttest probability excludes the diagnosis of pulmonary embolism, whereas a very high posttest probability confirms the diagnosis.

3. Summary

a. A high-probability $\dot{V}/\dot{Q}$ scan generally **rules in** the diagnosis of pulmonary embolism.

b. A normal $\dot{V}/\dot{Q}$ scan generally **rules out** the diagnosis of pulmonary embolism.

c. An intermediate $\dot{V}/\dot{Q}$ scan is generally not helpful—the likelihood ratio is essentially 1, so this scan result does not affect the posttest probability.

d. A low-probability $\dot{V}/\dot{Q}$ scan is difficult to interpret. In this case, the pretest probability (clinical assessment) is essential for interpreting scan results. If the pretest probability is low, then pulmonary embolism is unlikely. However, if the pretest probability is intermediate or high, the probability of pulmonary embolism is substantial. Additional diagnostic testing should be undertaken.

G. Noninvasive lower extremity testing. Most pulmonary emboli arise from proximal lower extremity deep venous thromboses. Because the treatment of deep venous thrombosis and pulmonary embolism are generally the same, documentation of deep venous thrombosis is adequate reason to stop diagnostic testing and initiate anticoagulation therapy. Two noninvasive tests for detecting lower extremity deep venous thrombosis are available: **impedance plethysmography** and **Doppler ultrasound.**

1. In patients with **symptomatic** deep venous thrombosis (i.e., leg swelling or pain), both tests have very high sensitivity and specificity.

2. In **asymptomatic** patients, the sensitivity of these tests is much lower (in the 50% range).

3. In angiographically proven cases of pulmonary embolism, only 50% of patients have positive studies.

H. Computed tomography (CT) angiography is a specific chest CT protocol that is highly accurate for the diagnosis of **central pulmonary emboli.** The utility of spiral CT for peripheral emboli remains to be clarified. A benefit of CT angiography over $\dot{V}/\dot{Q}$ scanning is the ability to identify occult alternative diagnoses (e.g., pneumothorax, pneumonia, heart failure, rib fractures). It remains unclear how confidently a negative CT angiogram rules out pulmonary embolism; until further study is completed, negative CT angiograms should be interpreted with caution.

I. Pulmonary angiography. Pulmonary angiography is the **gold standard** for diagnosing pulmonary embolism; however, the associated risks of death, major complications, and minor complications are approximately 0.5%, 1%, and 5%, respectively. Major complications include contrast-induced renal failure, bleeding and pulmonary arterial rupture.

V **TREATMENT.** The treatment of pulmonary embolism is anticoagulation with heparin (either unfractionated or low-molecular weight), followed by warfarin for several months. Inferior vena cava (IVC) filter is an alternative, short-term management option for patients with absolute contraindications to anticoagulation.

A. **Anticoagulation** is the standard treatment for both deep venous thrombosis and pulmonary embolism.
  1. **Heparin,** either unfractionated or low-molecular weight, should be administered immediately. The recurrence of venous thromboembolism increases with delayed or inadequate anticoagulation, so rapid achievement of a partial thromboplastin time (PTT) of 1.5–2.0 times control is desirable. Heparin is usually continued until adequate oral anticoagulation with warfarin is achieved.
  2. **Oral warfarin** should be started when the diagnosis is made. The efficacy and safety of early warfarin initiation have been well documented. The duration of therapy is not completely certain, but most experts recommend approximately 4–6 months of anticoagulation at an international normalized ratio (INR) of 2.0–3.0.
B. **IVC filter.** For patients with absolute contraindications to anticoagulation and lower extremity clot, an IVC filter may be placed percutaneously via the femoral vein. For patients with short-term contraindication to anticoagulation (e.g., trauma, recent stroke), temporary filters may be placed and removed once anticoagulation is achieved. IVC filters prevent lower extremity thrombus from traveling to the lungs and have been shown to lower the risk of early recurrent pulmonary embolization. Importantly, they show no benefit in long-term prevention of pulmonary embolism and are associated with higher rates of recurrent venous thrombosis.
C. **Thrombolytic agents** (e.g., urokinase, tissue plasminogen activator) dissolve clot, resulting in more rapid resolution of perfusion abnormalities than standard heparin therapy. Thrombolytics improve initial hemodynamics in massive pulmonary embolism but do not improve mortality rates. Furthermore, there is a substantial risk of bleeding associated with these agents. For these reasons, thrombolytic agents are not used routinely in the treatment of pulmonary embolism. In patients with massive pulmonary embolism characterized by hemodynamic instability, thrombolytics may be beneficial.

References

Value of the ventilation/perfusion scan in acute pulmonary embolism. Results of the prospective investigation of pulmonary embolism diagnosis (PIOPED). The PIOPED Investigators. JAMA 1990;263(20):2753–2759 (classic article).

Goldhaber SZ. Pulmonary embolism. N Engl J Med 1998;339(2):93–104.

Kelly J, Rudd A, Lewis RR, Hunt BJ. Plasma D-dimers in the diagnosis of venous thromboembolism. Arch Intern Med 2002;162(7):747–756.

Wolfe TR, Hartsell SC. Pulmonary embolism: making sense of the diagnostic evaluation. Ann Emerg Med 2001;37(5):504–514.

24. Pleural Effusion

I INTRODUCTION

A. Because pleural effusions **commonly complicate many medical conditions,** health-care providers need a straightforward approach to diagnosis and management.

B. The fluid can consist of anything from simple serous liquid to complicated pleural infections and hemorrhage.

II CLINICAL MANIFESTATIONS

A. History
   1. Patients with pleural effusions typically present with **dyspnea and pleuritic chest pain,** although they can be **asymptomatic.**
   2. Symptoms may be **indolent or rapidly progressive** depending on the rate of fluid accumulation.
   3. **Fevers, chills, and night sweats** can occur when effusions become **infected.**
B. Physical examination
   1. The physical examination generally reveals **dullness to percussion, absent or diminished breath sounds,** and **decreased tactile fremitus.**
   2. There is often a **horizontal band of egophony just above the area of dullness,** caused by compressive atelectasis of the overlying lung by the effusion.

III CAUSES

A. Because there are many causes of pleural effusions, the most clinically useful approach is to **categorize the effusion as "transudative" or "exudative"** (Table 24-1).
   1. **Transudative effusions** are fluid collections usually due to an **alteration in systemic factors influencing pleural fluid formation** (i.e., plasma osmotic and hydrostatic pressure). These usually resolve with treatment of the underlying disorder (e.g., heart failure, cirrhosis).
   2. **Exudative effusions** are more concerning as they **reflect primary pleural disease.** They often require removal (either via thoracentesis or tube thoracostomy) to prevent scarring and infection from developing.

TABLE 24–1. Common Causes of Pleural Effusions

Transudative Effusions	Exudative Effusions
Congestive heart failure	Infections (bacterial pneumonia, tuberculosis, fungal disease, viral disease)
Cirrhosis	Collagen-vascular disease
Nephrotic syndrome	Neoplasm (mesothelioma, bronchogenic lung cancer, metastatic disease, lymphoma)
Hypoalbuminemia	Gastrointestinal disease (pancreatitis, esophageal rupture, subdiaphragmatic abscess)
Myxedema	Trauma
Pulmonary embolism	Pulmonary embolism
	Miscellaneous (e.g., following coronary artery bypass surgery, asbestos-related)

> **HOT KEY**
> The three most common causes of pleural effusion in the United States are (in order): 1) congestive heart failure; 2) pneumonia; and 3) malignancy.

IV APPROACH TO THE PATIENT

A. Chest radiograph. The chest radiograph is the first test to order when evaluating a patient with suspected pleural effusion. Effusions of more than 200 cc should be visible on the PA view. Smaller effusions will be visible on a lateral radiograph only.

1. Small effusions cause blunting of the costophrenic angle (where the ribs meet the diaphragm).
2. Larger effusions will opacify the lower lung fields.
3. At times it is difficult to distinguish an effusion from a consolidative process in the lung. Lateral decubitus radiographs can help distinguish between the two by demonstrating dependent layering of pleural fluid.
4. Occasionally, pleural effusions do not layer clearly, and additional imaging (ultrasound or chest CT scan) is required.

B. Diagnostic thoracentesis

1. **When to perform a diagnostic thoracentesis.** Once a pleural effusion is identified, diagnostic thoracentesis should gener-

ally be performed, especially if the cause is unknown. If a patient has clear evidence of congestive heart failure with bilateral effusions of relatively equal size and no evidence of infection, it is reasonable to attempt diuresis and perform diagnostic thoracentesis if the effusions persist.

2. **Distinguishing between a transudate and exudate.** Pleural fluid should be sent to the laboratory for chemical and microbiological analysis to determine if it is transudative or exudative and if it appears infected (Table 24-2). If certain specific etiologies are suspected, additional studies should be performed (Table 24-3).

   a. Comparison of pleural and serum levels of **total protein** and **lactate dehydrogenase (LDH)** allow for distinction between transudative and exudative effusions (Table 24-2).

HOT
▶
KEY

The pleural fluid is considered exudative if **any** of the following three criteria (i.e., Light's criteria) are met:
1. Fluid LDH to serum LDH ratio > 0.6.
2. Fluid LDH $> 2/3$ of upper limit of normal of serum LDH.
3. Fluid protein to serum protein ratio > 0.5.

---

   b. Pleural fluid **glucose, pH, cell count with differential,** and **Gram stain with culture** should be performed on all pleural fluid (Table 24-2).
   c. Pleural fluid levels of **amylase, triglyceride,** and **creatinine; acid-fast staining** and **culture;** and **cytology** should be ordered when specific diagnoses are entertained (Table 24-3).

HOT
▶
KEY

Occasionally, some patients who have a transudative effusion will be misclassified as having an exudative effusion based on Light's criteria. If a transudative effusion is clinically probable yet the effusion is classified as "exudative" based on Light's criteria, calculating the serum to pleural fluid albumin gradient can be useful. Almost all patients with a serum albumin level 1.2 g/dl more than the pleural fluid albumin level have a transudative effusion.

V **TREATMENT.** Treatment is based on whether the effusion is a transudate or exudate, whether there is any evidence that the effusion is infected, or if the effusion appears to be loculated or have another complication.

TABLE 24-2. Basic Pleural Fluid Analysis

Study	Transudate	Exudate	Comment
Lactate dehydrogenase (LDH)	Less than 60% serum value; less than $^2/_3$ of upper limit of normal serum value	Greater than 60% serum value; greater than $^2/_3$ of upper limit of normal serum value	Draw serum LDH at the time of thoracentesis to compare values
Total protein	Less than 50% of serum value	Greater than 50% of serum value	Draw serum total protein at the time of thoracentesis to compare values
Glucose	Normal	Normal or low (below 60 mg/dl)	Very low in empyema and rheumatoid arthritis
pH	Normal	Normal or low (below 7.20)	Must be drawn into heparinized syringe and kept on ice
Cell count	WBC < 1000 (poor accuracy)	WBC > 1000 (poor accuracy)	RBC > 100,000 suggests trauma, malignancy, or pulmonary embolism
Differential	Neutrophil predominance	Neutrophil, occasionally lymphocyte predominance	Lymphocytic predominance (> 50%-80%) suggests malignancy or tuberculosis
Gram stain and culture	No organisms	No organisms unless empyema	

TABLE 24-3. Additional Pleural Fluid Studies Often Required and Associated Condition(s)

Study	Associated conditions
Amylase	Pancreatitis, esophageal rupture, malignancy
Triglyceride	Chylothorax
Creatinine	Urinothorax
Acid-fast stain and culture	Mycobacterial disease
Cytology	Malignancy

A. **Transudative effusions** rarely require drainage unless they are causing significant discomfort or hypoxemia. Treatment of transudative effusions should generally be **directed at the underlying cause.**

B. **Infected effusions,** or **empyema,** should be surgically **drained,** either by tube thoracostomy or with a thoracoscope. The **diagnosis of empyema** is made by **positive Gram stain, purulent fluid, or significant chemical abnormalities** (Table 24-4). Empyema requires **antibiotics** directed at the causative organism.

C. **Exudative effusions** that are not obviously infected **may still require surgical drainage** if they are frankly purulent, if they appear loculated (the fluid is trapped into multiple noncommunicating pockets), or if they have significant chemical or microbiologic abnormalities that suggest that loculation or infection is likely (Table 24-4).

TABLE 24-4. Indications for Surgical Treatment (Tube Thoracostomy or Thoracoscopy)

1. Frank pus on thoracentesis
2. Positive Gram stain
3. pH < 7.00
4. Glucose < 40 mg/dl
5. LDH > 1000 (isolated elevated LDH can be treated with serial thoracentesis in some cases)
6. Evidence of loculation on chest radiograph, ultrasound, or chest CT scan

References
Colice GL, Curtis A, Deslauriers J, et al. Medical and surgical treatment of parapneumonic effusions: an evidence-based guideline. Chest 2000;118(4):1158–1171.
Light RW. Clinical practice: pleural effusion. N Engl J Med 2002;346:1971–1977.
Light RW, Macgregor MI, Luchsinger PC, Ball WC Jr. Pleural effusions: the diagnostic separation of transudates and exudates. Ann Intern Med 1972;77(4):507–513 (classic article).

25. Respiratory Failure

I **INTRODUCTION.** Respiratory failure is a common admitting diagnosis in the intensive care unit (ICU). There are two underlying mechanisms of respiratory failure:

A. Failure to oxygenate. The patient's PaO_2 is less than 60 mm Hg while breathing room air.

B. Failure to ventilate. The patient's $PaCO_2$ is greater than 50 mm Hg.

II **CAUSES OF RESPIRATORY FAILURE**

A. Failure to oxygenate (see Chapter 17 III). Of the following five mechanisms of **hypoxemia,** the last two rarely cause respiratory failure.
  1. **Ventilation—perfusion ($\dot{V}/\dot{Q}$) mismatch**
  2. **Diffusion defect**
  3. **Hypoventilation**
  4. **Right-to-left shunt**
  5. **Low inspired partial pressure of oxygen**

B. Failure to ventilate. Hypercapnia is caused by impaired ventilation. Causes may be organized anatomically, starting with the brain (the breathing center) and moving to the alveoli (where carbon dioxide is excreted). Any problem along the way can result in impaired ventilation and hypercapnia. Causes include:
  1. **Central nervous system (CNS) depression,** most commonly from drugs (opiates and benzodiazepines), rarely from brain tumors or strokes.
  2. **Neuromuscular disorders** (e.g., botulism, Guillain-Barré syndrome, amyotrophic lateral sclerosis, myxedema)
  3. **Chest wall disorders** (e.g., obesity, kyphoscoliosis)
  4. **Upper airway obstruction** (e.g., epiglottitis, laryngospasm, obstructive sleep apnea)
  5. **Lower airway obstruction** [e.g., asthma, chronic obstructive pulmonary disease (COPD)]
  6. **Dead space ventilation.** Significant parenchymal damage [e.g., infection or post-acute respiratory distress syndrome (ARDS)] can increase dead space ventilation and cause hypercarbia.

III **APPROACH TO THE PATIENT**

A. Assess the urgency of the situation.
  1. If respiratory failure is acute, evaluate the patient quickly and decide on therapy. The rest of this chapter deals primarily with acute respiratory failure.

    2. If respiratory failure is chronic, there is less urgency to treatment.

B. Assess the need for intubation.

    1. If the patient has any of the following signs, be prepared to intubate:

       a. A significantly elevated respiratory rate (> 30 respirations/min)

       b. Fatigue and labored respiration

       c. Use of the accessory muscles to breathe

       d. Stridor (suggests impending upper airway obstruction)

       e. Depressed level of consciousness and inability to protect the airway

    2. Indications for intubation are discussed in Chapter 14. In general, if you think a patient might need to be intubated, they probably do!

C. Attempt to define the cause of the respiratory failure.

    1. Patient history. Ask about onset, additional symptoms, preceding events, and comorbid conditions.

    2. Physical examination

       a. Obtain a full set of vitals (including oxygen saturation).

       b. Note the presence or absence of the following:

          (1) Alteration in mental status, gag reflex

          (2) Expiratory wheezes, rales, diminished or absent breath sounds, dullness to percussion

          (3) Third heart sound (S_3) with a sustained point of maximal impulse (PMI), elevated jugular venous pressure, dependent edema

          (4) Abdominal tenderness, bowel sounds

          (5) Peripheral edema and cyanosis

    3. Diagnostic studies. The following studies should be performed immediately in most patients with acute respiratory failure:

       a. Chest radiograph

       b. 12-Lead electrocardiogram (ECG)

       c. Arterial blood gas analysis [to assess serum pH, oxygenation (PaO_2), and ventilation ($PaCO_2$)]

HOT **KEY** An arterial blood gas is essential to distinguish failure to oxygenate from failure to ventilate:
Low PaO2 → failure to oxygenate
High PaCO2 → failure to ventilate

---

       d. Complete blood count (CBC), serum electrolytes, blood urea nitrogen (BUN), and **creatinine**

IV TREATMENT. General therapeutic measures for patients in acute respiratory failure are outlined in Chapter 14. A general approach to mechanical ventilation is described in Chapter 26.

References

International Consensus Conferences in Intensive Care Medicine: noninvasive positive pressure ventilation in acute respiratory failure. Am J Respir Crit Care Med 2001;163(1):283–291.

Pierson DJ. Indications for mechanical ventilation in adults with acute respiratory failure. Respir Care 2002;47(3):249–262.

26. Mechanical Ventilation

I INTRODUCTION

A. **Definition.** A ventilator is simply a pump that delivers a set volume or pressure of mixed gas (usually oxygen and nitrogen).

B. **Phases of ventilatory support.** The three main phases of ventilatory support can be compared to a plane flight: **initiation** (take off), **maintenance** (cruising), and **liberation** (landing).

   1. **Initiation.** Chapter 14 describes guidelines for making the decision to intubate.

   2. **Maintenance.** The goal is to achieve a balance between making the patient comfortable and allowing enough awareness to allow assessment of neurologic status and pain. Any of the modes of ventilation detailed in this chapter may be appropriate.

   3. **Liberation (also called weaning)** is often the trickiest part (as is landing an airplane). The method should be tailored to the patient, depending on the patient's underlying disease, mental status, and degree of comfort.

II MODES OF POSITIVE-PRESSURE VENTILATION

A. **Volume-cycled modes**

   1. **Synchronized intermittent mandatory ventilation (SIMV).** The ventilator delivers a set tidal volume at a set rate but delivers no tidal volume for patient-initiated breaths above the set rate. Ventilator breaths are synchronized with patient-initiated breaths, but the ventilator also delivers a breath when the patient does not initiate one. Pressures vary.

      a. **Advantages.** SIMV offers maximum control of ventilation.

      b. **Disadvantages**

         (1) It is difficult for the patient to overcome resistance of the tubing when breathing over the set rate.

         (2) High pressures may be needed to deliver the set tidal volume.

   2. **Assist control (AC).** The ventilator delivers a set tidal volume at a set rate and delivers the same tidal volume for patient-initiated breaths above the set rate. Ventilator breaths are synchronized with patient breaths. Pressures vary.

      a. **Advantages.** The patient receives assistance for every breath.

b. Disadvantages
   (1) The patient may develop respiratory alkalosis because every patient-initiated breath receives a full tidal volume.
   (2) High pressures may be needed to deliver the set tidal volume.

B. Pressure-cycled modes. In the **pressure control (PC) mode,** the ventilator delivers a constant pressure at a set rate and delivers the same pressure for patient-initiated breaths above the set rate. Tidal volumes vary.

   1. Advantages. This mode can be used when peak airway pressures are too high (e.g., > 40 cm H_2O) on SIMV or AC.
   2. Disadvantages. The patient may not receive adequate tidal volumes.

C. Flow-cycled modes

   1. Pressure support (PS). The ventilator delivers a set pressure only when the patient initiates a breath. Pressure support ceases when flow decreases to 25% of maximum inspiratory flow.
      a. Advantages. Because this method is more physiologic than many of the others, patient comfort is enhanced.
      b. Disadvantages
         (1) The patient must trigger every respiration.
         (2) The patient may not receive adequate tidal volumes.

   2. Noninvasive positive-pressure ventilation (NPPV). Ventilation is delivered through a face mask rather than through an endotracheal tube. NPPV is triggered by air flow and delivers a constant pressure throughout inspiration.
      a. Advantages
         (1) Patients with hypercapnic ventilatory failure [e.g., an acute exacerbation of chronic obstructive pulmonary disease (COPD)] may respond well to this mode of ventilation.
         (2) NPPV may help delay or avoid endotracheal intubation.
      b. Disadvantages
         (1) The face mask may be uncomfortable for the patient.
         (2) It is difficult to deliver high levels of oxygen.

D. Combined modes. In **SIMV+PS,** the ventilator delivers a set tidal volume at a set rate and delivers a set pressure for patient-initiated breaths above the set rate.

   1. Advantages. This mode maintains control of ventilation with SIMV while maximizing patient comfort with pressure-supported breaths.
   2. Disadvantages. The patient may develop respiratory alkalo-

sis because every patient-initiated breath receives pressure
support assistance.

E. Liberation modes

    1. Continuous positive airway pressure (CPAP). The ventilator
delivers a continuous pressure, usually 5 cm H_2O, throughout
inspiration and expiration.

        a. Advantages. The patient does the work of breathing (the
low level of support theoretically overcomes the resistance of the ventilator tubing).

        b. Disadvantages. It still provides some positive pressure
support and may not completely predict success with normal ventilation.

    2. T-piece. The endotracheal tube is attached to a T-shaped
piece of tubing that delivers only oxygen. The patient is not
attached to a ventilator.

        a. Advantages. The patient does the work of breathing with-
out positive pressure support.

        b. Disadvantages. Because the patient is not attached to a
ventilator, no alarms will sound if the patient becomes
tachypneic or apneic.

III **INITIAL VENTILATOR SETTINGS** are summarized in Table
26-1.

IV **LIBERATION**

A. Methods. Weaning can be accomplished in several ways.

    1. SIMV. The set rate is turned down gradually.

    2. PS. The level of pressure support is turned down gradually.

    3. CPAP. The patient is placed on CPAP for a limited time
each day. This method has been shown to shorten length of
intubation compared with the above methods without increasing the rate of reintubation.

B. Criteria

    1. Reversal or improvement of the condition causing respira-
tory failure

    2. Awake patient able to protect the airway

    3. Fraction of inspired oxygen (FIO_2) ≤ 0.4 [with an arterial
oxygen tension (PaO_2) > 60 mm Hg]

    4. Positive end-expiratory pressure (PEEP) ≤ 5 cm H_2O

    5. Rapid shallow breathing index (RSBI). This is the most pre-
dictive measure of successful extubation. The RSBI is the
spontaneous respiratory rate/spontaneous tidal volume (VT)
in liters while off positive inspiratory pressure (only PEEP). A
ratio of less than < 100 is predictive of successful extubation.

TABLE 26-1. Initial Ventilator Settings

	Settings	Normal lung (e.g., overdose, general anesthesia, neuromuscular disease)	Increased FRC (e.g., COPD, asthma, central airway tumors)	Decreased FRC (e.g., ARDS, pulmonary edema, pneumonia, atelectasis)
Ordered by physician	Mode	SIMV	SIMV	AC
	Rate	10–12 breaths/min	6–10 breaths/min	12–16 breaths/min
	Tidal volume (VT)	10–12 cc/kg	6–10 cc/kg	6–12 cc/kg
	FiO$_2$	1.0	1.0	1.0
	PEEP	5	0	5–10
	Pressure support	5	5	N/A
	I:E ratio	1:3	1:4	1:2
Set by respiratory therapist	Inspiratory flow (VT/ inspiratory time)	600 cc/sec (depending on I:E ratio and rate)	600 cc/sec (depending on I:E ratio and rate)	600 cc/sec (depending on I:E ratio and rate)
	Trigger sensitivity	−1 to −2 cm H$_2$O	−1 cm H$_2$O	−2 cm H$_2$O
	Peak flow	60 L/min	100 L/min	60 L/min

AC = assist control mode; ARDS = acute respiratory distress syndrome; COPD = chronic obstructive pulmonary disease; I:E ratio = inspiration: expiration ratio; FiO$_2$ = fraction of inspired oxygen; FRC = functional residual capacity; PEEP = positive end-expiratory pressure; SIMV = synchronized intermittent mandatory ventilation mode.

6. Minute ventilation[1] (VE) ≤ 15 L/min
7. Maximum inspiratory force (MIF) > −20 cm H_2O

Most Important Weaning Criteria ("WEANS NOW")

Wake (patient must be able to protect the airway!)
Electrolytes OK (i.e., no hypomagnesemia or hypophos-
    phatemia)
Acidosis (metabolic) or **A**lkalosis (metabolic) absent
Neuromuscularly intact (beware of prolonged aminogly-
    coside or steroid use or neuromuscular blockade)
Suctioning/**S**ecretions controlled

Nutritionally intact
Obstruction of the airways reduced
Weaning parameters
    Rapid shallow breathing index < 100 breaths/L
    MIF > −20 cm H2O
    VE ≤ 15 L/min

V VENTILATOR EMERGENCIES

HOT
KEY

Always disconnect the patient from the ventilator and bag the
patient with 100% oxygen until the problem is resolved.

VI

A. Low airway pressure alarm. Differential diagnoses include the
following:
  1. Disconnected tubing
  2. Air leak around the cuff (e.g., balloon rupture or tracheal di-
    latation)
  3. Extubation (e.g., tube has slipped into the oropharynx)
  4. Tracheo-esophageal fistula
B. High airway pressure alarm. Differential diagnoses include the
following:

---

[1]VE = tidal volume (VT) × respiratory rate.

1. Kinked tube
2. Tube out of position (e.g., right main-stem bronchus intubation)
3. Tube or airway is obstructed by secretions (e.g., mucous plug)
4. Pneumothorax
5. Bronchospasm
6. Worsening of parenchymal lung disease (increasing compliance)
7. Patient resistance to the ventilator (agitation)
C. **Apnea alarm.** Differential diagnoses include the following:
1. Sedatives
2. Central nervous system (CNS) depression
3. Muscle weakness
4. Neurologic defect

References
Evidence-based guidelines for weaning and discontinuing ventilatory support: a collective task force facilitated by the American College of Chest Physicians; the American Association for Respiratory Care; and the American College of Critical Care Medicine. Chest 2001;120(Suppl 6):375S-95S.
Tobin MJ. Advances in mechanical ventilation. N Engl J Med 2001;344(26):1986–1996.

PART IV

GASTROENTEROLOGY

27. Abdominal Pain

I INTRODUCTION

A. The evaluation of a patient with abdominal pain is complicated by the overabundance of potential diagnoses, the frequency of nonspecific signs and symptoms, and the limitations of radiographic studies.

B. Life-threatening conditions can easily "hide" in the abdomen, initially causing few, if any, symptoms. The consequences of wrongly attributing the pain to a benign condition (e.g., gastritis) can be catastrophic. Remember, **"Always respect the belly."**

II CAUSES OF ABDOMINAL PAIN.
The list of diseases that can cause abdominal pain is almost endless and includes diseases of the liver, gallbladder, pancreas, spleen, kidneys, abdominal aorta, and the entire gastrointestinal tract (including the appendix). Pain can also be referred from the thorax (e.g., myocardial infarction or pneumonia) and pelvis [e.g., pelvic inflammatory disease (PID), testicular torsion]. A thorough approach to abdominal pain consists of the following three steps:

A. **Consider the abdominal organs.** By remembering that **infection, obstruction,** or **ischemia** may cause abdominal pain in any intra-abdominal organ, you will form a broad differential diagnosis.

B. **Rule out referred pain from the thorax and pelvis.**

C. **Consider metabolic** and **systemic causes of abdominal pain.** These can be remembered using the following mnemonic.

Metabolic and Systemic Causes of Abdominal Pain ("Puking **My BAD LUNCH**")

Porphyria
Mediterranean fever
Black widow spider bite
Addison's disease or **A**ngioedema
Diabetic ketoacidosis

Lead poisoning
Uremia
Neurogenic (impingement of spinal nerves or roots, diabetes, syphilis)
Calcium (hypercalcemia)
Herpes zoster

III APPROACH TO THE PATIENT

A. Patient history
1. **Epidemiologic factors** have an important impact on the likelihood of a particular diagnosis (e.g., intravenous drug use suggests hepatitis; alcohol abuse suggests pancreatitis or alcoholic hepatitis; hypertension suggests myocardial ischemia or abdominal aneurysm).
2. **Time course.** The progression of certain symptom complexes is critical. For instance, in appendicitis, pain almost always precedes nausea and vomiting.
3. **Symptoms**
   a. **Pain**
      (1) **Quality.** Judgments regarding the quality of pain are often misleading or useless, given the significant variation and overlap among diagnoses. However, acute abdominal pain is often more of a cause for concern than chronic pain, and the chances of finding pathology are significantly higher.
      (2) **Location.** The location of the pain is extremely important and may help order the differential diagnosis (Table 27-1). Because there is a great deal of overlap, you can never be faulted for being too careful (e.g., checking a urinalysis in a patient who has upper quadrant symptoms but lacks the classic costovertebral angle tenderness).

TABLE 27-1. Differential Diagnoses for Abdominal Pain as Suggested by Location

Location of Pain	Associated Organs	Common Diseases
Right upper quadrant	Liver, gallbladder	Hepatitis, hepatic tumor or abscess, cholecystitis, choledocholithiasis, ascending cholangitis, AIDS cholangiopathy
Epigastric	Stomach, pancreas, duodenum, abdominal aorta	Gastritis, peptic ulcer disease, pancreatitis, abdominal aortic aneurysm, biliary disease, cardiac disease
Left upper quadrant	Spleen	Splenic enlargement, infarct, or abscess
Left or right lower quadrant	Appendix, intestines, ovary, fallopian tubes, testes, kidney, ureters	Appendicitis,* right- or left-sided diverticulitis, ovarian cyst or torsion, ectopic pregnancy, pelvic inflammatory disease, epidydimitis, testicular torsion, nephrolithiasis, pyelonephritis
Periumbilical	Small intestine, appendix, abdominal aorta	Small bowel obstruction, gastroenteritis, appendicitis, abdominal aortic aneurysm, ischemic bowel†
Suprapubic	Bladder, uterus, ovaries, fallopian tubes	Urinary tract infection, pelvic inflammatory disease, endometriosis, ovarian cyst, ectopic pregnancy

*Although the pain of appendicitis eventually localizes to the right lower quadrant, it usually begins in the periumbilical region.
†The location of pain from ischemic bowel is variable.

HOT KEY The pattern of pain migration may help in making the proper diagnosis. For example, pain from appendicitis often begins in the periumbilical region and then shifts and remains in the right lower quadrant.

   b. Other symptoms. Common symptoms and associated organs or organ systems are summarized in Table 27-2. Remember to ask about cardiac, pulmonary, and pelvic symptoms as well.
B. Physical examination
   1. Auscultation may not provide much information, because the presence or absence of bowel sounds usually does not narrow the differential diagnosis.
   2. Palpation. Always move gently toward the area of the patient's complaint.
   3. Rectal and **pelvic examination.** Always perform a rectal examination (with stool guaiac) and a pelvic examination in patients with abdominal pain. Pain during rectal or pelvic examination may indicate pelvic pathology or a disorder involving a lower intraabdominal structure (e.g., a retrocolic appendix).
C. Diagnostic tests
   1. Basic tests. The results of the following tests provide a starting point for narrowing the list of possible diagnoses.
      a. Complete blood count (CBC). Look for leukocytosis or anemia.
      b. Renal panel. Electrolyte disturbances can be the cause or result of the illness. Elevated blood urea nitrogen (BUN) and creatinine levels may suggest volume depletion or renal pathology.
      c. Liver function tests screen for liver or biliary pathology.
      d. Amylase. Evaluating the lipase level in addition to the amylase level may increase the sensitivity and specificity for pancreatitis.

TABLE 27-2. Symptoms and Associated Organ Systems	
Symptom	**Likely Site of Pathology**
Dysuria, frequency	Kidney, bladder
Nausea, vomiting, diarrhea	Gastrointestinal tract
Jaundice, pruritis	Liver, gallbladder
Pain that decreases upon sitting up	Pancreas
Abrupt onset of midline pain that is out of proportion to the exam	Mesenteric vessels

   e. Urinalysis is helpful to rule out diabetic ketoacidosis and renal pathology.
   f. Urine pregnancy test. If the patient is a woman of child-bearing age, a pregnancy test should be performed regardless of how probable pregnancy seems to the patient.
   g. Coagulation studies. Prothrombin time (PT) and partial thromboplastin time (PTT). Although these add little information regarding the etiology of acute abdominal pain, it is worthwhile performing these for anyone who may need an invasive procedure.
2. **Ancillary tests.** Given your initial diagnostic impressions, the following tests may be indicated.
   a. Serum calcium. This test can rule out hypercalcemia as a possible diagnosis.
   b. Serum albumin. A low value may increase suspicion of an intraabdominal malignancy.
   c. Fecal white blood cell (WBC) count. A fecal WBC count should be performed to screen for bowel inflammation in any patient with diarrhea.
   d. Radiologic examination of the abdomen. Flat and upright views are useful for evaluating bowel obstruction or the presence of kidney stones.
   e. Radiologic examination of the chest. Posterior-anterior (PA) and lateral views are indicated when the patient is experiencing upper abdominal pain (to rule out a lower lobe pneumonia) or when there is any suspicion of peritonitis (to rule out free air).
      (1) A lateral radiograph sometimes demonstrates free air not seen on the PA film. The patient should remain upright for at least 5 minutes before PA and lateral radiographs to increase the sensitivity for detecting air beneath the diaphragm. In a patient who cannot sit up (e.g., because of pain or hypotension), a **left lateral decubitus view** can be used to evaluate for free air.
      (2) Enlargement of the aortic or cardiac silhouette may suggest an abdominal aortic aneurysm or a cardiac cause of the pain.
   f. Abdominal ultrasound is often the best way of evaluating gallbladder, biliary, and renal pathology; diseases in the liver, spleen, pancreas, abdominal aorta, and some intraabdominal abscesses can also be detected.
   g. Abdominal computed tomography (CT) scan. An abdominal CT scan is better than ultrasound for evaluating most intraabdominal structures (except for the biliary tree and perhaps the kidney). Triple-contrast studies (intravenous, oral, and rectal) are usually performed, yielding much finer detail. For patients with elevated crea-

tinine levels, intravenous contrast can sometimes be avoided if the bowel is of primary concern; however, abscesses will often be missed unless intravenous contrast is used. [Abdominal magnetic resonance imaging (MRI) is an option for patients in whom radiocontrast dye is contraindicated.]

   h. Paracentesis. If the patient has ascites, you should always perform a paracentesis to rule out peritonitis.

   i. Electrocardiography. Every patient with a history of cardiac disease or risk factors and abdominal pain (especially upper abdominal pain) should have an electrocardiogram (ECG) to rule out myocardial ischemia. Inferior wall myocardial ischemia is the type of ischemia most likely to cause abdominal pain.

D. General guidelines for the management of a patient with abdominal pain

   1. The patient should have nothing by mouth during the initial evaluation because surgery may be necessary.

   2. Associated conditions (e.g., severe volume depletion or electrolyte imbalances) should be corrected while the diagnostic workup is proceeding.

   3. In the past, it was thought that the use of painkillers (e.g., opiates) during evaluation of the patient would "mask" potential diagnoses. However, it is now generally considered inappropriate to withhold medication in a patient with severe pain. The use of short-acting opiates (e.g., fentanyl) allows careful titration, which helps prevent hypotension.

   4. A nasogastric tube is indicated in patients with severe vomiting or bowel obstruction.

   5. Early consultation with a surgeon when certain disorders are suspected clinically (e.g., appendicitis, peritonitis, cholecystitis) can prevent long delays and unnecessary tests.

   6. When an etiology is not apparent and the patient appears ill (e.g., fever, diaphoresis, resting tachycardia, abdominal tenderness), observation in the hospital is usually necessary. In these situations, there is no substitute for frequent follow-up exams and the tincture of time. In addition, advanced imaging (CT scan with contrast) may be extremely helpful.

References

Dang C, Aguilera P, Dang A, Salem L. Acute abdominal pain. Four classifications can guide assessment and management. Geriatrics 2002;57(3):30–42.

DeBanto JR, Varilek GW, Haas L. What could be causing chronic abdominal pain? Anything from common peptic ulcers to uncommon pancreatic trauma. Postgrad Med 1999;106(3):141–146.

Suleiman S, Johnston DE. The abdominal wall: an overlooked source of pain. Am Fam Physician 2001;64(3):431–438.

28. Liver Tests

I INTRODUCTION

A. The liver has been called "the custodian of the milieu interieur." Hepatic disorders, therefore, have far-reaching effects on homeostasis. Fortunately, there are several tests that can help determine the cause of the injury and allow assessment of the liver's remaining synthetic capacity.

B. The blood tests used to assess the liver are commonly called liver function tests (LFTs). Whereas some of these measures reflect the actual function of the liver (e.g., albumin, bilirubin, prothrombin time), many only reflect injury [e.g., aspartate aminotransferase (AST), alanine aminotransferase (ALT), and alkaline phosphatase].

II GENERAL APPROACH

A. Synthetic function

1. **Albumin.** The liver is an important site of protein synthesis. Assessment of albumin levels can tell us how well the liver is making proteins in general. If dietary intake is constant and the liver fails, it can take several weeks for albumin levels to fall. Therefore, in a patient with acute liver failure, the albumin level may be normal. Conversely, in patients with high levels of metabolic stress (sepsis, shock), albumin levels may drop quickly despite adequate liver function.

2. **Prothrombin time (PT).** The PT is a function of plasma levels and the activity of factors I, II, V, VII, and X. The half-lives of some of these proteins are much shorter than that of albumin; therefore, the PT increases within hours of a significant decrease in the synthetic function of the liver.

3. **Total bilirubin levels** can also be used to assess liver function. Clinical jaundice is usually apparent with bilirubin levels that exceed 3 mg/dl. A complete discussion of bilirubin formation and elimination is beyond the scope of this chapter, but, briefly, bilirubin is formed by the breakdown and cleavage of the heme ring. The bilirubin is then glucuronidated (conjugated) in the liver and excreted in the bile. Elevations can be thought of as being predominantly **unconjugated** or **conjugated.** Most are a mix of both.

   a. Unconjugated (indirect). Levels of unconjugated bilirubin increase if production increases (e.g., as a result of hemolysis or hematoma) or hepatic uptake or conjugation decrease (as seen in Gilbert's syndrome and Crigler-Najjar syndrome).

H O T

The most common cause of unconjugated hyperbilirubinemia in an otherwise healthy person is Gilbert's syndrome.

K E Y

---

    b. Conjugated (direct). Levels of conjugated bilirubin increase with decreased secretion of bilirubin into bile canaliculi (as seen in Dubin-Johnson syndrome and Rotor's syndrome). Biliary epithelial damage (as a result of hepatitis, toxins, or cirrhosis) or ductal obstruction (as a result of biliary stones, cholangitis, or pancreatic cancer) can also increase conjugated bilirubin levels.

  4. Glucose levels may be decreased in patients with severe liver dysfunction secondary to disruptions in glycolysis and gluconeogenesis.

B. Injury pattern. The two predominant patterns of liver injury are **cholestatic** and **hepatocellular**.

  1. Cholestatic pattern. The cholestatic pattern is characterized by elevations in **alkaline phosphatase** and **γ-glutamyl transpeptidase (GGT)**.

    a. Alkaline phosphatase is an enzyme that hydrolyzes organic phosphate esters. Alkaline phosphatase is found primarily in liver and bone, but may also be found in the small intestine, kidney, placenta, and leukocytes. In the liver, alkaline phosphatase is found primarily on the surface of the bile canalicular membrane. Disproportionate elevations of alkaline phosphatase occur with any disease that obstructs bile flow (e.g., biliary stones, cholangitis, pancreatic cancer) or diseases that infiltrate the liver causing micro-obstruction or damage (e.g., tuberculosis, sarcoidosis, metastatic cancer).

    b. GGT is an enzyme found in many tissues, but notably, not bone. Therefore, it is most useful for evaluating the cause of an elevated alkaline phosphatase level. If both enzymes are elevated, the liver is a likely source, whereas elevation of alkaline phosphatase with a normal GGT suggests a bone source. GGT is also elevated in patients with alcoholic liver disease.

  2. Hepatocellular pattern. The hepatocellular pattern is associated with elevations in **aspartate aminotransferase [AST, serum glutamate oxaloacetate transaminase (SGOT)]**, **ala-**

TABLE 28-1. Common Liver Function Test Abnormalities*

Disease	AST	ALT	Alkaline Phosphatase	Bilirubin	Comments
Cholelithiasis	N	N	N	N	Usually asymptomatic; may cause postprandial pain
Choledocholithiasis	N/↑	N/↑	↑↑	↑	Biliary colic; may lead to cholangitis
Cholecystitis	N/↑	N/↑	N/↑	N/↑	Positive Murphy's sign; fever; elevated WBC count
Cholangitis	↑↑	↑↑	↑↑↑	↑↑	Charcot's triad (fever, right upper quadrant pain, jaundice)
Viral hepatitis	↑↑↑↑	↑↑↑↑	↑	↑↑↑↑	ALT > AST
Alcoholic hepatitis	↑↑	↑↑↑	↑↑	↑↑↑	AST > ALT; AST usually <300 IU/L unless in combination with another insult
Congestive hepatopathy	↑↑↑	↑↑↑	↑↑↑	↑↑	PT often rises early
Metastatic disease	↑↑	↑↑	↑↑↑	N	Consider this diagnosis with isolated increased alkaline phosphatase

ALT = alanine aminotransferase; AST = aspartate aminotransferase; N = normal; PT = prothrombin time; WBC = white blood cell.
*These disorders often present with variable liver function test abnormalities.

nine aminotransferase [**ALT,** serum glutamate pyruvate transaminase (SGPT)], and **lactate dehydrogenase (LDH).**

a. AST is an enzyme found in the cytosol and mitochondria of hepatocytes. It is also found in cardiac muscle; renal, brain, pulmonary, and pancreatic tissue; leukocytes; and erythrocytes. AST is a sensitive indicator of hepatic injury but is not specific.

b. ALT is an enzyme found in the cytosol of hepatocytes. Because it is found only in the liver, ALT is a very specific indicator of hepatocellular injury.

c. LDH is an enzyme that is found in many tissues; isoenzyme 5 (LDH-5) is found in the liver. LDH levels increase with any hepatocellular injury.

Causes of Significantly Increased (> 1000 U/L) AST and ALT Levels ("Tainted Mushrooms Can Cause Bad Hepatitis, So Watch Out!")

Tylenol or Tetracycline toxicity
Mushrooms (*Amanita phalloides*)
Carbon tetrachloride toxicity (rare)
Congestive hepatopathy
Budd-Chiari syndrome
Hepatitis (viral)
Shock liver (due to hypotension of any cause)
Wilson's disease (subtype associated with fulminant hepatic necrosis)
Other toxins (e.g., halothane, valproic acid, vitamin A)

 III **COMMON LIVER FUNCTION TEST ABNORMALITIES** are summarized in Table 28-1.

References

Gopal DV, Rosen HR. Abnormal findings on liver function tests. Interpreting results to narrow the diagnosis and establish a prognosis. Postgrad Med 2000;107(2): 100–110.

Pratt DS, Kaplan MM. Evaluation of abnormal liver-enzyme results in asymptomatic patients. N Engl J Med 2000;342(17):1266–1271.

29. Acute Diarrhea

I **INTRODUCTION.** Although we might think of diarrhea as primarily a nuisance, more than 5 million deaths per year worldwide can be attributed to this ailment.

A. Definition. Diarrhea is the excretion of more than 300 g of stool per day. Diarrhea is not a subjective experience of increased frequency or quantity of stool.

B. Classification. Diarrhea can be classified as acute (< 3 weeks in duration) or chronic (> 3 weeks in duration). Because acute diarrhea is seen more often in hospitalized patients, it is the focus of this chapter.

II **CAUSES OF ACUTE DIARRHEA**

A. Infection. Diarrhea of an infectious etiology is by far the most common type.

B. Inflammation. Diarrhea resulting from an inflammatory process (e.g., inflammatory bowel disease, ischemic bowel disease) often presents with blood and pus in the stool. An infectious etiology must be ruled out to make this diagnosis.

C. Drugs, including laxatives, antacids containing magnesium, antibiotics, and colchicine, are an often overlooked cause of diarrhea.

D. Toxins, including heavy metals, seafood toxins, and mushroom toxins, can cause acute diarrhea.

III **APPROACH TO THE PATIENT**

A. Evaluate volume status. Physical examination findings suggestive of dehydration include resting tachycardia, orthostatic hypotension, dry mucous membranes, and skin tenting.

B. Most cases of acute, infectious diarrhea are self-limited and do not need workup, only supportive care. Figure 29–1 can help you differentiate which patients need a diagnostic workup and which patients need antimicrobial treatment.

IV **TREATMENT**

A. Bland diet. Dairy foods, spicy foods, and caffeine should be avoided. The patient should follow the BRAT diet: **b**ananas, **r**ice, **a**pplesauce, and **t**oast.

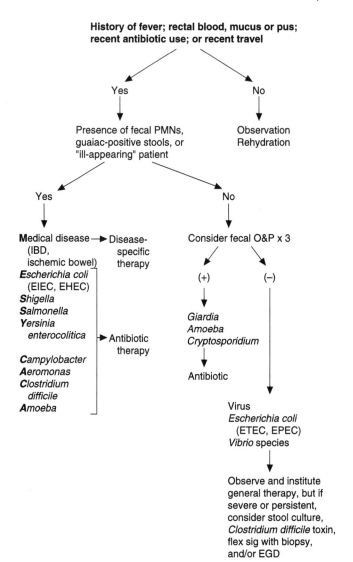

FIGURE 29-1. Algorithm for evaluating patients with acute diarrhea. *IBD* = inflammatory bowel disease; *O&P* = ova and parasites; *PMNs* = polymorphonuclear neutrophils; *EGD* = esophagogastroduodenoscopy; *EIEC* = enteroinvasive *Escherichia coli*; *EHEC* = enterohemorrhagic *E. coli* (serotype O157:H7); *EPEC* = enteropathogenic *E. coli*; *ETEC* = enterotoxigenic *E. coli*; flex sig = flexible sigmoidoscopy.

B. Rehydration. Intravenous fluids may be necessary if the patient is unable to take liquids orally.

C. Pharmacologic therapy

1. **Antimotility agents.** In some patients with infectious diarrhea, antimotility agents pose a theoretical risk of toxic megacolon and prolongation of illness.

2. **Bismuth subsalicylate** has antisecretory and antimicrobial properties and can be useful for traveler's diarrhea or viral diarrhea.

3. **Antibiotics,** if necessary, are usually given in 5- to 7-day courses.

References

Bartlett JG. Clinical practice. Antibiotic-associated diarrhea. N Engl J Med 2002;346 (5):334–339.

Schiller LR. Diarrhea. Med Clin North Am 2000;84(5):1259–1274.

Yassin SF, Young-Fadok TM, Zein NN, Pardi DS. Clostridium difficile-associated diarrhea and colitis. Mayo Clin Proc 2001;76(7):725–730.

30. Acute Gastrointestinal Bleeding

I **INTRODUCTION.** Gastrointestinal (GI) bleeding is both a common and serious problem in the United States.

A. **Classification.** GI bleeding is traditionally classified as **"upper"** or **"lower,"** depending on whether the bleed originates above or below the ligament of Treitz.

B. **Definitions**
  1. **Hematemesis** is blood, including "coffee grounds," in the vomitus. Hematemesis clearly represents an upper GI source.
  2. **Hematochezia** is red or maroon-colored blood in the stool. Hematochezia can occur with lower GI bleeds and rapidly bleeding upper GI bleeds.

HOT KEY

In 10% of patients with hematochezia, the source of bleeding is the upper GI tract.

  3. **Melena** is black, tarry stool resulting from digested blood. Melena usually indicates an upper GI bleed because the blood has been digested to hematin, but small bowel and right-sided colonic hemorrhages can also produce melena. Melena has three characteristics that help to distinguish it from other causes of dark stool: a) it is dark black, b) it has a characteristic odor (patients say it smells far worse than normal stool), and c) it has a consistency that is loose and tarry/oily.

HOT KEY

Bismuth subsalicylate, iron, spinach, and charcoal can also produce black stools.

II **CAUSES OF GI BLEEDING**

A. **Upper GI source.** There are many causes of upper GI tract bleeding; the most common can be remembered easily using the mnemonic, "GUM BLEEDING." (The first three causes are the most common.)

Gastrointestinal Bleeding—Upper Gastrointestinal Sources
("GUM BLEEDING")

Gastritis [secondary to nonsteroidal anti-inflammatory drugs
(NSAIDs), alcohol, or stress]
Ulcers (often caused by Helicobacter pylori or NSAIDs)
Mallory-Weiss tear (often secondary to excessive vomiting)

Biliary (hemobilia, usually secondary to trauma)
Large varices (seen in patients with portal hypertension)
Esophagitis or Esophageal ulcer
Enteroaortic fistula (usually seen in patients with aortic
grafts)
Duodenitis or Dieulafoy's lesion (an ectatic artery in the
stomach)
Inflammatory bowel disease (upper tract Crohn's disease)
Neovascularization (arteriovenous malformation), usually
seen in the elderly; more commonly causes lower GI
bleeding
Gastric cancer

B. Lower GI source. Use the following mnemonic to remember
the causes of lower GI tract bleeding—you may need a
"DRAIN" to collect the blood.

Gastrointestinal Bleeding—Lower Gastrointestinal Sources
("DRAIN")

Diverticulosis
Radiation colitis
Arteriovenous malformation (angiodysplasia)
Ischemia, Inflammation, or Infection
Neoplasm

1. **Diverticulosis** is the most common cause of lower GI bleeding. The disorder is painless and is almost never a cause of chronic blood loss.
2. **Radiation colitis** can occur at any time following radiation therapy. Most commonly seen after radiation of the prostate (men) or cervix/uterus (women).
3. **Arteriovenous malformations (angiodysplasia)** occur primarily in the elderly and may cause both acute and chronic blood loss.
4. **Ischemia.** In mesenteric ischemia, for example, the patient experiences pain out of proportion to the examination.
5. **Inflammatory bowel disease** is usually accompanied by diarrhea and rarely causes massive bleeding.

6. **Infectious colitis** is also usually accompanied by diarrhea.
7. **Neoplasms** (benign or malignant) usually cause chronic, rather than acute, blood loss.

III APPROACH TO THE PATIENT

A. **Patient history.** The history is helpful for distinguishing between an upper and lower source of bleeding, but poor for determining the exact cause of the bleeding. It is important to inquire about the following:
   1. Number of episodes
   2. Most recent episode
   3. Use of NSAIDs and aspirin
   4. Use of anticoagulants
   5. Cirrhosis
   6. Alcohol abuse
   7. Vomiting before hematemesis
   8. Presence and location of abdominal pain
   9. Prior aortic surgery
   10. Previous history of GI bleeding
B. **Physical examination**
   1. **Vital signs.** Check orthostatics—if your patient "tilts" (i.e., moving from a supine position to an upright position causes his or her pulse to increase by more than 20 beats/min or systolic blood pressure to decrease by more than 10 mm Hg), then intravascular volume is 10%–20% below normal. Patients taking β blockers might have a "normal" pulse rate, despite a large volume loss.
   2. **HEENT.** Check for scleral icterus, which may indicate liver disease with associated varices. Rule out epistaxis and oral lesions as a source of upper GI tract bleeding.
   3. **Lungs and heart.** Check for evidence of left ventricular dysfunction, which can affect fluid administration.
   4. **Abdomen.** Given the cathartic nature of blood, the absence of bowel sounds may suggest an intraabdominal catastrophe. Look carefully for rigidity, involuntary guarding, and rebound tenderness, which may suggest peritonitis. Presence of borborygmi (bowel sounds heard without a stethoscope) is caused by increased motility from blood in the small bowel (typically suggesting an upper GI source).
   5. **Rectum.** Palpate for rectal masses. A stool guaiac should be performed if the stools are not clearly bloody.
   6. **Neurologic examination.** Check for asterixis (evidence of liver disease).
   7. **Skin.** Look for signs of liver disease, such as jaundice, spider angiomata, and palmar erythema.
C. **Diagnostic tests.** Important initial tests to run include:
   1. Blood typing and cross-matching

2. Complete blood count (CBC) with platelets
3. Electrolyte panel
4. Blood urea nitrogen (BUN) and creatinine levels
5. Liver tests
6. Prothrombin time (PT) and partial thromboplastin time (PTT)
7. Chest and abdominal radiographs
8. Electrocardiogram (ECG)
D. General guidelines for the management of a patient with GI bleeding. In a patient with GI bleeding, **do not delay management because you have not figured out the cause of the bleeding!** GI bleeding is one situation in internal medicine in which the initial management is usually the same regardless of the exact cause.
   1. Ensure that the ABCs (airway, breathing, circulation) are in place.
   2. Begin fluid replacement. Intravenous access should be obtained immediately, preferably with two large-bore (18-gauge or larger) intravenous lines.
   3. Insert a nasogastric tube if there is any possibility of an upper GI bleed. Bolus with 500 cc of water, then withdraw; keep a tab of how much water it takes for the aspirate to become almost clear.
      a. The nasogastric tube aspirate may be negative, even in the presence of upper GI bleeding, if:
         (1) The source of the bleeding is below the end of the nasogastric tube (e.g., if the nasogastric tube ends in the stomach, bleeding from a duodenal ulcer may not be apparent in the aspirate).
         (2) The bleeding is transient.
      b. The tube should be kept in place if there is active bleeding or signs of small bowel obstruction.
   4. Hold antihypertensive or diuretic therapy. In addition, the patient should receive nothing by mouth.
   5. Decide whether to admit the patient to the intensive care unit (ICU).
      a. If your patient needs to take a trip to the ICU, he or she will need a "VISA." Patients generally require admission if any of the following criteria are met:

Criteria for Admittance to ICU with a Gastrointestinal Bleed ("VISA")

Variceal bleeding (suspected or confirmed)
Instability of vital signs
Serious comorbid conditions [e.g., coronary artery disease, chronic obstructive pulmonary disease (COPD)]
Active GI bleeding

b. All patients admitted to the ICU should be seen by a gastroenterologist immediately.

6. Stabilize the patient. No diagnostic testing (endoscopic or radiologic imaging) can be performed until the patient is adequately resuscitated.

    a. Transfusion

        (1) Elderly patients or those with coronary artery disease are usually transfused to keep their hematocrit greater than 30%. At least 2 units of typed and cross-matched packed red blood cells (RBCs) should be kept in the blood bank at all times.

        (2) In a patient with active bleeding, consider a platelet transfusion if the patient's platelet count is less than 50,000/mm³. Fresh frozen plasma should be used if the patient's international normalized ratio (INR) is greater than 1.5.

    b. Intravenous H₂ blockers are traditionally administered. However, proton pump inhibitors given intravenously may be more effective.

    c. Vitamin K should be administered if the patient's PT or PTT is abnormal.

HOT

A unit of blood entering or leaving the body should change the patient's hemoglobin level by approximately 1 g/dl.

KEY

---

7. Perform ancillary tests if necessary.

    a. After resuscitation, patients with evidence of ongoing upper GI bleeding will typically undergo upper endoscopy within a few hours. This "urgent" endoscopy will not only assess the source of bleeding but will also attempt to achieve hemostasis. In patients with no clear ongoing bleeding, endoscopy should typically be performed within 12–24 hours.

    b. A technetium-99 (T⁹⁹)—labeled red blood cell scan can be performed if a slow (i.e., 0.1–1 ml/min) lower GI bleed is present.

    c. An angiogram may be indicated when a rapid (i.e., > 1 ml/min) lower GI bleed is suspected.

References
Dallal HJ, Palmer KR. ABC of the upper gastrointestinal tract: upper gastrointestinal haemorrhage. BMJ 2001;323(7321):1115–1117.
Fallah MA, Prakash C, Edmundowicz S. Acute gastrointestinal bleeding. Med Clin North Am 2000;84(5):1183–1208.
Sharara AI, Rockey DC. Gastroesophageal variceal hemorrhage. N Engl J Med 2001;345(9):669–681.

31. Splenomegaly

I INTRODUCTION

A. Splenomegaly is enlargement of the spleen.
  1. A normal spleen is 12 cm × 7 cm and weighs less than 200 g. It is surrounded by a thin capsule. The spleen is usually not palpable unless it is enlarged; therefore, **a palpable spleen is always abnormal.**
  2. At times the spleen may be difficult to palpate, but dullness to percussion in the 11th left intercostal space (Traube's space) suggests splenic enlargement.
  3. **Massive splenomegaly** occurs when the spleen weighs more than 3000 g.
B. Hypersplenism is the term given to any clinical situation in which the **spleen inappropriately removes excess amounts of leukocytes, platelets,** or **erythrocytes** from the circulation.
  1. **Hypersplenism and splenomegaly are not synonymous.** Patients with hypersplenism all have splenomegaly; however, only a small percentage of those with splenomegaly have hypersplenism.
  2. **Characteristics** of hypersplenism include the following:
     a. Splenomegaly
     b. Splenic destruction/sequestration of one or more cell lines
     c. Normal or hyperplastic bone marrow
     d. Reversal of the cytopenia following splenectomy

II CLINICAL MANIFESTATIONS OF SPLENOMEGALY

A. Nonacute splenomegaly is most common. Clinical presentations include:
  1. **Early satiety** (because of impaired gastric filling); may lead to weight loss
  2. **Cytopenia** (as a result of hypersplenism); may lead to infections, bleeding, or fatigue
  3. **Symptoms of the underlying disease**
  4. Many patients have no symptoms referable to splenomegaly.
B. Acute splenomegaly
  1. **Clinical signs** include the sudden onset of left upper quadrant pain and a tender, enlarged spleen.
  2. **Differential diagnoses:**
     a. Subcapsular hematoma
     b. Splenic rupture due to trauma (even remote) or an in-

fectious process (e.g., malaria, mononucleosis, typhoid fever)
  c. Splenic infarct due to embolism or sickle cell disease
  d. Hemorrhage into a splenic cyst

III CAUSES OF SPLENOMEGALY

A. Congestive causes. This category includes any disease that leads to disordered splenic blood flow, so that the blood "backs up" in the spleen. Think of causes that anatomically head away from the spleen.
  1. **Splenic vein obstruction**
  2. **Portal vein obstruction**
  3. **Hepatic schistosomiasis**
  4. **Cirrhosis**
  5. **Hepatic vein obstruction**
  6. **Constrictive pericarditis**
  7. **Congestive heart failure (CHF)**
B. Reactive causes. This category includes those diseases that lead to splenic hyperplasia. Because the spleen is a lymphoid gland, many diseases that cause a systemic immunologic response can cause splenomegaly. In addition, blood disorders that lead to hemolysis can also cause the spleen to enlarge.
  1. **Infections**
    a. **Bacterial** (e.g., endocarditis, tuberculosis, sustained bacteremia)
    b. **Viral** (e.g., mononucleosis, viral hepatitis)
    c. **Parasitic** (e.g., malaria, leishmaniasis, trypanosomiasis)
    d. **Fungal** (e.g., disseminated histoplasmosis)
  2. **Collagen vascular diseases**
    a. **Rheumatoid arthritis.** Felty's syndrome is the triad of granulocytopenia, rheumatoid arthritis, and splenomegaly.

HOT KEY
Rheumatoid arthritis—like congestive heart failure, systemic lupus erythematosus, and endocarditis—usually causes mild splenomegaly.

---

  b. **Systemic lupus erythematosus (SLE)**
  3. **Serum sickness.** This immune complex disorder—usually caused by a drug hypersensitivity reaction—occurs 1–3 weeks following primary exposure (or within 36 hours of reexposure) to an offending agent.

Clinical Manifestations of Serum Sickness ("SALT")

Skin rash (morbilliform, urticarial, or palpable purpura)
Arthralgias or **A**rthritis
Lymphadenopathy
Temperature increase

  4. Work hypertrophy can be caused by hemolysis.
C. Infiltrative causes
  1. Benign
    a. Sarcoidosis
    b. Amyloidosis
    c. Gaucher's disease, an autosomal recessive disorder characterized by an accumulation of sphingolipid within phagocytic cells throughout the body
  2. Malignant
    a. Lymphomas
    b. Leukemias
    c. Myeloproliferative disorders
    d. Primary splenic tumors
    e. Metastatic tumors

Causes of Massive Splenomegaly ("**H**opefully, **My** **M**edical **S**tudents **C**an **L**earn **G**astroenterology")

Hairy cell leukemia (uncommon, resembles chronic lymphocytic leukemia)
Malaria
Myeloid metaplasia with myelofibrosis (one of four myeloproliferative disorders)
Sarcoidosis
Chronic myelogenous leukemia (another myeloproliferative disorder)
Lymphoma (primarily splenic lymphoma)
Gaucher's disease

IV APPROACH TO THE PATIENT

A. Patient history. When taking the history, focus on searching for an underlying cause. Things to look for include:
  1. Alcohol use or **cirrhosis**
  2. CHF

3. **Febrile illness (current or recent)**
4. **Arthralgias, arthritis, or joint stiffness**
5. **Fever, weight loss, diaphoresis, or lymph node swelling**
6. **Family history of anemia** or **splenomegaly**

B. **Physical examination.** Look for evidence of hepatomegaly, lymphadenopathy, skin rash, subcutaneous nodules, CHF, liver disease, or an infectious process.

C. **Laboratory tests** usually include a **complete blood count (CBC) with platelets** and analysis of the peripheral smear and **liver tests.**

D. Other tests. Blood cultures may be warranted. An ultrasound is useful to confirm the presence of splenomegaly and evaluate liver size. **Bone marrow biopsy, lymph node biopsy, serologies, exploratory laparotomy,** and **other imaging studies** may also be performed.

References

Carr JA, Shurafa M, Velanovich V. Surgical indications in idiopathic splenomegaly. Arch Surg 2002;137(1):64–68.

Grover SA, Barkun AN, Sackett DL. Does this patient have splenomegaly? JAMA 1993:270(18):2218–2221 (classic article).

32. Ascites

INTRODUCTION. Ascites is the accumulation of excess fluid within the peritoneal cavity.

CAUSES OF ASCITES. Ascites may occur as part of anasarca (generalized edema) or as an isolated fluid collection.

A. Anasarca. The causes of a generalized edematous state can be remembered as the **"osis group"—nephrosis, cirrhosis, cardiosis, and hypothyroidosis.**

B. Isolated fluid collection. There are three primary mechanisms of ascites production. In addition, there are miscellaneous disorders that cause ascites by various mechanisms.

  1. Increased hydrostatic pressure in the splanchnic capillaries may result from diseases that produce elevated venous pressure. One way of thinking about the causes of increased hydrostatic pressure is to trace the venous blood from the heart down.

   a. Cardiac. Right-sided heart failure and **constrictive pericarditis** lead to elevated venous pressure and can cause ascites.

   b. Hepatic

   (1) Postsinusoidal obstruction includes inferior vena cava obstruction, hepatic vein obstruction (i.e., **Budd-Chiari syndrome**), or hepatic venule obstruction (i.e., **veno-occlusive disease**).

   (2) Sinusoidal obstruction is the most common cause of ascites and usually results from **cirrhosis.**

   (3) Presinusoidal obstruction may be caused by **schistosomiasis** or **portal vein thrombosis.** (Portal vein thrombosis may cause variceal bleeding but only rarely produces ascites.)

  2. Decreased oncotic pressure may result from decreased albumin intake (i.e., **starvation**), decreased albumin production (i.e., **severe liver disease**), or increased loss of albumin (e.g., **nephrotic syndrome, protein-losing enteropathy**).

  3. Increased capillary permeability may occur with **infection** (e.g., tuberculosis) or **malignancy.**

  4. Miscellaneous causes

   a. Hypothyroidism. Myxedema usually produces anasarca, not isolated ascites.

b. Pancreatitis may cause **pancreatic ascites.**

c. Lymphatic obstruction from **trauma, tumor,** or **infection** (e.g., filariasis, tuberculosis) may cause **chylous ascites.**

III APPROACH TO THE PATIENT

A. Patient history and physical examination. A complete history and physical examination (including rectal and pelvic examinations) are necessary. By remembering the underlying mechanisms, you can systematically pursue the diagnosis.

1. **Increased hydrostatic pressure**
   a. **Right-sided heart failure** or **constrictive pericarditis.** Ask about symptoms of left-sided heart failure (the most common cause of right-sided heart failure). Perform a careful cardiac examination and evaluate the jugular venous pressure. Assess the patient for evidence of hepatojugular reflux.
   b. **Budd-Chiari syndrome** may be suggested by right upper quadrant pain and an enlarged liver in a patient with a myeloproliferative disorder.
   c. **Hepatic veno-occlusive** disease should be considered in patients with ascites and a history of chemotherapy or bone marrow transplantation.
   d. **Cirrhosis** is the most common cause of ascites. Inquire about risk factors, including alcohol consumption and hepatitis exposures (e.g., intravenous drug use). Look for signs of chronic liver disease (see Chapter 34).
2. **Low oncotic pressure** in the absence of severe liver disease may be suggested by a history of starvation or by the presence of nephrotic syndrome.
3. **Increased capillary permeability** may be suggested by a history of fevers or weight loss, which could suggest infection or malignancy.
4. **Miscellaneous mechanisms**
   a. **Pancreatic ascites** should be considered whenever pancreatitis or pancreatic ductal disruption is a possibility.
   b. **Lymphatic obstruction** is suspected on the basis of the "milky" appearance of chylous ascites.
   c. **Myxedema.** If myxedema is the etiology, the patient will usually have other symptoms of hypothyroidism (see Chapter 80).

B. Laboratory tests. Routinely performed laboratory tests include a complete blood count (CBC) with differential, an electrolyte panel, blood urea nitrogen (BUN) and creatinine levels, prothrombin time (PT) and partial thromboplastin time (PTT), and liver function tests with serum albumin. A urine dipstick test for protein and thyroid function tests are also frequently performed, especially when anasarca is present.

C. Diagnostic paracentesis is almost always needed to make a diagnosis. Even when the diagnosis seems apparent, diagnostic paracentesis is still indicated to rule out secondary processes [e.g., spontaneous bacterial peritonitis (SBP)].

1. Procedure

    a. Make sure the patient has emptied his or her bladder before the procedure. Alternatively, a Foley catheter may be inserted.

    b. A midline approach (i.e., 1–2 cm directly below the umbilicus) may be preferable because this region is avascular. However, prior midline surgery often necessitates a lateral approach because the bowel may be adherent to the peritoneal wall.

    c. A small needle (19-gauge or smaller) is usually used.

2. Evaluation. A cell count with differential, bacterial Gram stain and cultures, and an albumin level should be obtained on the fluid sample. Lactate dehydrogenase (LDH) and glucose levels may provide additional information. An amylase or triglyceride level should be ordered if there is a possibility of pancreatic or chylous ascites, respectively. In patients in whom malignancy is a concern, cytology can be performed on the fluid (the larger volume assessed, the higher the yield).

HOT

KEY
Remember to order a serum albumin level at approximately the same time the ascitic fluid is obtained.

---

3. Interpretation. Table 32-1 contains likely etiologies of ascites and their characteristic fluid findings. Remember that the findings given are only generalizations and will not apply in all cases. Furthermore, the presence of two or more disorders may skew the fluid analysis.

    a. Cell count. The cell count can be used to evaluate the possibility of SBP, tuberculosis, or malignancy.

        (1) SBP. Treatment of SBP is usually indicated when the absolute neutrophil count exceeds **250 cells/µl.** Counts greater than 500 cells/µl are more specific but less sensitive for SBP.

        (2) Tuberculosis or **malignancy.** A cell count that exceeds 250 cells/µl and is lymphocyte predominant often implies tuberculous or malignant ascites (however, SBP can also occasionally have a lymphocyte predominant pattern).

    b. Serum—ascites albumin gradient. Subtract the ascitic fluid albumin value from the serum albumin value.

TABLE 32-1. Characteristic Fluid Findings

Disorder	Serum-Ascites Albumin Gradient	Cell Count (Cells/μl)	Total Protein*	Other Findings
Cirrhosis	≥1.1	< 250 (mesothelial)	Moderate	Abnormal liver function tests
Spontaneous bacterial peritonitis (SPB)	≥1.1	> 250 (PMNs)	Moderate	Culture may be positive
Congestive heart failure	≥1.1	< 1000 (mesothelial)	High	Elevated neck veins, gallops, abnormal ECG
Hypothyroidism	≥1.1	< 250 (variable)	Variable	Decreased free T_4, increased TSH
Liver malignancy (primary or secondary)	≥1.1	Variable	Moderate	Elevated serum AFP with primary malignancy
Nephrotic syndrome	<1.1	< 250 (mesothelial)	Low	Positive urine dipstick and 24-hour collection for protein
Tuberculous ascites	<1.1	> 1000 (variable)	High	Ascitic acid-fast bacillus stain occasionally positive
Secondary peritonitis	<1.1	> 250 (PMNs)	Moderate	Very low ascitic glucose, polymycrobial
Pancreatic ascites	<1.1	> 1000 (PMNs)	Moderate	Increased serum and fluid amylase
Peritoneal malignancy	<1.1	> 1000 (variable)	High	Cytology, CT scan, peritoneal biopsy may be useful

AFP = α-fetoprotein; ECG = electrocardiogram; PMNs = polymorphonuclear neutrophils; T_4 = thyroxine; TSH = thyroid-stimulating hormone.
*Total protein is considered low if it is less than 1 g/dl, moderate if it is 1–3 g/dl, and high if it is > 3 g/dl.

(1) If the result is greater than or equal to 1.1, portal hypertension is implicated (i.e., a hydrostatic etiology is responsible).

(2) If the value is less than 1.1, capillary permeability is probably abnormal (i.e., infection or malignancy may be implicated).

HOT

KEY

If portal hypertension is accompanied by another disorder that produces increased capillary permeability, the gradient will usually remain greater than or equal to 1.1. SBP usually occurs in patients with portal hypertension; therefore, the gradient is usually greater than or equal to 1.1 in these patients.

   c. Gram stain and **culture** of ascitic fluid should be performed if peritonitis is suspected.

   d. LDH and **glucose levels.** An elevated LDH or low glucose level may indicate tuberculosis or malignancy.

   e. Amylase and **triglyceride levels.** Elevated amylase or triglyceride levels may indicate pancreatic or chylous ascites, respectively.

D. Additional testing may be necessary when the ascitic fluid contains an elevated cell count with a lymphocyte predominance, increasing suspicion for tuberculous or malignant ascites.

   1. Purified protein derivative (PPD) test. A positive PPD test will increase suspicion for tuberculous peritonitis.

   2. Acid-fast bacillus stain and **culture of ascitic fluid.** These are relatively insensitive tests, but sending a large volume of fluid (e.g., 1 L) may increase the yield.

   3. Abdominal computed tomography may reveal an intraabdominal malignancy.

   4. Laparoscopy with **peritoneal biopsy** is often performed to make an expedient diagnosis.

 TREATMENT. The general management of ascites is discussed in Chapter 35; other specific therapies are tailored to the underlying etiology and will not be discussed here.

References

Runyon BA. Management of adult patients with ascites caused by cirrhosis. Hepatology 1998;27(1):264–272.

Wongcharatrawee S, Garcia-Tsao G. Clinical management of ascites and its complications. Clin Liver Dis 2001;5(3):833–850.

33. Acute Pancreatitis

I **INTRODUCTION.** **Pancreatitis implies inflammation of the pancreas.**

A. **Acute pancreatitis** results from the leakage of pancreatic enzymes into pancreatic tissue, leading to autodigestion. Because acute pancreatitis is more common than chronic pancreatitis, acute pancreatitis is the focus of this chapter.

B. **Chronic pancreatitis.** Causes are varied and ultimately lead to destruction of the pancreatic tissue. The process usually starts with multiple episodes of acute pancreatitis which subsequently leave the patient with a damaged pancreas.

II **CLINICAL MANIFESTATIONS OF ACUTE PANCREATITIS**

A. **Symptoms** usually include the abrupt onset of epigastric pain that lasts for hours to days and radiates to the back, nausea and vomiting, sweating, weakness, and anxiety. The patient typically feels better when sitting up and leaning forward.

B. **Physical examination findings**
   1. The patient may be febrile, tachycardic, tachypneic, and hypotensive.
   2. The skin of the periumbilical area may be discolored **(Cullen's sign),** or flank ecchymoses **(Turner's sign)** may be present.
   3. The abdomen is hypoactive with mild distention (because of ileus). Upper abdominal tenderness (usually without rebound or rigidity) is present.

C. **Laboratory findings**
   1. **Elevated serum amylase** and **lipase** are the hallmarks of acute pancreatitis.
   2. Other findings may include leukocytosis (12,000–15,000/mm^3), hypoalbuminemia, hyperglycemia, and elevated aspartate aminotransferase (AST, SGOT), alkaline phosphatase, and bilirubin.

III **CAUSES OF ACUTE PANCREATITIS.** There are numerous causes of pancreatitis. The simplest way to remember the most important of these causes is with the mnemonic, "BAD HITS." (HINT: If you move the "S" in front of the "H," the mnemonic will be easier to remember but more difficult to utter in public.)

Common Causes of Acute Pancreatitis ("BAD HITS")

Biliary stones
Alcohol abuse
Drugs

Hyperlipidemia or Hypercalcemia
Idiopathic or Infectious
Trauma
Surgery (post-ERCP or intraabdominal surgery) or Scorpion sting

A. **Biliary stones** are the most common cause of acute pancreatitis in suburban hospitals.
B. **Alcohol abuse** is the most common cause in urban hospitals.
C. **Drugs.** Many drugs can cause acute pancreatitis, including thiazide diuretics, sulfa antibiotics, pentamidine, and some antiretroviral agents.
D. **Hyperlipidemia (types I, IV, V).** Pancreatitis usually does not occur in hyperlipidemic patients until their serum triglyceride level exceeds 1000 mg/dl.
E. **Idiopathic causes.** In 15% of patients, no obvious cause of pancreatitis is identified; however, many authors implicate pancreas divisum (a congenital defect) as the cause.
F. **Infectious etiologies** include mumps, cytomegalovirus (CMV), human immunodeficiency virus (HIV), and infections caused by *Escherichia coli.*
G. **Trauma.** Blunt, rather than penetrating, trauma is most often responsible.
H. **Surgical.** Postsurgical pancreatitis occurs in 3% of patients undergoing endoscopic retrograde cholangiopancreatography (ERCP).
I. **Scorpion stings.** This cause is really only important to know for resident's report or on attending rounds.

IV **APPROACH TO THE PATIENT.** The diagnosis is based on finding elevated serum amylase or lipase levels in the context of an appropriate clinical setting. Imaging studies that may be helpful include abdominal ultrasound and computed tomography (CT). When a patient presents with pancreatitis, you should:

A. **Determine the cause** of the pancreatitis.
B. **Assess the severity** and **estimate the prognosis.** Because the serum amylase and lipase levels do not correlate with severity, **Ranson's criteria** are used to assess severity and prognosis.

1. Ranson's criteria are assessed at admission and during the initial 48 hours.

Ranson's Criteria at Admission ("WAGLS")

White blood cell (WBC) count > 16,000/mm³
Age > 55 years
Glucose > 200 mg/dl
Lactate dehydrogenase (LDH) > 350 U/L
Serum glutamate oxaloacetate transaminase (SGOT) > 250 U/L

Ranson's Criteria During the Initial 48 Hours ("**BaCH** wasn't an **SOB**")

Base deficit > 4 mEq/L
Calcium < 8 mg/dl
Hematocrit decrease > 10%
Sequestration of fluid > 6 L
Oxygen < 60 mm Hg
Blood urea nitrogen (BUN) increase of > 5 mg/dl

2. In general, as the number of criteria increases, so does the mortality rate.

V **TREATMENT** is primarily supportive and includes bowel rest, volume resuscitation, pain control, and management of respiratory distress and renal failure. Nasogastric tubes are used for gastric decompression in patients with persistent vomiting. If gallstones are thought to be the cause, endoscopic retrograde cholangiopancreatography (ERCP) may be indicated. Cholecystectomy should only be considered once the patient recovers from the acute episode.

VI **COMPLICATIONS**

A. Pancreatic abscess should be suspected when patients worsen after initial improvement. Radiology-guided drainage or surgical intervention is often necessary in this group of patients.
B. Pancreatic pseudocyst occurs in 10%-20% of patients and usually does not require specific treatment unless it has been pres-

ent for longer than 6 weeks, is greater than 5 cm in diameter, or is accompanied by significant symptoms.

C. Renal failure and **respiratory failure** are the two most common systemic complications.

References

Mergener K, Baillie J. Acute pancreatitis. BMJ 1998;316(7124):44–48.

Warshaw AL, Banks PA, Fernandez-Del Castillo C. AGA technical review: treatment of pain in chronic pancreatitis. Gastroenterology 1998;115(3):765–776.

34. Alcoholic Liver Disease

I INTRODUCTION

A. The amount of alcohol required to produce liver disease in a given patient is variable. Women appear to be more susceptible than men, but men are more often affected because of higher alcohol consumption rates.

B. Most authorities believe that a susceptible person must drink 60–80 g of alcohol per day for at least 10 years before developing cirrhosis. Many women, however, develop cirrhosis with much lower alcohol intake. Patients with additional liver disease (e.g., viral hepatitis, non-alcoholic liver disease) are more susceptible to alcoholic liver injury.

C. Alcohol contents of common beverages: 1) beer: 11.5 g in 12 oz (1 can), 2) wine: 11.5 g in 4 oz (1 glass), and 3) hard liquor: 10.3 g in 1 oz (1 shot).

D. There are three degrees of alcoholic liver disease. These three syndromes often overlap in a given patient.

   1. Fatty liver
   2. Alcoholic hepatitis
   3. Micronodular (Laënnec's) cirrhosis

HOT **KEY** Approximately all heavy drinkers (i.e., those who consume at least 60 g of alcohol per day) develop fatty liver, whereas less than one-third develop alcoholic hepatitis and less than 20% develop cirrhosis.

II CLINICAL MANIFESTATIONS OF ALCOHOLIC LIVER DISEASE.
Table 34-1 summarizes the clinical findings that accompany the various degrees of alcoholic liver disease.

III APPROACH TO THE PATIENT

A. Fatty liver is usually diagnosed in patients with a history of alcohol consumption accompanied by mildly abnormal liver function tests, hepatomegaly, or both. A definitive diagnosis may be made by biopsy but is rarely necessary. Other possible causes of fatty liver include obesity, diabetes, hyperlipidemia, steroids (endogenous or exogenous), starvation, parenteral nutrition, and toxins (e.g., carbon tetrachloride).

TABLE 34-1: Clinical Findings in Alcoholic Liver Disease

Syndrome	Symptoms	Signs	Laboratory Findings
Fatty liver	None	None, or possibly hepatomegaly with or without tenderness	AST mildly elevated
Alcoholic hepatitis	Subjective fever, right upper quadrant pain, nausea, vomiting	Fever, tender hepatomegaly, jaundice (common), splenomegaly, ascites, peripheral edema, encephalopathy (in severe cases)	AST: ALT ratio >2:1, with AST < 300 IU/L; elevated PT, alkaline phosphatase* and bilirubin levels; low hematocrit, platelet count, and albumin
Cirrhosis	Anorexia, weight changes, jaundice, variceal bleeding, encephalopathy	Jaundice, liver size is variable (but usually small), ascites, splenomegaly, palmar erythema, spider angiomas, testicular atrophy, gynecomastia, Dupuytren's contractures, asterixis, altered mental status	Same as for alcoholic hepatitis; prerenal azotemia may also be seen

ALT = alanine aminotransferase; AST = aspartate aminotransferase; PT = prothrombin time.
*But usually less than 3 times normal.

B. Alcoholic hepatitis can be very mild or life-threatening. The patient often presents with the signs and symptoms summarized in Table 34-1 after a "drinking binge"; often the onset of symptoms coincides with the cessation of drinking (patients quit drinking because they feel so poorly). Although alcoholic hepatitis is a common disease in alcoholics, other diseases (e.g., cholecystitis and cholelithiasis) may mimic alcoholic hepatitis quite closely. To avoid missing other pathologies, have a low threshold for getting an abdominal ultrasound in an alcoholic patient with right upper quadrant pain. In addition, alcoholic patients who come in with significantly elevated transaminase levels have something in addition to alcohol-related disease (e.g., acetaminophen toxicity, viral infection).

C. Cirrhosis. Alcoholism is one of the most common causes of cirrhosis in the United States. The diagnosis is usually obvious clinically once the patient develops decompensated liver disease (see Table 34-1). It is important to evaluate the alcoholic patient for other common causes of liver disease. Many patients who develop chronic alcoholic liver disease also have other disease affecting the liver (e.g., hepatitis C).

IV TREATMENT

A. Fatty liver. Abstinence is the mainstay of therapy. **Exercise** and **nutritional counseling** are advisable for patients with obesity, diabetes, or hyperlipidemia.

B. Alcoholic hepatitis. The long-term prognosis depends on liver function and the patient's ability to abstain from consuming alcohol.

    1. Supportive therapy includes correction of fluid and electrolyte status and observation for alcohol withdrawal, seizures, and delirium tremens. Patients with alcoholic hepatitis are often significantly malnourished and need aggressive vitamin, mineral, and calorie supplementation.

    2. Steroid therapy may benefit some patients with extensive liver dysfunction.

C. Cirrhosis. Abstinence is critical to prevent worsening of liver function.

HOT KEY

Many patients with alcohol-related liver disease have the potential for dramatic improvement in liver function with abstinence from alcohol and supportive care. It is not uncommon for patients with alcoholic hepatitis and ascites (or even encephalopathy) to have complete clinical resolution with long-term abstinence.

References

Hill DB, Kugelmas M. Alcoholic liver disease. Treatment strategies for the potentially reversible stages. Postgrad Med 1998;103(4):261–268.

Menon KV, Gores GJ, Shah VH. Pathogenesis, diagnosis, and treatment of alcoholic liver disease. Mayo Clin Proc 2001;76(10):1021–1029.

35. Liver Failure

I INTRODUCTION

A. Acute liver failure is defined by the presence of **encephalopathy** and **coagulopathy associated with acute hepatic disease.** It is often classified as fulminant or subfulminant, depending on whether it develops within 2 months of, or as many as 6 months after, the onset of illness.

B. Chronic liver failure occurs over a longer period. It is characterized by evidence of hepatic synthetic dysfunction and clinical signs such as ascites, encephalopathy, and muscle wasting.

II CLINICAL MANIFESTATIONS OF LIVER FAILURE

A. Acute liver failure is characterized by the rapid development of nonspecific symptoms (e.g., nausea, malaise), jaundice, and altered mental status, usually in a previously healthy patient.

   1. Central nervous system (CNS) signs

   a. Altered mental status. Encephalopathy produces an alteration in mental status that ranges from mild obtundation (grade I or II encephalopathy) to stupor or coma (grade III or IV encephalopathy). Patients may also present with agitation and delusions, which are uncommon in chronic liver failure. Unlike chronic liver disease, acute liver failure may not be clinically obvious; it is therefore important to consider hepatic failure in all patients with altered mental status.

   b. Asterixis is frequently noted on examination.

   c. Cerebral edema accompanies hepatic encephalopathy in the majority of acute liver failure patients with grade IV encephalopathy (coma). Significant cerebral edema can lead to brain herniation and is a common cause of death in patients with acute liver failure. **Cushing's reflex (hypertension and bradycardia), abnormal pupillary reflexes,** and **increased muscle tone progressing to decerebrate posturing** are signs of increasing **cerebral edema.** Cerebral edema occurs more commonly with fulminant liver failure, whereas renal failure and ascites are more often associated with a subfulminant course.

   2. Hematologic signs. Elevation of the prothrombin time (PT) is universally present and may be accompanied by an elevated partial thromboplastin time (PTT). Thrombocytopenia may also occur.

199

3. **Cardiovascular signs** may include hypovolemia, a decrease in systemic vascular resistance associated with hypotension, and an increase in cardiac output. Because these findings may also indicate sepsis, infection should be considered and ruled out.

4. **Metabolic changes**

   a. **Hypoglycemia** may aggravate the alteration in mental status. Patients with profound liver injury can develop refractory hypoglycemia. Blood glucose levels should be monitored frequently.

   b. **Hypokalemia** can result from respiratory alkalosis induced by liver failure.

   c. **Hyponatremia** and **hypophosphatemia** may also occur.

5. **Complications**

   a. **Hemorrhage.** Thrombocytopenia is a strong risk factor for gastrointestinal or other bleeding.

   b. **Infections.** Defects in neutrophil function as well as humoral and cell-mediated immunity may result in bacterial or fungal infections. Early use of broad-spectrum antibiotics are encouraged in patients with acute liver failure who have evidence of infection.

   c. **Renal failure** is an ominous complication.

      (1) **Hepatorenal syndrome** should be considered in patients with severe liver disease, declining renal function, and prerenal physiology (i.e., a low urinary sodium level). Hepatorenal syndrome is distinguished from hypovolemia by the patient's failure to respond to a fluid challenge. Hepatorenal syndrome must also be distinguished (on the basis of clinical criteria) from other causes of kidney failure that result in prerenal physiology (see Chapter 37).

      (2) **Acute tubular necrosis** may also occur.

   d. **Hepatopulmonary syndrome.** Intrapulmonary shunting of blood leads to hypoxia. Typically, patients are more symptomatic when they are sitting up, as opposed to lying down (i.e., they are platypneic), because sitting up increases blood flow to the lower lobes where more shunting is known to occur. This complication is most commonly seen in chronic liver failure.

B. **Chronic liver failure.** Clinical manifestations of chronic liver failure are summarized in Table 34-1.

III CAUSES OF LIVER FAILURE

A. **Acute liver failure**

1. **Infection**

   a. **Viral hepatitis** is one of the most common causes of acute liver failure (along with acetaminophen toxicity).

(1) Hepatitis A is a rare cause of fulminant hepatitis and never produces chronic disease.

(2) Hepatitis B causes fulminant liver failure in approximately 1% of infected patients.

(3) Hepatitis C usually causes only chronic disease but at a high rate (greater than 70%).

(4) Hepatitis D causes coinfection or superinfection only in the presence of hepatitis B surface antigen (HBsAg) and may account for more than 50% of cases of fulminant disease caused by hepatitis B.

(5) Hepatitis E is endemic in Mexico and parts of Asia; the mortality rate is high among pregnant women.

(6) Epstein-Barr virus, cytomegalovirus (CMV), and **herpesvirus** occasionally cause acute liver failure.

2. **Drugs and toxins**
   a. **Drugs**
      (1) Direct hepatotoxicity
         (a) Acetaminophen overdose. Alcoholics and malnourished patients have a higher risk of hepatotoxicity as a result of acetaminophen overdose.

HOT KEY

Remember the **"rule of 140s"** when confronted with the possibility of acetaminophen overdose: the approximate toxic dose is 140 mg/kg, a blood level that exceeds 140 μg/ml 4 hours after ingestion may be toxic, and the first dose of acetylcysteine (the antidote) is 140 mg/kg orally or by nasogastric tube (often followed by 70 mg/kg every 4 hours for 17 doses).

         (b) Heavy metals, phosphorus, vitamin A, valproic acid, and **tetracyclines** may also be directly hepatotoxic.
      (2) Idiosyncratic reactions may also result in acute liver failure. **Isoniazid, halothane, phenytoin,** and **sulfonamides** are some examples of drugs that can cause idiosyncratic hepatotoxicity.
   b. **Toxins.** *Amanita phalloides* (the death-cap mushroom) and **carbon tetrachloride** (found in industrial cleaning solvents) can both produce acute liver failure.
3. **Vascular abnormalities**
   a. **Inadequate arterial supply,** as a result of cardiac pathology (e.g., cardiac arrest, myocardial infarction, cardiomyopathy), infiltrating malignancies, or sepsis, may cause liver failure.

    b. Venous obstruction
       (1) Veno-occlusive disease. Intrahepatic obstruction of
       the hepatic venules may be associated with bone mar-
       row transplantation, chemotherapy, or oral contra-
       ceptive use.
       (2) Inferior vena cava obstruction or **hepatic vein ob-**
       struction (i.e., **Budd-Chiari syndrome**) often results
       from thrombosis associated with a myeloproliferative
       disorder or hypercoagulable state or from direct tu-
       mor invasion.
  4. Inherited metabolic disorders. Wilson's disease usually pre-
    sents in younger patients (20–40 years of age) and may result
    in acute or chronic liver failure.
  5. Miscellaneous causes
    a. Pregnancy. Both acute **fatty liver** and the **HELLP (He-**
    molysis, Elevated Liver enzymes, Low Platelets) **syn-**
    drome may complicate pregnancy.
    b. Reye's syndrome. Children younger than 15 years may
    develop Reye's syndrome, which is usually associated
    with viral illness and concomitant salicylate use.
B. Chronic liver failure
  1. Infections, including **viral hepatitis** (primarily hepatitis B
    and C), **schistosomiasis,** and **toxoplasmosis**
  2. Drugs and **toxins. Alcoholism** accounts for almost 50% of all
    cases of chronic liver failure.
  3. Vascular abnormalities (e.g., as a result of cardiac failure, tu-
    mors, or venous obstruction)
  4. Inherited metabolic disorders, including Wilson's disease,
    hemochromatosis, α_1-antitrypsin deficiency, and glycogen
    storage disease
  5. Miscellaneous causes
    a. Primary biliary cirrhosis. Women between the ages of 40
    and 60 years are most often affected. Pruritus, signifi-
    cantly elevated serum alkaline phosphatase, and the pres-
    ence of antimitochondrial antibody are typical features
    (antimitochondrial antibody is noted in 95% of cases).
    b. Secondary biliary cirrhosis may result from stones or stric-
    tures causing chronic biliary tract obstruction.
    c. Autoimmune hepatitis is most common in young women.
    Patients may have other manifestations of autoimmunity;
    antinuclear and anti-smooth muscle antibodies are found
    in 20%-40% and 60%-80% of patients, respectively.

IV APPROACH TO THE PATIENT

A. Patient history. A thorough history is critical if a drug or toxin
exposure is thought to be the cause of the liver failure. Vascu-

lar disorders may also be suggested by the history (e.g., right upper quadrant pain may imply Budd-Chiari syndrome; weight loss may suggest an intraabdominal malignancy).

B. Laboratory tests

1. General tests. The following tests are usually performed to evaluate liver function and screen for associated metabolic or hematologic derangements and complications (e.g., bleeding, infection, or renal failure):

   a. Complete blood count (CBC) with differential and platelets

   b. Electrolyte panel with blood urea nitrogen (BUN), creatinine, and glucose levels

   c. Evaluation of PT and PTT

   d. Liver tests [i.e., aspartate aminotransferase (AST), alanine aminotransferase (ALT), alkaline phosphatase, total bilirubin]

2. Specific tests can be used to help determine the etiology.

   a. Hepatitis serologies, including hepatitis A and C antibodies, HBsAg, and hepatitis B surface and core antibodies are often ordered.

   b. Acetaminophen level. An acetaminophen level should be obtained in all patients with signs of acute liver failure. A **salicylate level** and **toxicology screen** are also commonly performed.

   c. Serum ceruloplasmin. Wilson's disease should be considered in patients younger than 50 years who have acute or chronic liver failure. A low serum ceruloplasmin level is a sign of Wilson's disease; other findings include a high urinary copper level or the presence of Kayser-Fleischer rings on slit-lamp examination.

   d. Transferrin saturation and **ferritin levels** are high in patients with hemochromatosis, a cause of chronic liver failure. These levels may be artificially elevated in acute liver injury; they respond as acute phase reactants.

   e. α_1-Antitrypsin level. Deficiency may result in chronic liver failure.

   f. Antibody tests. Antinuclear, anti-smooth muscle, and antimitochondrial antibodies may be studied to evaluate the possibility of autoimmune hepatitis or primary biliary cirrhosis.

C. Liver biopsy or **imaging studies** may be performed when the diagnosis is still in question.

 TREATMENT

A. Identify and treat any treatable causes

1. Acute liver failure

   a. Acetaminophen overdose can be treated with N-acetylcysteine. Early treatment is desirable, and empiric therapy may be indicated when a toxic dose is suspected. Patients may benefit even when the ingestion occurred as many as 36 hours before therapy.

b. Mushroom poisoning may be treated with penicillin, silybin, or both.

c. Pregnancy-related liver failure is often resolved by delivering the baby.

2. Chronic liver failure. Regardless of etiology, chronic liver failure is usually not reversible. If administered early in the course of the disease, however, specific treatments may prevent the progression to chronic liver failure. For example:

a. Hemochromatosis may be treated with phlebotomy or deferoxamine chelation therapy.

b. Wilson's disease may be treated with penicillamine chelation therapy.

c. Autoimmune hepatitis is extremely sensitive to steroid therapy.

d. Chronic hepatitis B or **C** may be treated with anti-viral therapy.

B. Prevent or **treat complications**

1. Infections, such as **spontaneous bacterial peritonitis (SBP),** must be treated aggressively. **A third-generation cephalosporin** is often the initial therapy and is administered for at least 5 days. Following therapy, **norfloxacin** may be used to decrease the rate of recurrent spontaneous bacterial peritonitis. Every attempt should be made to avoid potentially nephrotoxic drugs such as gentamicin in patients with liver disease.

2. Hemorrhage

a. Patients who are not actively bleeding are usually administered **vitamin K** subcutaneously in case vitamin deficiency is partially responsible for the coagulopathy.

b. Fresh frozen plasma and blood products may be required for patients with active bleeding (see Chapter 66).

3. Bleeding esophageal varices

a. Treatment

(1) Pharmacologic treatment involves the intravenous administration of **octreotide** or **vasopressin plus nitroglycerin.** Octreotide is currently the standard of care.

(2) Injection sclerotherapy and **band ligation** are effective procedures but may not be technically feasible in all patients.

(3) Transjugular intrahepatic portosystemic shunting (TIPS) or **surgical shunting** may be used for refractory bleeding.

b. Prophylaxis. Propranolol (20–80 mg orally twice daily) is often given to patients who are stable after a variceal bleed (usually days later) and to those with very large varices.

4. **Ascites** and **edema** are often treated with a **sodium-restricted diet** and **diuretics.**

   a. The primary method of treating ascites in patients with chronic liver disease is sodium restriction. Patients should ingest less than 2 g of sodium per day. Fluid does not need to be limited except in patients with significant hyponatremia. (Up to 20% of patients with ascites can be completely controlled with sodium restriction alone.)

   b. Spironolactone. The initial dose is often 50–100 mg orally once daily; this amount is increased by 100 mg/day every few days while following the serum and urine electrolytes. Reversal of the normal urinary sodium and potassium concentrations (i.e., urinary sodium exceeds urinary potassium) indicates an aldosterone antagonist effect and should prompt frequent evaluations for hyperkalemia. Spironolactone will take several days before maximal benefit occurs.

   c. Furosemide may also be added to the regimen to increase diuresis. Careful monitoring of volume status and electrolytes is always required.

   d. Large-volume paracentesis is often necessary for patients with massive ascites whose conditions are refractory to medical therapy or are symptomatic (80% of patient with ascites can be controlled with sodium restriction and diuretics alone). Intravenous albumin is often given just before large-volume paracentesis is performed to maintain the intravascular volume (especially in patients without peripheral edema).

   e. TIPS is being increasingly used for patients with refractory ascites.

5. **Hepatic encephalopathy** may be precipitated by infections, overly aggressive diuresis, electrolyte abnormalities, gastrointestinal bleeding, or drugs (e.g., sedative-hypnotics, narcotics). Management usually involves treating precipitating factors and administering **lactulose** (often 30 ml orally three times daily or by nasogastric tube, titrated to maintain three loose stools per day). In patients with acute liver failure, cerebral edema may occur and can be treated with **mannitol** (usually 0.3–0.4 g/kg body weight) or hyperventilation.

HOT KEY Intracerebral hemorrhage is always a possibility in patients with coagulopathy and altered mental status and may require further evaluation [e.g., with computed tomography (CT)].

6. **Hepatorenal syndrome.** No therapy has been shown to have a consistent benefit; renal vasodilators, including low-dose dopamine and calcium channel blockers, are still sometimes tried.

7. **Metabolic derangements**
   a. **Hypoglycemia** may require intravenous administration of a 10% glucose solution.
   b. **Hypokalemia** and **hypophosphatemia** may require electrolyte replacement.
   c. **Hyponatremia** may require free water restriction.

C. **Consider the appropriateness of liver transplantation.** Liver transplantation may be performed in patients with acute or chronic liver failure.
   1. In the acute setting, liver transplantation is usually indicated when a variety of prognostic factors (e.g., PT, grade of encephalopathy, etiology) suggest a poor chance of survival without it. Because safe transport to a specialized facility is easier when patients have low-grade encephalopathy, a liver transplant should be considered as soon as possible following a diagnosis of acute liver failure.
   2. The 5-year survival rate after liver transplantation may be as high as 60%-80%.

References

Gill RQ, Sterling RK. Acute liver failure. J Clin Gastroenterol 2001;33(3):191–198.
Lee WM. Acute liver failure. N Engl J Med 1993;329(25):1862–1872.
Riordan SM, Williams R. Treatment of hepatic encephalopathy. N Engl J Med 1997; 337(7):473–479.

PART V

RENAL/ACID-BASE

36. Overview of Nephrology

I INTRODUCTION

A. In nephrology, there are many syndromes, each with a set of causative diseases. Specific diseases are often capable of causing more than one syndrome.

 HOT KEY

In medicine, a "syndrome" refers to a set of clinical manifestations occurring together.

B. Know the clinical manifestations and lab data that correspond to each renal syndrome and then think of the diseases that could cause that syndrome. The differential diagnoses for most of the renal syndromes are easy to remember; just match the diagnosis with the patient's complaints and data and you'll be off to the right start.

II RENAL SYNDROMES. The renal syndromes are discussed in more detail in Chapters 37–40. Table 36-1 provides an overview.

References
Haugh M, Fouque D. Evidence-based nephrology. Nephrol Dial Transplant 1999; (Suppl 14)3:38–41.
Tomson CR. Recent advances: nephrology. BMJ 2000;320(7227):98–101.

TABLE 36-1: Overview of Renal Syndromes

Syndrome	Key to the Diagnosis	Examples of Causes
Acute renal failure	Classify the cause as pre-, post-, or intrarenal	Dehydration, shock, toxins, interstitial nephritis, obstruction due to enlarged prostate, HUS/TTP
Nephrotic syndrome	Classify the cause as renal or systemic	Primary renal diseases (e.g., membranous glomerulonephritis); systemic diseases (e.g., diabetes, amyloid, SLE)
Nephritic syndrome	Classify the cause as normocomplementemic or hypocomplementemic	MPGN, RPGN, various infections (e.g., post-steptococcal), SLE, vasculitis
Renal tubular acidosis	Classify the acidosis as type 1, 2, or 4	Amyloid, multiple myeloma, drugs (e.g., ampho-tericin), diabetes, Addison's disease

HUS/TTP= hemolytic-uremic syndrome/thrombotic thrombocytopenic purpura; MPGN = membranoproliferative glomerulonephritis; RPGN = rapidly progressive glomerulonephritis; SLE = systemic lupus erythematosus.

37. Acute Renal Failure

I Introduction

A. Definition. Acute renal failure is defined as a rapid decrease in glomerular filtration that results in abnormal fluid and electrolyte balance and inappropriate nitrogen waste accumulation (azotemia). Because nitrogen accumulation is initially asymptomatic, the diagnosis is commonly made when the serum creatinine level rises abruptly (e.g., by 0.5 mg/dl or more) during a 24-hour period.

> **HOT**
>
> **KEY**
>
> Although serum creatinine (SCr) is almost solely filtered and therefore provides a good estimate of the glomerular filtration rate (GFR), it is actually slightly secreted. Some drugs (e.g., cimetidine) can block this secretion, raise the SCr, and cause an underestimation of the actual GFR and, therefore, renal function.

B. Epidemiology. Approximately 5% of all hospitalized patients are diagnosed with acute renal failure; the incidence can be as high as 30% in the intensive care unit (ICU).

C. Clinical manifestations. Symptoms of acute renal failure are usually present when the **blood urea nitrogen (BUN) exceeds 100 mg/dl,** but may occur at lesser values. Clinical manifestations include **cardiovascular complications** (e.g., arrhythmias, volume overload, pericarditis), **neurologic abnormalities** (e.g., altered mental status, seizures), or **gastrointestinal complications** (e.g., bleeding, nausea, vomiting).

II CAUSES OF ACUTE RENAL FAILURE. The causes of

acute renal failure can be conveniently classified as **prerenal, intrinsic renal**, or **postrenal** failure (Figure 37–1).

A. Prerenal causes account for more than half of acute renal failure cases. Prerenal is actually preglomerular. Any disease state that results in a **decrease in blood flow to the glomerulus** will result in decreased glomerular filtration and, consequently, an elevated serum creatinine level. One way to remember the prerenal causes of acute renal failure is to begin with the filling of the left ventricle and work your way distally toward the glomerulus.

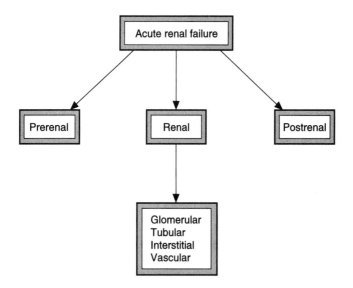

FIGURE 37-1. The causes of acute renal failure can be categorized as prerenal, intrinsic renal, or postrenal.

1. **Decreased filling of the left ventricle** results in decreased cardiac output and, therefore, decreased flow to the glomerulus. **Hypovolemia** is the most common cause, but right ventricular failure and mitral stenosis can also result in poor left ventricular filling and subsequent prerenal azotemia.
2. **Decreased left ventricular function** results in decreased cardiac output even with normal or elevated left ventricular filling.
3. **Aortic stenosis.** Even with normal left ventricular filling and function, critical aortic stenosis can block forward flow to the kidney.
4. **Renal artery stenosis** from fibromuscular dysplasia or atherosclerotic disease decreases flow to the glomerulus. (Fibromuscular dysplasia, most often seen in young women, is much less common than atherosclerotic disease.)
5. **Narrowing of the afferent arteriole** from vasoconstriction, inflammation, or thrombosis can result in prerenal azotemia.
   a. **Sepsis** can lead to constriction of the afferent arteriole via inflammatory mediators.
   b. **Nonsteroidal anti-inflammatory drugs (NSAIDs)** can lead to narrowing of the afferent arteriole by inhibiting prosta-

glandins, which normally dilate the vessel. This most often occurs in states of volume depletion.
  c. **Contrast dye** can also lead to constriction of the afferent arteriole and cause a prerenal picture.
  d. **Microangiopathic hemolytic anemias** (see Chapter 62) are rare causes of a prerenal azotemia.
  e. **Hepatorenal syndrome,** through unclear mechanisms, shunts blood away from the afferent arteriole, causing prerenal azotemia.
B. **Postrenal causes** account for approximately 5–10% of all cases of acute renal failure. Because one kidney can adequately compensate for the other, renal failure will only occur if both kidneys are not functioning properly.
  1. **Bladder neck obstruction** is the most common postrenal cause of acute renal failure. Common causes of bladder neck obstruction include:
    a. **Prostatic hypertrophy** or **malignancy**
    b. **Neurologic disorders** (e.g., neuropathy)
    c. **Anticholinergic medications**
  2. **Ureteral obstruction**
    a. **Unilateral ureteral obstruction** (e.g., from stones, blood clots, or pus) can result in acute renal failure in a patient with only one kidney.
    b. **Bilateral ureteral obstruction** may result from retroperitoneal fibrosis, malignancy, or lymphadenopathy.
C. **Intrinsic renal causes.** Think of the causes as anatomic components of a kidney (i.e., glomeruli, tubules, interstitium, vessels).
  1. **Acute glomerulonephritis** affects the glomeruli. The many causes of acute glomerulonephritis are discussed in Chapter 39 II.
  2. **Acute tubular necrosis (ATN)** affects the tubules.
    a. **Ischemia** and **shock** from all causes, but particularly septic shock, can lead to ATN.
    b. **Contrast dye agents** used for radiographic studies are toxic to the tubules, but most commonly result in renal failure in patients with underlying renal disease (particularly diabetic patients).
    c. **Endogenous pigments** (e.g., **myoglobin, hemoglobin**), **crystals,** and **proteins.** Myoglobinuria (from rhabdomyolysis) or hemoglobinuria (from intravascular hemolysis), uric acid deposition (from tumor lysis), and Bence Jones proteins (from multiple myeloma) can all cause tubule injury and result in ATN.
    d. **Medications** (e.g., aminoglycosides) and **toxins** (e.g., heavy metals) can be directly nephrotoxic.
    e. **Surgery** or **trauma.** Ischemic injury (as a result of hypoten-

sion and inflammatory mediators), tissue destruction (from myoglobin), or a combination of the two can lead to ATN.

HOT KEY The most common causes of ATN are sepsis, contrast dye agents, and nephrotoxic drugs.

3. **Acute interstitial nephritis** affects the interstitium. **Medications** (e.g., β-lactam antibiotics, sulfa antibiotics, furosemide, thiazide diuretics, NSAIDs) are the most common causes of acute interstitial nephritis.
4. **Vasculitis** and **microangiopathic hemolytic anemias** affect the blood vessels (see Chapters 62 and 76). Do not be confused by the fact that many of the vasculitides are listed as causes of glomerulonephritis (i.e., inflammation of the glomerulus); because the glomerulus contains a capillary bed, vasculitis can result in glomerulonephritis.

 APPROACH TO THE PATIENT. Using data gleaned from the patient history, physical examination, and basic laboratory tests and procedures, the cause is classified as primarily prerenal, postrenal, or renal.

HOT KEY The same disorder may cause more than one type of acute renal failure.

A. **Obtain a patient history**
1. **Prerenal.** A history of congestive heart failure (CHF), dehydration, or of new or increased use of diuretics or NSAIDs often signifies a prerenal etiology.
2. **Postrenal.** A history of benign prostatic hypertrophy, kidney stones, nephrectomy, anticholinergic medication use, or a retroperitoneal malignancy may alert you to postrenal causes.
3. **Renal**
   a. **Glomerulonephritis.** The causes of glomerulonephritis can help guide your questions regarding relevant symptoms. For example, a recent sore throat or skin infection may suggest postinfectious glomerulonephritis.
   b. **ATN** or **acute interstitial nephritis.** The medication history (including use of over-the-counter NSAIDs) may suggest a tubular or interstitial etiology.

    c. Vasculitis. Ask about rashes, arthralgias, and fevers (see Chapter 76).

B. Perform a physical examination. Always assess the vital signs, oxygen saturation, and urine output.

    1. Blood pressure. Hypotension often denotes a prerenal cause; **hypertension** may be a sign of glomerulonephritis. Additional evaluation and treatment are aimed at the underlying etiology.

    2. Temperature. High or **low temperatures** often indicate sepsis (although interstitial nephritis, glomerulonephritis, or vasculitis may also be associated with temperature abnormalities).

    3. Oxygen saturation. Hypoxemia may signal impending pulmonary edema (e.g., from renal failure with volume overload).

    4. Urine output measurements will help you classify the renal failure as **oliguric (< 400 ml/day)** or **nonoliguric (> 400 ml/day).** Nonoliguric renal failure is associated with lower mortality and dialysis rates. In patients with oliguric ATN, increased urine output heralds the return of renal function.

    5. Heart and lung examination. A complete physical examination is important, with special attention given to the heart and lungs. Heart and lung examination may provide information about the cause of the acute renal failure (e.g., critical aortic stenosis, severe left ventricular dysfunction) and also permits assessment of some of the consequences of the renal failure (e.g., volume overload, pericarditis).

    6. Auscultation. Renal bruits may indicate renal artery obstruction.

    7. Palpation. Increased bladder size and tenderness often signify postrenal obstruction.

C. Rule out obstruction

    1. Postvoid residual (PVR). A PVR is often performed before laboratory tests because if obstruction is the cause, a diagnosis can be made quickly and an extensive workup is avoided. This procedure is especially useful in older men, in whom obstruction from benign prostatic hypertrophy is not uncommon. The PVR is measured by catheterization after the patient has "emptied" the bladder.

        a. If the PVR is greater than 200–250 ml, obstruction is diagnosed and a Foley catheter should be left in place.

        b. If the patient already has an indwelling catheter, make sure to flush the catheter to evaluate obstruction by encrusted materials or blood clots.

    2. Ultrasound. The PVR does not help you evaluate the upper urinary tract. In patients with one kidney or suspected bilateral obstruction, renal ultrasound should be performed early in the workup. Occasionally, a computed tomography (CT) scan will be performed first depending on the patient's history.

D. Perform laboratory studies to help determine the diagnosis and the consequences of the renal failure.

1. **Complete blood count (CBC) with platelets.** The white blood cell (WBC) count helps assess the possibility of infection or interstitial nephritis. Anemia may indicate more chronic renal failure or bleeding from uremia.

2. **Electrolyte panel** (including Na^+, K^+, Cl^-, HCO^-_3, Ca^{2+}, PO_4, Mg^{2+}, and glucose). Common electrolyte or metabolic derangements include hyponatremia, hyperkalemia, hypocalcemia, hyperphosphatemia, and hypermagnesemia as well as a mixed anion and non-anion gap acidosis.

3. **Blood urea nitrogen:creatinine (BUN:Cr) ratio.** A normal BUN:Cr ratio is 10. In prenal states, urea gets reabsorbed from the proximal tubules while creatinine does not; therefore, a BUN:Cr ratio higher than 10 (and certainly one greater than 20) supports a prerenal diagnosis.

4. **Urinalysis.** A urinalysis is an essential part of the evaluation because an active urinary sediment implies an intraparenchymal cause of renal failure.

   a. **Red blood cell (RBC) casts** or **dysmorphic red cells** often imply glomerulonephritis or vasculitis.

   b. **WBC casts** are usually a sign of infection (i.e., pyelonephritis) or inflammation (i.e., interstitial nephritis).

   c. **Coarse granular** or **"muddy" brown casts** may signify ATN.

5. **Urine electrolytes** are a useful diagnostic test in patients with acute renal failure.

   a. **Urinary sodium** and **chloride** can be used to help delineate a prerenal cause from an intrarenal one. Values less than 20 mEq/L imply a prerenal etiology; values lower than 10 mEq/L are even more specific.

      (1) Early obstruction and contrast dye nephropathy can also result in a low urine sodium or chloride level.

      (2) With a concomitant metabolic alkalosis, the urinary chloride is a better indicator of a prerenal state because sodium may be excreted with bicarbonate to maintain electroneutrality. In this situation, the urinary sodium may be falsely increased, although prerenal physiology is present.

   b. **Fractional excretion of sodium (FENa).** FENa is another way of diagnosing prerenal physiology and can also help evaluate tubulointerstitial dysfunction. To calculate the FENa, remember "UP . . . UP" with "sodium over creatinine":

$$FENa = \frac{\text{Urine Na}^+/\text{Plasma NA}^+}{\text{Urine Cr}/\text{Plasma Cr}} \times 100\%$$

Normal values are between 1% and 3%, depending on the amount of sodium ingested.

(1) A value less than 1% usually signifies prerenal physiology, whereas one greater than 3% usually indicates tubulointerstitial disease (because there is a defect in sodium reabsorption).

HOT KEY

Glomerulonephritis without tubular dysfunction will not produce an abnormal FENa, because sodium reabsorption is primarily a renal tubular function.

(2) A normal value provides no evidence of these entities but does not rule them out either (i.e., there may be a mixed disorder).

HOT KEY

Patients receiving diuretics may have an increased FENa despite being prerenal; on the other hand, a patient taking diuretics with a FENa less than 1% usually can be assumed to be severely volume depleted.

6. **Creatine kinase.** Evaluation of the creatine kinase level is helpful **if the urine dipstick is positive for blood, but no or few RBCs** are noted microscopically. This implies that urinary myoglobin (from **rhabdomyolysis**) or hemoglobin (from **intravascular hemolysis**) is present. **Evaluate the possibility of rhabdomyolysis first;** then consider working up intravascular hemolysis. Creatine kinase levels **greater than 6000 IU** (and often more than 15,000 IU) are usually needed to cause tubular necrosis; however, creatine kinase levels may be normal if the rhabdomyolysis and ATN occurred a few days before the workup.

7. **Ancillary tests.** If glomerulonephritis or vasculitis is suspected or diagnosed, additional tests need to be ordered (see Chapters 39 and 76). Liver function tests are ordered when the hepatorenal syndrome is suspected, but the clinical diagnosis is usually obvious.

E. **Perform additional diagnostic studies** if the diagnosis remains unclear.

1. **Renal ultrasound.** In addition to ruling out **obstruction,** renal ultrasound helps to **distinguish acute from chronic renal failure.**
   a. The kidneys are usually normal in size in patients with acute renal failure.
   b. They are **usually small in patients with chronic renal failure.** It is easy to remember the chronic diseases that lead to enlarged kidneys because the SHAPE is large:

Chronic Diseases that Lead to Enlarged Kidneys ("SHAPE")

Scleroderma
HIV-associated nephropathy
Amyloidosis/infiltrative diseases
Polycystic kidney disease
Endocrinopathy (i.e., diabetes mellitus)

---

2. **Renal biopsy** is usually unnecessary but is indicated for unresolving acute renal failure of unknown etiology or to define the need for potentially toxic treatment of glomerulonephritis.

IV TREATMENT

A. **Disease-specific**
   1. **Prerenal causes**
      a. **Fluids** are usually indicated because hypovolemia is the predominant prerenal cause of acute renal failure.

HOT KEY

Remember—if the cause of acute renal failure is cardiac in origin (e.g., CHF, critical aortic stenosis), giving fluids may not be appropriate. Consider these possibilities before giving fluids!

---

   (1) Administration of **small, defined boluses** (e.g., 250 ml of 0.9% saline) can prevent volume overload.
   (2) **Reevaluate the patient frequently.** The goal urine output is at least 30 ml/hour. Boluses can be continued with that goal in mind as long as the oxygen saturation is maintained and the lungs remain clear (i.e., there is no evidence of pulmonary edema).
      b. **Other treatments** tailored to the specific etiology may also be necessary (e.g., discontinuing medications, administering antibiotics for sepsis).

2. Postrenal causes
a. Catheterization. A Foley catheter should be placed, if one has not been placed already.
   (1) Clamp the catheter if more than 750 cc drains acutely to prevent the patient from becoming hypotensive. If, after 30 minutes, no hypotension develops, you can allow more drainage while monitoring blood pressure.
   (2) Observe for postobstructive diuresis. If the blockage has been present for a few days, a postobstructive diuresis often ensues. This may result from urea accumulation with an osmotic diuresis as well as salt accumulation with a physiologic diuresis. Although this diuresis is partly a physiologic phenomenon, transient tubular dysfunction can contribute to severe volume depletion unless fluids are replaced.
      (a) Fluid replacement. It is customary to give back approximately two-thirds of the urinary losses with half normal saline. Giving normal saline will only exacerbate the problem by adding to the volume overload.
      (b) Electrolyte replacement. Depletion of electrolytes, particularly potassium and magnesium, occurs frequently.
b. Percutaneous drainage through a percutaneous nephrostomy tube may be needed in cases of upper tract obstruction.
3. Renal causes are treated based on the specific pathology, but there are general treatments that are common to all.
a. General measures
   (1) Fluid restriction. Fluids may need to be restricted to 1 L/day. Volume status should be monitored using daily weights and input/output measurements.
   (2) Diet. The diet should be low-salt, low-potassium, and low-phosphorous.
   (3) Adjust medication dosages. The dosages of medications that are excreted renally should be adjusted. Magnesium- and phosphorous-containing medications should be avoided.
b. Specific measures
   (1) Glomerulonephritis. Treatment is discussed in Chapter 39.
   (2) ATN
      (a) Fluids may help prevent oliguric renal failure (by "washing out" tubular casts that may precipitate in the nephron) and may also dilute the effects of certain toxins (i.e., myoglobin, contrast dye).
      (b) Furosemide in high doses is sometimes successful in converting oliguric to nonoliguric renal failure;

however, maintaining volume status and appropriate renal blood flow is critical, and the patient should never be "on the dry side."

(c) Mannitol is an antioxidant and osmotic diuretic. It may precipitate CHF, however, and should be avoided in susceptible patients.

(3) Acute interstitial nephritis is usually treated by discontinuing offending medications and administering fluids as tolerated. A short course of corticosteroids (1 week with a rapid taper) is occasionally used.

(4) Vasculitis. Treatment is discussed in Chapter 76.

B. Acute dialysis. The following indications are usually applicable regardless of the cause of renal failure.

Indications for Acute Dialysis ("AEIOU")

Acidosis
Electrolytes (e.g., hyperkalemia)
Intoxication
Overload
Uremia

1. **Acidosis.** Dialysis is usually necessary when the patient is experiencing complications of a metabolic acidosis (e.g., arrhythmias, left ventricular dysfunction) or if the serum pH starts to fall below 7.2. Sodium bicarbonate is sometimes used as a temporizing measure until dialysis can be initiated.

2. **Severe, refractory hyperkalemia** (usually > 6.5–7 mEq/L) or hyperkalemia with persistent electrocardiogram (ECG) changes is an indication for acute dialysis. Temporizing measures include the following: 1) intravenous calcium, which acts as a cardiac membrane stabilizer; and 2) sodium bicarbonate, albuterol nebulizers, or insulin and glucose, which cause potassium to move intracellularly. Sodium polystyrene sulfonate is an exchange resin that can be given orally or rectally to decrease potassium levels over several hours. However, as potassium is bound, sodium is released; thus, caution should be used when giving this medication to patients with CHF.

3. **Intoxication.** Dialysis may be necessary when acute renal failure results from a dialyzable, toxic ingestion (e.g., salicylates, ethylene glycol).

4. **Overload.** Volume overload that is refractory to diuretics is an indication for dialysis. Temporizing measures include ni-

trates and furosemide (which cause venodilation and may therefore decrease pulmonary edema).

5. **Uremia.** Altered mental status, seizures, pericarditis, intractable nausea and vomiting, and uncontrolled bleeding from platelet dysfunction are all indications for acute dialysis.

References

Albright RC Jr. Acute renal failure: a practical update. Mayo Clin Proc 2001;76(1): 67–74.

Block CA, Manning HL. Prevention of acute renal failure in the critically ill. Am J Respir Crit Care Med 2002;165(3):320–324.

Vanholder R, Sever MS, Erek E, Lameire N. Rhabdomyolysis. J Am Soc Nephrol 2000;11(8):1553–1561.

38. Nephrotic Syndrome

I. INTRODUCTION

A. Pathophysiologic mechanism. Nephrotic syndrome results from increased glomerular permeability to serum proteins via changes in either charge-selective or size-selective properties of the glomerular basement membrane.

B. Clinical manifestations of nephrotic syndrome. Onset is insidious, and renal function may be normal. Gross hematuria and red blood cell (RBC) casts occur infrequently but are seen with some diseases that traditionally cause nephrotic syndrome (i.e., diabetic nephropathy). Clinical findings include proteinuria, low serum albumin, hyperlipidemia, and edema. (These patient may look "PALE" because they are excreting so much protein—this is not really so, but it makes the mnemonic easier to remember.)

Characteristics of the Nephrotic Syndrome ("PALE")

Proteinuria (> 3.5 g/24 hours)
Albumin (low)
Lipids (often elevated)
Edema

II. CAUSES OF NEPHROTIC SYNDROME

HOT KEY

Diabetic nephropathy is the most common cause of nephrotic-range proteinuria.

A. Primary glomerular disease. Among patients without diabetes, nephrotic syndrome is caused by primary glomerular disease in the vast majority. Specific etiologies change frequency by age (i.e., the frequency of minimal change disease decreases while that of membranous nephropathy increases with age). Primary glomerular diseases associated with nephrotic syndrome in adults include:

1. **Membranous nephropathy**
2. **Minimal change disease**
3. **Focal segmental glomerulosclerosis (FSGS)**
4. **Membranoproliferative glomerulonephritis**
5. **Rapidly progressive glomerulonephritis**
B. **Secondary causes.** Commonly, nephrotic syndrome occurs secondary to systemic disease. Although there is a long list of possible secondary causes, most can be remembered easily using the mnemonic, "THIS LAD HAS nephrotic syndrome."

> Secondary Causes of Nephrotic Syndrome
>
> **T**umors
> **H**eroin, **H**eavy metals, and toxins/medications
> **I**nfection
>   **H**epatitis B and C
>   **A**IDS
>   **S**ubacute bacterial endocarditis, **S**yphilis, **S**chistosomiasis
> **S**ystemic disorders
>   **L**upus
>   **A**myloid
>   **D**iabetes

1. **Tumors.** Many cancers can cause nephrotic syndrome. In elderly patients with unexplained nephrotic syndrome, an underlying malignancy is a real concern. Both hematologic malignancies (e.g., lymphoma, leukemia, multiple myeloma) and solid tumors (e.g., cancer of the colon, lung, or breast) can cause nephrotic syndrome.
2. **Heroin, heavy metals,** and **toxins/medications.** "Street" heroin, organic gold, mercury, antitoxins, contrast media, lithium, nonsteroidal anti-inflammatory drugs (NSAIDs), and angiotensin-converting enzyme (ACE) inhibitors can cause nephrotic syndrome.
3. **Infections.** There are many infections that can cause nephrotic syndrome; some important ones are **hepatitis B and C, AIDS, subacute bacterial endocarditis, syphilis,** and **schistosomiasis.**
4. **Systemic disorders.** Major causes of nephrotic syndrome include **systemic lupus erythematosus (SLE), amyloid,** and **diabetes mellitus.**

 HOT KEY The incidence of diabetes mellitus is increasing dramatically in the general U.S. population; thus, diabetic nephropathy is increasing as well (accounts for more than 40% of patients starting hemodialysis).

III **APPROACH TO THE PATIENT.** Once it has been determined
that a patient has nephrotic syndrome, the search for the underlying cause begins. A thoughtful history and physical examination should be performed, looking for symptoms and signs
of diseases listed above. Depending on the suspected cause, the
following laboratory tests and procedures can be useful:

A. **Serum chemistries,** including blood urea nitrogen (BUN), cre-
atinine, glucose, and liver function test measurements
B. **Complete blood count (CBC)**
C. **Antinuclear antibody (ANA) assays**
D. **Hepatitis serologies**
E. **Rapid plasma reagin (RPR)** or **Venereal Disease Research
Laboratory (VDRL) test** for syphilis
F. **HIV test**
G. **Fat pad** or **rectal biopsy** (to look for amyloidosis)
H. **Blood cultures** (to rule out endocarditis)
I. **Chest radiograph**
J. **Serum and urine protein electrophoresis**
K. **Renal biopsy**

IV **TREATMENT** focuses on the underlying disorder. General
management strategies include:

A. **ACE inhibitors** to slow progression of renal disease to decrease
proteinuria, and to treat hypertension
B. Specific **therapy for hyperlipidemia** (e.g., HMG CoA reductase
inhibitors)
C. A **diet** low in sodium and saturated fat
D. Strict **treatment of hypertension** with a goal blood pressure of
less than 125/75 mm Hg.
E. **Fluid restriction** and **diuretics** (if hyponatremia and/or edema
are present)
F. **Protein restriction** (0.6–0.8 g/kg/day) to slow the rate of disease
progression is controversial.

V **COMPLICATIONS**

A. **Infections.** Patients with nephrotic syndrome are prone to peritonitis, sepsis, and cellulitis due to urinary losses of immunoglobulins and complement.
B. **Thrombosis** (both arterial and venous) can occur with loss of
antithrombin III, protein C, and protein S in the urine.
C. **Hypovolemia** may be a consequence of overdiuresis.
D. **Wasting** results from protein depletion, although monitored
protein restriction may be beneficial.
E. **Atherosclerosis** may result from hyperlipidemia.

References

Madaio MP, Harrington JT. The diagnosis of glomerular diseases: acute glomeru-lonephritis and the nephrotic syndrome. Arch Intern Med 2001;161(1):25–34.

Orth SR, Ritz E. The nephrotic syndrome. N Engl J Med 1998;338(17):1202–1211.

Schwarz A. New aspects of the treatment of nephrotic syndrome. J Am Soc Nephrol 2001;(Suppl 12)17:S44-S47.

39. Nephritic Syndrome

I **CLINICAL MANIFESTATIONS OF ACUTE NEPHRITIC SYNDROME (ACUTE GLOMERULONEPHRITIS).** Acute nephritic syndrome is characterized by the sudden onset of hematuria, proteinuria (usually < 3 g/24 hours), rising creatinine levels, and salt retention with accompanying hypertension. (Compare with the clinical manifestations of nephrotic syndrome, described in Chapter 38 I B.)

A. The presence of **red blood cell (RBC) casts** or **dysmorphic RBCs** is usually diagnostic. White blood cells (WBCs) or WBC casts may also appear in the urine as a sign of inflammation.

B. **Hematuria** may be microscopic but is often macroscopic (patients complain of dark or "smoky" urine).

C. **Edema** usually appears initially in areas of low tissue pressure (e.g., the periorbital region or scrotum) but may progress to pleural effusions and ascites.

D. **Hypertension** results from salt and water retention.

II **CAUSES OF ACUTE NEPHRITIC SYNDROME**

A. **Hypocomplementemic acute nephritic syndrome.** Activation of the complement system by immune complexes is the cause of low complement (C3) levels.

1. **Systemic diseases**
   a. **Systemic lupus erythematosus (SLE).** Complement levels are decreased in 75%-90% of patients with SLE. Other manifestations of lupus are usually present as well.
   b. **Subacute bacterial endocarditis.** More than 90% of patients have low complement levels. Blood cultures confirm the diagnosis.
   c. **"Shunt" nephritis** is usually caused by infection of a ventriculoperitoneal shunt used to relieve hydrocephalus. As with bacterial endocarditis, sustained bacteremia is the cause of nephritis.
   d. **Cryoglobulinemia.** Complement levels are decreased in 85% of these patients. Serum cryoglobulin levels confirm this diagnosis.

2. **Renal causes**
   a. **Post-infectious glomerulonephritis** (most commonly due to streptococcal infection) is the prototype for acute glomerulonephritis. Nephritis usually occurs 1–2 weeks

after a pharyngeal or cutaneous infection with a group A
(β-hemolytic) streptococcus. Ninety percent of patients
recover fully.

  b. **Membranoproliferative glomerulonephritis (MPGN)** is a
     disease of children and young adults.

     (1) It can be classified as **type I** (the most common type,
     usually with more nephritic-type manifestations) or
     type II (which has a higher incidence of hypocomple-
     mentemia).

     (2) MPGN can also present as nephrotic syndrome and
     has a variable clinical course.

Causes of Hypocomplementemic Acute Nephritic
Syndrome ("She Saw Sally Cook Poisoned Macaroni")

SLE
Subacute bacterial endocarditis
Shunt nephritis
Cryoglobulinemia
Post-infectious glomerulonephritis
MPGN

B. Normocomplementemic acute nephritic syndrome
  1. Systemic diseases
    a. Vasculitis syndromes (see Chapter 76). **Polyarteritis
       nodosa, hypersensitivity vasculitis** (including Henoch-
       Schönlein purpura), and **Wegener's granulomatosis** can
       cause acute glomerulonephritis.
    b. Goodpasture's syndrome is characterized by the presence
       of anti-GBM antibodies, pulmonary hemorrhage, and
       acute glomerulonephritis. It is caused by serum antibod-
       ies that react with glomerular and alveolar basement
       membranes.
  2. Renal diseases
    a. IgA nephropathy (Berger's disease), the most common
       primary glomerular disease in the United States, is con-
       sidered a monosymptomatic form of Henoch-Schönlein
       purpura.
       (1) IgA nephropathy often presents as **gross hematuria**
       (lasting 2–6 days) that occurs a few days after an upper
       respiratory tract or gastrointestinal infection, as op-
       posed to the hematuria that occurs with post-infectious
       glomerulonephritis (after 7-21 days).
       (2) Progression to renal failure occurs in 15% of patients

within 6 months and in up to 50% within 20 years. Up to one third of patients will fully recover renal function.

b. Rapidly progressive glomerulonephritis (RPGN) is the term applied to any glomerulopathy that is characterized by the combination of a **rapid decline in renal function** (due to acute glomerulonephritis) and extensive **crescent formation** in multiple glomeruli.

(1) RPGN may occur secondary to systemic diseases or may occur alone as a primary disorder.

(2) Primary RPGN affects older individuals (the average age is 60 years) and often has a prodrome that resembles a viral illness. Diagnosis is based on a characteristic renal biopsy.

(3) The prognosis is quite poor unless treatment is initiated early and aggressively.

III APPROACH TO THE PATIENT

A. Make the diagnosis. The most important aspect of making the diagnosis of acute glomerulonephritis (after taking the history and performing a physical examination) is to personally examine a **freshly voided urine** specimen, preferably before attending rounds! A spot urine protein to creatinine ratio is also important. A ratio of 1 is equivalent to 1 gram of proteinuria per day.

HOT KEY

The best way to increase the chance of finding RBC casts is to obtain an early morning specimen after the patient has placed a pillow behind the lumbar spine a few minutes after waking up.

B. Categorize and stage the glomerulonephritis. Once the diagnosis is made, the search for the underlying cause begins.

1. Laboratory studies. The **serum complement (C3) level** allows classification of the glomerulonephritis as hypocomplementemic or normocomplementemic. Other tests that may be useful, depending on the clinical setting, include antistreptolysin O (ASO), antinuclear antibody (ANA), antiglomerular basement membrane (anti-GBM) antibody, antineutrophil cytoplasm antibody (ANCA) titers, serum cryoglobulin, blood cultures, liver function tests, hepatitis serologies (B and C), and erythrocyte sedimentation rate (ESR).

2. Renal biopsy is the definitive procedure for diagnosing acute glomerulonephritis.

IV TREATMENT

> **HOT KEY**
>
> Acute glomerulonephritis is a renal emergency!

A. **Inflammatory renal disorders** should be treated with steroids and cytotoxic agents. If the glomerulonephritis is secondary to a systemic disease, the primary disorder should be treated as well.

B. Indications for **hemodialysis** are given in Chapter 37 IV B.

C. The patient's electrolyte status [including blood urea nitrogen (BUN) and creatinine levels], volume status, and blood pressure should be monitored frequently. Hypertension should be treated.

References

Couser WG. Glomerulonephritis. Lancet 1999;353(9163):1509–1515.

Donadio JV, Grande JP. IgA nephropathy. N Engl J Med 2002;347(10):738–748.

Hricik DE, Chung-Park M, Sedor JR. Glomerulonephritis. N Engl J Med 1998;339 (13):888–899.

40. Renal Tubular Defects

I INTRODUCTION

A. The various diseases, **congenital** and **acquired,** that cause renal tubular defects have one thing in common: they tend to affect the tubules to a greater extent than the glomeruli.

B. Defects may be **anatomic** or **physiologic.**

   1. Diseases that cause **anatomic defects** are usually hereditary and include polycystic renal disease, medullary sponge kidney, and medullary cystic disease. Anatomic defects can be diagnosed by intravenous pyelography or ultrasound.

   2. Diseases that cause **physiologic** defects in tubular transport usually present as polyuria, electrolyte imbalance, or a non-gap metabolic acidosis. This chapter focuses on the most confusing aspect of physiologic tubular defects, **renal tubular acidosis.**

II RENAL TUBULAR ACIDOSIS

A. Definition. Renal tubular acidosis results from a net decrease in tubular hydrogen secretion or bicarbonate reabsorption, causing a non-gap (or hyperchloremic) metabolic acidosis.

B. Classification. Most patients with a non-gap metabolic acidosis who do not have diarrhea or an anatomic gastrointestinal abnormality will have one of the three types of renal tubular acidosis (Table 40-1).

   1. Type 1 renal tubular acidosis occurs as a result of defective hydrogen ion secretion; therefore, urinary pH will be elevated. Hypokalemia occurs as potassium secretion is enhanced to accompany the bicarbonate excreted in the urine (the body always tries to retain electroneutrality).

   2. Type 2 renal tubular acidosis occurs as a result of decreased bicarbonate reabsorption in the proximal tubule. Initially, the urinary pH will be elevated because of bicarbonate loss; with continued bicarbonate loss, however, the serum bicarbonate and, thus, the urine bicarbonate concentrations will decrease. Then, all urine bicarbonate can be reabsorbed by the distal tubule, and urinary pH will fall. Patients are hypokalemic for the same reason as described in type I RTA.

   3. Type 4 renal tubular acidosis is usually caused by aldosterone deficiency or resistance. Hyperkalemia occurs for the same reason hyperaldosterone states cause hypokalemic meta-

TABLE 40-1: Overview of Renal Tubular Acidosis			
	Type 1 (Distal)	Type 2 (Proximal)	Type 4
Defect	Decrease in hydrogen secretion	Decrease in bicarbonate reabsorption	Aldosterone deficiency or resistance
Serum [K+]	Decreased	Decreased	Increased
Urinary pH	> 5.3	< 5.3	< 5.3
Major causes	Amphotericin toxicity, hyper-parathyroidism, obstructive uropathy, sickle cell anemia, cirrhosis	Fanconi's syndrome, drugs, Wilson's disease, vitamin D deficiency, amyloidosis, multiple myeloma, renal transplant	Diabetes mellitus, nephrosclerosis from hypertension, renal insufficiency, chronic interstitial nephritis, Addison's disease, ACE inhibitors, heparin
Treatment	Bicarbonate and K+	Bicarbonate and K+*	Mineralocorticoids and potassium restriction

ACE = angiotensin-converting enzyme; K+ = potassium.
*But not in Fanconi's syndrome.

bolic alkalosis. Relative hypoaldosteronism from hyporeninemic states can be seen in diabetic nephropathy, hypertensive nephropathy, tubulointerstitial diseases, and AIDS.

C. **Determination of the type of renal tubular acidosis** (Figure 40–1).

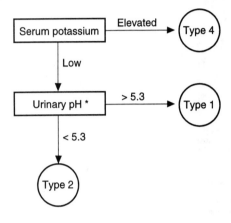

* Urinary pH determination should
be performed immediately after
obtaining a urine specimen.

FIGURE 40-1. Algorithm for determining the type of renal tubular acidosis.

References

Adrogue HJ, Madias NE. Management of life-threatening acid-base disorders. First of two parts. [Erratum appears in N Engl J Med 1999;340(3):247.] N Engl J Med 1998;338(1):26–34.

Adrogue HJ, Madias NE. Management of life-threatening acid-base disorders. Second of two parts. Ne Engl J Med 1998;338(2):107–111.

Kurtzman NA. Renal tubular acidosis syndromes. South Med J 2000;93(11):1042–1052.

41. Urinary Tract Infections (UTIs)

I **INTRODUCTION.** Urinary tract infections (UTIs) are extremely common and include cystitis, pyelonephritis, and urosepsis.

A. Etiology. *Escherichia coli* accounts for approximately 80% of all infections. *Staphylococcus saprophyticus, Klebsiella* species, *Proteus mirabilis, Enterococcus* species, and other bacteria account for the rest.

B. Epidemiology
  1. Women are more susceptible than men to UTIs because the female urethra is shorter, facilitating bacterial access to the bladder.
      a. Sexual intercourse and the use of diaphragms and spermicide are predisposing factors.
      b. In postmenopausal women, estrogen deficiency may predispose patients to acute cystitis (from increased colonization with *E. coli*).
  2. Uncircumcised men are at higher risk than circumcised men.

II **CLINICAL MANIFESTATIONS OF UTIs**

A. Dysuria (i.e., pain or burning with urination) is usually present and is commonly associated with other irritative symptoms (i.e., urinary frequency, urgency, and nocturia). Although dysuria often indicates acute cystitis, it is important to remember that other disorders may also present with dysuria. There is a FUND of irritative symptoms that may indicate the presence of a UTI:

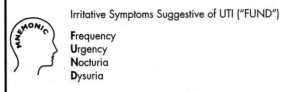

Irritative Symptoms Suggestive of UTI ("FUND")

Frequency
Urgency
Nocturia
Dysuria

B. Suprapubic or costovertebral angle pain or **tenderness** is usually indicative of cystitis or pyelonephritis, respectively.

C. Fever usually indicates pyelonephritis. **Hypotension** and **altered mental status** may indicate urosepsis.

III DIFFERENTIAL DIAGNOSES OF DYSURIA. Dysuria does not always signal acute cystitis. It is especially important to consider the alternative causes of dysuria in men, because acute cystitis is less common in men than in women. Non-UTI causes of dysuria include the following:

A. Women
 1. **Infectious causes**
    a. **Urethritis** (e.g., from *Neisseria gonorrhea, Chlamydia trachomatis,* or herpes simplex virus) may also cause dysuria. Compared with the dysuria of acute cystitis, the dysuria of urethritis usually evolves gradually, is less severe, and is less often accompanied by urinary frequency and urgency. A history of vaginal discharge or a new sexual partner also raises suspicion for urethritis.
    b. **Vaginitis** (e.g., from *Candida* or *Trichomonas*) usually presents with a malodorous vaginal discharge. The patient may also complain of dyspareunia.
 2. **Noninfectious causes**
    a. **Interstitial cystitis** presents with dysuria, urinary leukocytes, and a negative urine culture.
    b. **Chemotherapy** and **pelvic irradiation** may cause symptoms that mimic UTI.

B. Men
 1. **Bladder pathology** may result in dysuria in both men and women, but the relative paucity of UTIs in men increases the likelihood that some other diagnosis is responsible. Both bladder stones and tumors should be considered.
 2. **Prostate syndromes.** With the exception of acute bacterial prostatitis, which usually results in dysuria that is accompanied by significant systemic toxicity, prostate syndromes may be easily confused with cystitis. Laboratory testing is usually needed to differentiate among these disorders (see V F in this chapter).
 3. **Urethritis** from gonorrhea or chlamydia is often associated with penile discharge.

IV LABORATORY STUDIES. Not all the following tests need to be obtained in every patient. The indications for tests are discussed in part V of this chapter.

A. Urine dipstick testing allows for the determination of urinary pH, leukocyte esterase, nitrite, blood, and protein levels.

1. **Urinary pH.** An alkaline urine may indicate a urease-splitting organism (e.g., *Proteus*).
2. **Leukocyte esterase** usually indicates the presence of inflammatory cells [i.e., white blood cells (WBCs)], and therefore, infection. The sensitivity may exceed 75%. False-positive results may occur with urinary contamination.
3. **Nitrite** is detected when certain bacteria are present. The sensitivity is relatively low, and false-positive results are noted with bacterial contamination.
4. **Blood** in the urine may indicate myoglobin, hemoglobin, or intact red blood cells (RBCs). Cystitis can cause hematuria, but other causes of bladder pathology should also be considered (e.g., a malignancy anywhere along the urinary tract).
5. **Protein** in the urine may indicate a glomerulopathy, although low levels of proteinuria are seen with bladder irritation. Large numbers of WBCs may lead to a falsely positive protein determination.

B. **Urine microscopic analysis.** The presence of more than 5 leukocytes per high-power field denotes pyuria and is indicative of some urinary tract abnormality. Gram staining may also be performed but is not a sensitive test for UTI. **Sterile pyuria** (i.e., pyuria with a negative urine culture) may occur with contained bacterial infections (renal abscesses), systemic bacterial infections (endocarditis), nonbacterial infections (miliary tuberculosis), inflammatory processes (interstitial nephritis), and partially treated UTI.

C. **Urine culture** provides the gold standard for diagnosing UTI. Previously, a colony count of 10^5 was considered the cut-off point for diagnosing a UTI, but more than 50% of symptomatic women have a lower colony count. In fact, the presence of as few as 100 colonies may signal infection in a symptomatic woman.

D. **Prostatic secretion analysis.** Prostatic secretions may be elicited through prostatic massage. In elderly men with possible chronic prostatitis, a urinalysis with culture is often sent before and after prostatic massage.

E. **Urine pregnancy test.** Because pregnant patients are often treated with different antibiotics and with a longer course of therapy, a urine pregnancy test should be obtained in all patients for whom pregnancy is a possibility.

F. **Renal imaging (ultrasound or CT scan).** In patients who are systemically ill, and especially in those with a history of kidney stones or a presentation compatible with urolithiasis, an ultrasound may be obtained to rule out "pus under pressure" (i.e., an infection behind an obstruction that mimics an abscess).

V APPROACH TO THE PATIENT

A. **Uncomplicated cystitis**
1. **Women.** Empiric treatment is one possible approach in healthy, non-pregnant women who present with the classic symptoms of acute UTI without any evidence of pyelonephritis (i.e., no systemic symptoms such as fever, costovertebral angle pain, or nausea) or another cause of dysuria (urethritis, vaginitis). Another option is to obtain a **urinary dipstick,** which is usually the only test that is required. If the urinary dipstick is negative or the patient has pelvic pain or abnormal vaginal discharge, a **pelvic examination** and a **urine culture** are often indicated as well.
2. **Men.** A **urine dipstick** and **culture** is generally performed before therapy.
B. **Uncomplicated pyelonephritis.** Patients usually present with **irritative symptoms** associated with **fever, costovertebral angle pain** or **tenderness,** or both. The **urinary dipstick** is usually positive, and a **urine culture** is usually sent for definitive diagnosis and to ascertain the antimicrobial sensitivities of the causative organism.
C. **Recurrent cystitis** (e.g., three or more episodes per year) is much more common in women than men. Before diagnosing recurrent cystitis, **rule out relapse.**
1. **Relapses** typically occur early after the completion of therapy. The same species and strain of organism is isolated, and additional urologic evaluation is usually necessary.
2. **Recurrences** typically occur later. A different organism is usually isolated, and additional evaluation is often unnecessary.
D. **Complicated UTIs** may occur in men or women and are often suspected in patients whose conditions relapse or do not improve with initial therapy. A complicated infection results when a patient has an anatomic or functional abnormality of the urinary tract or a resistant infection. Urinary catheter-related infection (see Chapter 4) is considered to be complicated. A urine culture is always recommended.
E. **Asymptomatic bacteriuria.** In most patients, screening for asymptomatic bacteriuria is unnecessary. Exceptions include the following.
1. Pregnant women are often screened and treated if the bacteria count is 10,000 or more (to decrease the risk of pyelonephritis).
2. Patients undergoing urologic surgery also benefit from screening.
F. **Prostate syndromes.** The presence of obstructive symptoms (i.e., hesitancy, difficulty starting and stopping the stream, de-

creased urinary flow) may favor a diagnosis of chronic prostatitis or prostatodynia. Of note, prostate tenderness on examination is not a sensitive marker for these disorders. If a prostate syndrome is suspected, a urine sample is obtained for urinalysis and culture, and then a second sample is obtained following prostate massage.

1. **Chronic bacterial prostatitis.** An increase in leukocytes usually occurs with massage; culture of prostatic secretions is positive.

2. **Chronic nonbacterial prostatitis** usually demonstrates an increase in leukocytes after massage, but the culture is negative. *Ureaplasma* or *Chlamydia* may be the cause.

3. **Prostatodynia** (a misleading term because the prostate is normal) is a diagnosis of exclusion that is made when the patient has typical symptoms, but no increase in leukocytes with massage and a negative culture.

VI TREATMENT

A. **Uncomplicated cystitis.** Empiric therapy is generally appropriate when the urine dipstick test is positive. It may also be appropriate for patients with no alternative diagnosis and a high clinical suspicion for UTI.

1. **Trimethoprim (TMP)/sulfamethoxazole (SMX)** (e.g., TMP 160 mg/SMX 800 mg) is often administered orally twice daily for 3 days. A longer course of therapy (e.g., 7 days) may be appropriate in higher risk patients (e.g., patients with diabetes, elderly patients). Men are usually treated for 7 days.

2. **Fluoroquinolones.** A fluoroquinolone can be substituted if the patient has a sulfa allergy or if resistant strains have emerged in the local area.

3. **Amoxicillin** or **nitrofurantoin** is indicated if the patient is pregnant.

B. **Uncomplicated pyelonephritis**

1. **Outpatient treatment** is appropriate for many patients. TMP/SMX (TMP 160 mg/SMX 800 mg orally twice daily) may be prescribed for 14–21 days, unless resistant strains of bacteria have emerged in the area (in which case a fluoroquinolone would be an appropriate agent).

2. **Inpatient treatment** may be necessary for diabetic patients, the elderly, and in patients who appear severely ill or are unable to maintain hydration secondary to nausea and vomiting. Inpatient treatment is also recommended for pregnant patients. A **third-generation cephalosporin** or the **combination of ampicillin and gentamicin** is often used. The former may be more appropriate for patients with renal dysfunction, whereas the latter may be better suited for severely ill pa-

tients and those in whom an enterococcus species is suspected to be the causative organism.
C. Recurrent cystitis is often an indication for prophylaxis.
  1. General recommendations. Postmenopausal women may benefit from topical estrogen to help prevent *E. coli* colonization. Women who use diaphragms or spermicide should consider alternative methods of birth control. These measures may obviate the need for prophylaxis.
  2. Prophylaxis
    a. Postcoital prophylaxis is often used in patients who relate their UTIs to sexual intercourse. One tablet of TMP/SMX may be taken following intercourse, and patients should be advised to urinate soon after intercourse.
    b. Daily or three-times-per-week prophylaxis with TMP/SMX may be used in patients with recurrent UTIs unrelated to sexual intercourse.
    c. Early therapy may be preferred in patients who have infrequent recurrences (e.g., two episodes per year). Patients initiate their own 3-day treatment with the onset of symptoms.
D. Complicated UTIs. If a resistant infection is the cause, therapy is generally aimed at the organism and often given for an extended period (e.g., 10–14 days or longer). A fluoroquinolone is often given to outpatients, while broad-spectrum intravenous antibiotics may be required for initial inpatient therapy. If the infection is related to the use of a urinary catheter (see Chapter 4), urine culture and appropriate antimicrobial treatment for 7–14 days is usually required.

H O T
KEY

If a patient develops a Foley catheter-related infection and still requires an indwelling catheter, the catheter should be replaced before initiating antimicrobial treatment (biofilm development along the surface of the catheter harbors microorganisms and may "protect" these organisms from the antimicrobial agent).

E. Prostate syndromes
  1. Chronic bacterial prostatitis. Prolonged treatment (often with TMP/SMX for 6 weeks or more) is generally given.
  2. Chronic nonbacterial prostatitis. Empiric treatment against *Ureaplasma* or *Chlamydia* (e.g., with erythromycin) is often initiated for 2 weeks and should be continued for 3–6 weeks only if symptoms have improved.
  3. α-blocking agents may be helpful for bladder neck and urethral spasms.

References

Bent S, Nallamothu BK, Simel DL, Fihn SD, Saint S. Does this woman have an acute uncomplicated urinary tract infection? JAMA 2002;287(20):2701–2710.

Gupta K, Hooton TM, Stamm WE. Increasing antimicrobial resistance and the management of uncomplicated community-acquired urinary tract infections. Ann Intern Med 2001;135(1):41–50.

Lipsky BA. Prostatitis and urinary tract infection in men: what's new; what's true?. Am J Med 1999;106(3):327–334.

Lipsky BA. Managing urinary tract infections in men. Hosp Pract (Off Ed) 2000; 35(1):53–59.

Roberts JA. Management of pyelonephritis and upper urinary tract infections. Urol Clin North Am 1999;26(4):753–763.

Stamm WE, Hooton TM. Management of urinary tract infections in adults. N Engl J Med 1993;329(18):1328–1334 (classic article).

42. Approach to Acid–Base Disorders

I INTRODUCTION

A. All acid–base disorders can be placed in one of the following categories:
1. **Metabolic acidosis**
   a. **Nonanion gap**
   b. **Anion gap**
2. **Metabolic alkalosis**
   a. **Chloride-responsive**
   b. **Chloride-unresponsive**
3. **Respiratory acidosis**
4. **Respiratory alkalosis**

B. Often, there is more than one metabolic derangement, which can make interpretation more difficult. However, the approach discussed in this chapter will enable you to diagnose most acid–base disorders.

II STEPS IN THE EVALUATION OF ACID–BASE DISORDERS.[1]

An arterial blood gas and electrolyte panel are needed to fully evaluate all acid–base disorders.

A. Decide whether the patient is acidemic or alkalemic. Although a pH of 7.35–7.45 is considered "normal," mixed disorders or the body's compensatory mechanisms (see IV) may hide significant acid–base derangements within this range. It is therefore useful to decide on acidemia or alkalemia simply on the basis of whether the pH falls below or above 7.40.
   1. **Acidemia** is diagnosed when the pH is less than 7.40.
   2. **Alkalemia** is diagnosed when the pH is greater than 7.40.

B. Determine whether the acid-base abnormality has a metabolic or respiratory cause. You can make this determination by looking at the arterial carbon dioxide tension ($PaCO_2$). A high $PaCO_2$ causes an acidosis, whereas a low $PaCO_2$ causes an alkalosis.
   1. **Acidemia**
      a. If the patient is acidemic and the $PaCO_2$ is high, you have diagnosed **respiratory acidosis.** An **acute** respiratory acido-

---

[1]Modified with permission from Haber RJ. A practical approach to acid-base disorders. West J Med 1991;155(2):146–151.

sis will cause serum bicarbonate to rise about 1 meq/L per 10 mm Hg rise of $PaCO_2$. After 6–12 hours, the kidney can begin to generate more bicarbonate, and over days a patient can develop **chronic** respiratory acidosis with serum bicarbonate increasing about 3 meq/L per 10 mm Hg rise in $PaCO_2$.

    b. If the patient is acidemic and the $PaCO_2$ is low, you have diagnosed **metabolic acidosis** (because the $PaCO_2$ does not account for the acidosis). Pure metabolic acidosis results in about a 1.0–1.3 decrease in $PaCO_2$ per 1 meq/L decrease in serum bicarbonate.

  2. Alkalemia

    a. If the patient is alkalemic and the $PaCO_2$ is low, you have diagnosed **respiratory alkalosis.** Acute respiratory alkalosis will cause serum bicarbonate to fall about 2 meq/L per 10 mm Hg fall in $PaCO_2$. **Chronic** respiratory alkalosis will cause serum bicarbonate to fall about 5 meq/L per 10 mm Hg fall in $PaCO_2$.

    b. If the patient is alkalemic and the $PaCO_2$ is high, you have diagnosed **metabolic alkalosis.** Pure metabolic alkalosis results in about a 0.7 mm Hg increase in $PaCO_2$ for each 1 meq/L increase in serum bicarbonate.

C. Calculate the anion gap. The anion gap equals **the measured cations minus the measured anions** [i.e., $Na^+ - (Cl^- + HCO3^-)$]. Because the measured cations are normally more than the measured anions, the unmeasured anions must be greater than the unmeasured cations by exactly the same amount to maintain electroneutrality. Any disorder that increases unmeasured anions will decrease measured anions or increase cations and cause an increased anion gap.

  1. Normal is 8–12.

  2. If the anion gap is **more than 20, anion gap acidosis** is present. The body does not compensate for a respiratory alkalosis with an anion gap acidosis; therefore, the presence of an anion gap acidosis represents a primary abnormality (see III A 2).

  3. If the anion gap is 12–20, there still might be an underlying anion gap acidosis.

D. Calculate the corrected serum bicarbonate

  1. The purpose of this calculation is to determine what the serum bicarbonate would be if no anion gap existed (i.e., the corrected serum bicarbonate).

    a. If correcting the anion gap results in an elevated serum bicarbonate (i.e., > 28), the patient has an underlying metabolic alkalosis.

    b. If correcting the anion gap results in a reduced serum bicarbonate (i.e., < 23), the patient has an underlying non-anion gap acidosis.

c. If correcting the anion gap results in a normal serum bicarbonate, then the decreased serum bicarbonate is completely explained by the anion gap acidosis.

2. The following formula can be used to calculate the corrected serum bicarbonate:

$$CB = \text{Measured AG} - \text{Normal AG} + \text{Measured HCO}_3{}^-$$
$$(CB = \text{corrected bicarbonate and AG} = \text{anion gap})$$

By subtracting the normal anion gap from the measured anion gap, you have a measurement of the "extra acid" that is present. Because each extra acid titrates approximately one base, this calculation approximates the amount of bicarbonate consumed in titrating the anion gap acidosis. By adding this value to the measured bicarbonate value, you correct the bicarbonate for the effect of the anion gap acidosis.

HOT **KEY**

Steps for Determining Acid-Base Abnormalities
- Determine whether the pH is greater than or less than 7.4
- Look at the $PaCO_2$
- Calculate the anion gap
- Calculate the corrected serum bicarbonate

III DIFFERENTIAL DIAGNOSES. Once you have completed the four steps described in section II, you will have identified most possible acid-base disorders. Three disturbances simultaneously (the "triple ripple") is the maximum because respiratory alkalosis and respiratory acidosis cannot exist simultaneously. The following differentials can help you arrive at a cause for the patient's acid-base disorder or disorders.

A. Metabolic acidosis
  1. Nonanion gap. The common causes of nonanion gap acidosis include two renal, two gastrointestinal, and two "post" causes.
  a. Renal
    (1) Renal failure usually causes a mixed anion and nonanion gap acidosis.
    (2) Renal tubular acidosis (see Chapter 40)
  b. Gastrointestinal
    (1) Diarrhea. Bicarbonate loss can result in a nonanion gap metabolic acidosis.
    (2) Colovesicular fistula or **ileostomy** can also cause bicarbonate loss.
  c. "Post" disorders
    (1) Post-hyperventilation. The kidney compensates for a

respiratory alkalosis by "spilling" bicarbonate to generate a nonanion gap metabolic acidosis. If the respiratory alkalosis ceases (e.g., following treatment of heart failure), a nonanion gap acidosis may remain until the kidney can regenerate bicarbonate.

(2) **Post-anion gap acidosis.** For the kidney to maintain the body's electroneutrality, the increase in unmeasured anions that accompanies an anion gap acidosis is associated with chloride loss, producing hypochloremic acidosis. If a significant volume loss accompanies the anion gap acidosis (e.g., diabetic ketoacidosis with an osmotic diuresis from hyperglycemia), the kidney will try to correct by reabsorbing salt and water. In doing so, chloride is reabsorbed and a hyperchloremic (i.e., nonanion gap) acidosis may occur until the kidney can replace the consumed bicarbonate (this often takes a few days).

2. **Anion gap.** Metabolic anion gap acidoses result from an increase in unmeasured anions. Armed with the following mnemonic, "MUDPLIERS," you can zero in on the cause or causes of an anion gap acidosis.

Causes of Anion Gap Acidosis ("MUDPLIERS")

Methanol intoxication (through conversion into formic acid)
Uremia (urea is an anion)
Diabetic or alcoholic ketoacidosis
Paraldehyde (a medicine no longer in use)
Lactate (usually from anaerobic metabolism during shock or extensive tissue injury)
Isoniazid or Iron overdose
Ethylene glycol intoxication (antifreeze ingestion)
Rhabdomyolysis
Salicylate intoxication

---

a. **Uremia.** Check the blood urea nitrogen (BUN).
b. **Rhabdomyolysis.** Check creatine kinase.
c. **Diabetic ketoacidosis.** Diabetic ketoacidosis can be ruled out on the basis of a negative urine dipstick for ketones.
d. **Salicylate overdose.** A salicylate level should be obtained for all unexplained anion gap acidoses.
e. **Methanol** or **ethylene glycol intoxication. A simultaneous blood sample for osmolarity, serum electrolytes,** and eth-

anol level is especially important in patients with altered consciousness and in alcoholics with an anion gap acidosis because the probability of a methanol or ethylene glycol ingestion is increased.

(1) Calculate the osmolar gap. All alcohols (including ethanol, isopropyl alcohol, methanol, and ethylene glycol) can produce an osmolar gap (a difference between measured and calculated osmolarity), but only methanol and ethylene glycol lead to osmolar gaps with significant anion gap acidoses. Calculate the osmolar gap as follows:

Calculated osmolarity = 2 × Na + BUN/2.8 + glucose/18
Osmolar gap = Actual osmolarity − Calculated osmolarity

(2) Correct for ethanol. The ethanol level divided by 4.6 equals the amount of osmoles that ethanol is contributing to the gap.

(3) Calculate the remaining osmolar gap. Subtract the osmoles due to ethanol from the original osmolar gap. The remaining osmolar gap is still unexplained. A value greater than 5 mOsm/kg H_2O is concerning (but not specific) for a toxic ingestion of another alcohol (e.g., methanol or ethylene glycol). Other clinical evidence that may confirm your suspicion includes visual disturbances (with methanol ingestion) and urinary oxalate crystals (with ethylene glycol ingestion).

f. Lactate. Often a lactic acidosis is diagnosed on a clinical basis (e.g., obvious sepsis) or by exclusion. An elevated lactate level confirms your clinical suspicion.

g. Alcoholic ketoacidosis is probably much more common than we think and deserves to be a diagnosis of exclusion so that other potentially treatable and life-threatening conditions are not missed.

B. Metabolic alkalosis. To determine the cause of metabolic alkalosis, first obtain a urine chloride level. Causes are referred to as **chloride-responsive** or **chloride-unresponsive**.

1. Urine chloride < 20 mEq/L. Metabolic alkalosis resulting from the following causes **will correct with sodium chloride administration.**

a. Prerenal states (e.g., severe heart failure). Most metabolic alkaloses are generated by the kidney reacting to a decrease in renal blood flow. Any of the prerenal states (see Chapter 37 II A) can lead to metabolic alkalosis. **Mechanisms** by which a **prerenal state** produces a metabolic alkalosis include:

(1) Increased proximal bicarbonate reabsorption. Avid reabsorption of sodium in the proximal tubule induces increased bicarbonate reabsorption in order to maintain electroneutrality.

(2) Increased distal acid secretion. A prerenal state results in higher renin and aldosterone levels, which increases sodium uptake in the distal tubule while leading to potassium and hydrogen ion secretion.

b. Gastric fluid loss (from vomiting or a nasogastric tube) can lead to a metabolic alkalosis.

c. Prior diuretic therapy leading to volume depletion can result in metabolic alkalosis.

2. Urine chloride > 20 mEq/L. Metabolic alkalosis resulting from the following causes **will not correct with sodium chloride administration.** The most common causes can be remembered easily if you think of the first four letters of the alphabet:

Common Causes of Chloride-Unresponsive Metabolic Alkalosis ("ABCD")

Aldosteronism (primary)
Bartter's syndrome
Cushing's syndrome
Depletion of magnesium

a. Primary hyperaldosteronism increases excretion of potassium and hydrogen ion at the distal tubule, resulting in hypokalemia and alkalosis.

b. Bartter's syndrome results from defects in salt reabsorption in the thick ascending limb of the renal tubule. Salt and water loss trigger aldosterone production, which causes hypokalemia and alkalosis (hypomagnesemia may also be seen).

c. Cushing's syndrome may produce hypokalemia and alkalosis by mechanisms similar to those of primary hyperaldosteronism.

d. Depletion of magnesium may result in potassium wasting. Hypokalemia may cause hydrogen ions to shift intracellularly and may also result in increased excretion of hydrogen at the distal tubule; both mechanisms may lead to alkalosis.

HOT KEY Bartter's syndrome and magnesium depletion are generally associated with normal or low blood pressure, whereas primary hyperaldosteronism and Cushing's syndrome are generally associated with hypertension.

HOT KEY Diuretics often produce a confusing picture because although urinary chloride is > 20 mEq/L, metabolic alkalosis is usually responsive to sodium chloride administration.

C. Respiratory acidosis (hypoventilation). See Chapter 25 II.
D. Respiratory alkalosis (hyperventilation). There are eight common etiologies:
  1. **Primary central nervous system (CNS) disorders**
  2. **Pulmonary disease** (including all causes of hypoxemia)
  3. **Metabolic acidosis**
  4. **Sepsis**

HOT KEY Respiratory alkalosis can be the first acid-base abnormality seen in patients with sepsis.

  5. **Pregnancy**
  6. **Drugs** (e.g., salicylates)
  7. **Liver disease**
  8. **Pain or anxiety**

IV COMPENSATION

A. Clinicians look at compensatory mechanisms for two reasons:
  1. To determine whether compensation is occurring or if there is another primary abnormality
  2. To estimate the acuity of an acid-base abnormality
B. Compensation refers to the body's natural mechanisms of counteracting a primary acid-base disorder. For example, the lungs will compensate for the kidneys through hyperventilation during metabolic acidosis and, to a lesser extent, hypoventilation during metabolic alkalosis. The kidneys will compensate for the lungs by excreting or retaining bicarbonate when respiratory alkalosis or acidosis, respectively, is present.

HOT KEY For every change of 10 mm Hg in the $PaCO_2$ (up or down), the pH changes 0.08 if the process is acute and 0.03 if the process is chronic (in the opposite direction of the $PaCO_2$).

References

Adrogue HJ, Madias NE. Management of life-threatening acid-base disorders. First of two parts. [Erratum appears in N Engl J Med 1999;340(3):247.] N Engl J Med 1998;338(1):26–34.

Adrogue HJ, Madias NE. Management of life-threatening acid-base disorders. Second of two parts. N Engl J Med 1998;338(2):107–111.

Fall PJ. A stepwise approach to acid-base disorders. Practical patient evaluation for metabolic acidosis and other conditions. Postgrad Med 2000;107(3):249–250, 253–254, 257–258.

Gluck SL. Acid-base. Lancet 1998;352(9126):474–479.

Haber RJ. A practical approach to acid-base disorders. West J Med 1991;155(2): 146–151. (classic article)

43. Hyponatremia

I INTRODUCTION

A. Definition. Hyponatremia refers to a **serum sodium concentration of less than 135 mEq/L.** Hyponatremia is the most common electrolyte disturbance in hospitalized patients.

B. Action of antidiuretic hormone (ADH). Understanding the action of ADH is essential to understanding hyponatremia.

1. Normally, the body regulates serum osmolality very closely by increasing or decreasing ADH secretion. When the effective circulating volume (ECV) decreases, the body senses that there is a lack of intravascular fluid and secretes ADH to help expand intravascular volume at the expense of serum osmolality.

2. Hyponatremia is usually caused by either an:
   a. Appropriate increase in ADH (as seen with hypovolemic or some hypervolemic causes), or an
   b. Inappropriate increase in ADH [as seen in the syndrome of inappropriate ADH secretion (SIADH)]

C. Clinical manifestations of hyponatremia depend on the cause, level, and rapidity of hyponatremia; they include confusion, muscle cramps, nausea, and lethargy that may progress to seizures and coma.

D. Approach to the patient

1. The initial step in evaluating patients with hyponatremia is to check the **serum osmolality** to ensure that the patient does not have hypertonic or isotonic hyponatremia.
   a. **Hypertonic hyponatremia** is caused by hyperglycemia or hypertonic infusions [e.g., mannitol, total parenteral nutrition (TPN)]. For every 100 mg/dl of glucose above 100 mg/dl, serum sodium will decrease by about 1.6 meq/L.
   b. **Isotonic hyponatremia** can be caused by hyperlipidemia or hyperproteinemia **(pseudohyponatremia)** and is attributable to laboratory error. Isotonic hyponatremia can also be caused by hyperglycemia and hypertonic infusions, but to a lesser degree than what would cause a hypertonic state.

2. If the serum osmolality is low (< 280 mOsm), the next step is to evaluate the patient's **fluid status.** With this information, it is possible to narrow down the possible causes of the **hypotonic hyponatremia.**

▐▌ HYPOTONIC HYPONATREMIA

A. Hypovolemic

1. **Physical examination** will reveal signs of **volume depletion** (e.g., orthostasis, resting tachycardia, poor skin turgor, dry mucous membranes, low jugular venous pressure).

2. **Causes** are summarized in Table 43-1.

3. **Treatment** entails **intravascular fluid expansion** (usually with normal saline) and **treatment of the underlying cause.** The initial goal of treatment for any cause of hyponatremia is to increase the sodium only **halfway** during the first 24 hours, and no faster than 1–2 meq/L per hour. Overly rapid correction increases the risk for central pontine myelinolysis. Demyelination occurs when pontine brain cells undergo rapid shrinkage due to fluid shifts, which can cause neurologic deficits, coma, and death.

B. Hypervolemic

1. **Physical examination** reveals signs of **volume expansion** (e.g., peripheral edema, ascites, pleural effusions, pulmonary edema).

2. **Causes** are summarized in Table 43-2.

3. **Treatment** usually involves a combination of fluid restriction and diuretics.

C. Euvolemic

1. **Physical examination** is notable for the lack of signs indicative of volume depletion or expansion.

2. **Causes** of euvolemic hypotonic hyponatremia are summarized in Table 43-3.

3. **Treatment** involves fluid restriction plus treatment of the underlying cause.

TABLE 43-1: Causes of Hypotonic Hypovolemic Hyponatremia		
Common Causes	**FENa**	**Serum Uric Acid**
Skin loss	< 1%	> 5 mg/dl
Gastrointestinal loss	< 1%	> 5 mg/dl
Lung loss	< 1%	> 5 mg/dl
Third spacing of fluids	< 1%	> 5 mg/dl
Adrenal insufficiency	> 1%	> 5 mg/dl
Renal loss (diuretics, tubular damage)	> 1%	> 5 mg/dl

FENa = fractional excretion of sodium (see Chapter 37).

TABLE 43-2: Causes of Hypotonic Hypervolemic Hyponatremia		
Common Causes	**FENa**	**Serum Uric Acid**
Nephrosis (i.e., nephrotic syndrome)	< 1%	> 5 mg/dl
Cirrhosis	< 1%	> 5 mg/dl
Cardiosis (i.e., congestive heart failure)	< 1%	> 5 mg/dl

FENa = fractional excretion of sodium.

III SIADH is often a difficult but important diagnosis to make. Because the management of SIADH usually requires fluid restriction in a hospitalized patient (who may be NPO, febrile, or both), it is important to be fairly sure of the diagnosis to prevent dehydration. If a hyponatremic patient meets all (or at least most) of the following five criteria, you can feel reasonably confident about treating the patient for SIADH:

A. The patient should have an **underlying reason** to have SIADH. The most common causes are malignancies, central nervous system (CNS) and pulmonary disease, and various drugs.
B. The patient should be clinically **euvolemic** but is actually slightly hypervolemic.
C. The patient should have **normal renal, adrenal,** and **thyroid** function.
D. The patient's **urine osmolality** is inappropriately **increased** and is usually greater than the serum osmolality.
E. The patient may also have a **low serum uric acid level.** Of all the causes of hyponatremia, only two—SIADH and primary polydipsia—are characterized by hypouricemia. In these two

TABLE 43-3: Causes of Hypotonic Euvolemic Hyponatremia		
Common Causes	**FENa**	**Serum Uric Acid**
SIADH	> 1%	< 4 mg/dl
Water intoxication (polydipsia)	Variable	< 5 mg/dl
Hypothyroidism	Variable	> 5 mg/dl
Renal dysfunction	> 1%	> 5 mg/dl

FENa = fractional excretion of sodium; SIADH = syndrome of inappropriate antidiuretic hormone excretion.

disorders, the intravascular volume is actually expanded (even though the disorders are categorized as euvolemic). The kidney handles uric acid the same way it handles sodium; therefore, in states of intravascular expansion, sodium and uric acid elimination are enhanced.

References

Adrogue HJ, Madias NE. Hyponatremia. N Engl J Med 2000;342(21):1581–1589.

Kumar S, Berl T. Sodium. Lancet 1998;352(9123):220–228.

Milionis HJ, Liamis GL, Elisaf MS. The hyponatremic patient: a systematic approach to laboratory diagnosis. Can Med Assoc J 2002;166(8):1056–1062.

44. Hypernatremia

I INTRODUCTION

A. **Definition.** Hypernatremia refers to **serum sodium concentration greater than 145 mEq/L.**
B. **Severe hypernatremia** is rare if a patient has access to water and has an intact thirst mechanism. Those prone to hypernatremia include the very old, the very young, and the very sick.
C. **Plasma osmolality.** Unlike hyponatremia, hypernatremia is associated with only one state of serum osmolality: hyperosmolality.
D. Hypernatremia is usually due to **water loss out of proportion to electrolyte losses.**

II CLINICAL MANIFESTATIONS OF HYPERNATREMIA depend on the cause, level, and rapidity of changing serum sodium.

A. **Symptoms are** primarily neurologic in origin due to a contracted intracellular fluid volume, which leads to contracted brain cells, which undergo osmotic adaptation. Symptoms may include altered mental status, hyperthermia, delirium, seizures, and coma.
B. Polyuria and polydipsia may also be prominent.

III APPROACH TO THE PATIENT. The initial step in evaluating patients with hypernatremia is to check the **urine osmolality.** A high urine osmolality (> 400 mOsm/kg) ensures that renal water conservation is intact. Dilute urine (< 250 mOsm/kg) is characteristic of diabetes insipidus (DI).

A. **Hyperosmolar urine**
   1. **Nonrenal losses (e.g., due to excessive sweating, respiratory tract or gastrointestinal water loss).** Hypernatremia can occur if water intake cannot keep up with hypotonic fluid loss. Urine sodium is typically < 10 mEq/L due to appropriate attempts to conserve total body sodium.
   2. **Renal losses (e.g., due to diabetic hyperglycemia, mannitol use).** Progressive volume depletion occurs with the ensuing osmotic diuresis. During these conditions, renal sodium and water conservation is not present, and the urine sodium is typically > 20 mEq/L.

3. **Rarely, hypernatremia reflects an increased amount of total body sodium.** Causes include hypertonic fluid administration (e.g., during cardiopulmonary resuscitation with hypertonic fluids), sodium chloride tablet ingestion without adequate water, and primary hyperaldosteronism. In these cases, urine sodium is typically > 20 mEq/L.

B. **Hypo-osmolar urine** in the setting of hypernatremia indicates DI.

1. **Nephrogenic DI** stems from renal resistance to the action of ADH. Causes include drugs such as lithium and demeclocycline, chronic kidney disease affecting the collecting ducts (e.g., interstitial nephritis and ureteral obstruction), and electrolyte disorders (hypercalcemia and hypokalemia).

2. **Central DI** is most commonly caused by lack of ADH production in the posterior pituitary (e.g., brain surgery in the area of the pituitary or hypothalamus, head trauma, and idiopathic causes [50%]).

IV TREATMENT. Extracellular fluid (ECF) status and the speed of development of hypernatremia must be assessed. Before the steps described below are taken, the initial underlying disorder must be corrected. Intranasal desmopressin is used for central DI, and the concentrating defect in nephrogenic DI can be treated with a low-sodium diet and a thiazide diuretic.

A. **ECF depletion** should be corrected first with isotonic fluids until ECF is restored. Then, water or hypotonic fluids can be administered.

Free water deficit = current TBW × ([Na+] − 140)/140.
(TBW = total body weight = 0.6 × ideal body weight)

B. **ECF expansion** can be treated with diuretics. If renal failure is present, dialysis may be necessary.

C. **Chronic hypernatremia** should be corrected at 1–2 mOsm/hr over 24–48 hours.

References
Adrogue HJ, Madias NE. Hypernatremia. N Engl J Med 2000;342(20):1493–1499.
Kumar S, Berl T. Sodium. Lancet 1998;352(9123):220–228.

45. Hypokalemia

I INTRODUCTION

A. **Definition.** Hypokalemia refers to **serum potassium concentration < 3.5 mEq/L.**
B. **Maintenance of plasma potassium**
   1. Ninety-five percent of potassium is intracellular.
   2. Plasma potassium is maintained in a narrow range primarily via two mechanisms:
      a. Intracellular and extracellular shifts of potassium
      b. Renal potassium excretion
   3. Increased intracellular shifts and increased renal and gastrointestinal potassium losses lead to hypokalemia.

II CLINICAL MANIFESTATIONS primarily arise from alterations in membrane polarization.

A. **Cardiac.** Altered cardiac conduction is the most life-threatening abnormality. An electrocardiogram may display **flat T waves** and **prominent U waves.** Patients are at risk for significant ectopy, which does not always correlate with potassium levels.

> **HOT KEY**
> Hypokalemia predisposes patients to digoxin toxicity.

B. **Neuromuscular.** Patients can experience a range of abnormalities from **mild weakness to overt paralysis.** Paralysis is not typically seen with potassium levels > 2.0 mEq/L. Constipation and ileus can occur.

> **HOT KEY**
> Hypokalemia predisposes patients to rhabdomyolysis.

C. **Renal.** Hypokalemia leads to a decline in glomerular filtration rate and renal blood flow. It also leads to direct thirst stimulation and a urinary concentrating defect, which causes polydipsia and polyuria.

D. Endocrine. Aldosterone levels are depressed, and pancreatic insulin release is inhibited.

III CAUSES OF HYPOKALEMIA

A. **Hypokalemia with transcellular redistribution**
   1. **Alkalosis.** Metabolic alkalosis results in major total body potassium deficits up to 500 mEq; however, respiratory alkalosis typically induces much less of a potassium deficit.
   2. **Insulin excess** indirectly stimulates the transcellular Na^+, K^+-ATPase pump, which leads to muscle and liver cellular potassium uptake.
   3. **β-Adrenergic agonists** cause direct stimulation of the Na^+, K^+-ATPase pump.
   4. **Hypokalemic periodic paralysis** is a rare hereditary disorder leading to rapid recurrent attacks of flaccid paralysis, lasting from 4–24 hours, due to intracellular potassium shifts. Asians and patients with thyroid disease are particularly vulnerable to this entity.
   5. **Pseudohypokalemia** occurs in patients with very high white blood cell counts ($> 10^5$). Redistribution occurs with leukocyte uptake of potassium.
B. **Hypokalemia due to potassium depletion.** Urinary potassium can only be interpreted in a euvolemic patient. Otherwise, volume contraction may reduce urinary potassium excretion and obscure a state of hyperaldosteronism.
   1. **Extrarenal potassium loss.** Urinary potassium excretion should be < 20 mEq/day. Diarrhea, fistula drainage, and villous adenomas are usually easily diagnosed. Laxative use may be more difficult to diagnose, however, requiring stool electrolyte measurement. Inadequate potassium intake is a rare cause but can be seen in patients with eating disorders.
   2. **Renal potassium loss.** Urinary potassium excretion is > 20 mEq/day. The causes of hypokalemia in this setting are subdivided based on the patient's blood pressure.
      a. **Patients with elevated blood pressure.** Mineralocorticoid excess leads to potassium loss in these disorders.
         (1) **Hyperreninemic states** include hypertensive emergencies, renovascular hypertension, and rare renin-producing tumors.
         (2) **Hyporeninemic states** include primary hyperaldosteronism, Cushing's syndrome, excessive licorice ingestion, and congenital adrenal hyperplasia.
      b. **Patients with normal or low blood pressure.** These disorders can be categorized based on serum bicarbonate concentration.

(1) Low bicarbonate syndromes include renal tubular acidoses (see Chapter 40).

(2) High bicarbonate syndromes include diuretic use, Bartter's syndrome (genetic defects in the thick ascending limb of the loop of Henle), and magnesium depletion, all of which have urinary chloride excretions > 10 mEq/day. Vomiting typically causes volume depletion and metabolic alkalosis, leading to renal potassium wasting and urinary chloride excretion < 10 mEq/day.

 IV TREATMENT. The underlying disorder, if known, should be treated along with the serum potassium level.

A. Oral repletion is the preferred method.
   1. Intravenous (IV) administration can be considered with severe, symptomatic hypokalemia or if patients are unable to tolerate oral medication.
   2. Peripheral IV rates should not exceed 10 mEq/hr, with central IV rates not exceeding 20–40 mEq/hr.

H O T

 High rates of potassium repletion require continuous electrocardiographic monitoring.

K E Y

B. Hypomagnesemia, and glucose or alkali administration, can worsen hypokalemia and should be corrected before or during potassium administration.
C. Serum potassium levels should be followed very closely. For every 10 mEq of supplemental potassium given, serum potassium rises by 0.1 mEq/L; however, this approximation is less valid when serum potassium levels are less than 3.0 mEq/L.

References
Cohn JN, Kowey PR, Whelton PK, Prisant LM. New guidelines for potassium replacement in clinical practice: a contemporary review by the National Council on Potassium in Clinical Practice. Arch Intern Med 2000;160(16):2429–2436.
Gennari FJ. Hypokalemia. N Engl J Med 1998;339(7):451–458.
Halperin ML, Kamel KS. Potassium. Lancet 1998;352(9122):135–140.
Rastergar A, Soleimani M. Hypokalaemia and hyperkalaemia. Postgrad Med 2001; 77(914):759–764.

46. Hyperkalemia

I INTRODUCTION

A. **Definition.** Hyperkalemia refers to **serum potassium concentration > 5.0 mEq/L.**

B. **Maintenance of plasma potassium**
1. Plasma potassium is **maintained in a narrow range** primarily via two mechanisms:
   a. Intracellular fluid (ICF) and extracellular fluid (ECF) shifts of potassium
   b. Renal potassium excretion
2. **Increased potassium shifting to the extracellular space** and **decreased renal potassium losses** lead to hyperkalemia.
3. **Increased potassium intake** is rarely associated with hyperkalemia unless a patient is oliguric or has significant renal disease. [Typically, a glomerular filtration rate (GFR) > 20 ml/min is sufficient to maintain potassium balance.]

II CLINICAL MANIFESTATIONS. Symptoms primarily arise from **alterations in membrane polarization.**

A. **Cardiac**
1. **Altered cardiac conduction** is the most life-threatening abnormality.
2. An electrocardiogram (ECG) may first show **peaking of the T wave;** then **flattening of the P wave** and **prolongation of the PR interval;** then **widening of the QRS complex;** and finally a **deep S wave or sine wave,** heralding ventricular fibrillation and cardiac arrest.

B. **Neuromuscular.** A range of abnormalities from **mild weakness to tingling and paraesthesias** may occur. Rarely, flaccid paralysis takes place.

C. **Renal.** Hyperkalemia reduces renal ammoniagenesis and NH_4^+ reabsorption, leading to less net acid excretion and **metabolic acidosis.** The acidosis then worsens the degree of hyperkalemia.

D. **Endocrine.** Aldosterone, insulin, and glucagon release are stimulated. Plasma renin levels are suppressed.

III CAUSES OF HYPERKALEMIA

A. **Hyperkalemia with transcellular redistribution**
1. **Acidosis-induced hyperkalemia** occurs primarily due to **acidosis due to inorganic acids.** Cations move intracellu-

larly in exchange for potassium; potassium levels rise about 0.7 mEq/L for every decrease of 0.1 pH units. Respiratory acidosis causes a small rise in serum potassium levels.

 HOT KEY Metabolic acidosis from organic acids (e.g., lactic acid) **does not** typically result in hyperkalemia, because both the cation and organic anion are freely permeable across the cell membrane.

2. **Insulin deficiency and hypertonicity** (e.g., hyperglycemia) promotes potassium shift from the ICF to the ECF.
3. **β-Adrenergic antagonists** cause hyperkalemia but do not lead to life-threatening potassium levels.
4. **Hyperkalemic periodic paralysis** is a rare hereditary disorder leading to recurrent weakness or paralysis. Stimuli that lead to mild hyperkalemia (e.g., exercise) can precipitate an episode.
5. **Pseudohyperkalemia** occurs with redistribution of potassium out of cells after blood is drawn (the laboratory will usually report that the blood sample analyzed was a hemolyzed specimen).

B. **Decreased potassium excretion**
1. **Renal failure.** A GFR < 5 ml/min is usually accompanied by oliguria and hyperkalemia, whereas a GFR > 20 ml/min rarely leads to hyperkalemia.

 HOT KEY It is extremely important to educate patients with significant renal dysfunction about the high potassium content of certain foods, such as citrus fruits and juices, tomatoes, and salt substitutes.

2. **Renal secretory defects** associated with interstitial nephritis, sickle cell disease, obstructive uropathy, and renal transplantation all may lead to renal tubular defects and hyperkalemia.
3. **Drugs**
   a. **Heparin,** regardless of molecular weight, suppresses aldosterone excretion.
   b. **Spironolactone, triamterene,** and **trimethoprim** inhibit potassium excretion via sodium channels in the distal nephron.
   c. **Angiotensin-converting enzyme inhibitors** suppress aldosterone production.

   d. Nonsteroidal anti-inflammatory drugs cause a reversible
   form of hyporeninemic hypoaldosteronism.
   e. Cyclosporine and **tacrolimus** also cause renal potassium
   secretory defects.
4. **Mineralocorticoid deficiency** leads to a hyperchloremic
   metabolic acidosis and hyperkalemia. Causes include Addison's disease and hyporeninemic hypoaldosteronism, as seen
   in patients with type 4 renal tubular acidosis (see Chapter 40)
   or AIDS.

IV TREATMENT. As with hypokalemia, the underlying disorder, if known, should be treated along with the serum potassium level. The level should be confirmed with a repeat blood
draw, particularly in asymptomatic patients, by measuring
plasma levels rather than serum. This avoids the leakage of
potassium out of cells in the course of clotting.

A. **Antagonism of cardiac conduction abnormalities** can be accomplished with the administration of **calcium.**
   1. Give 10 ml of **10% calcium gluconate** administered intra-
      venously over 2–3 minutes.
   2. The onset of action is minutes, and the effect lasts for up to
      1 hour.

HOT **KEY**
Intravenous calcium does not lower serum potassium levels, but
this therapy should be used whenever there is any ECG evidence of hyperkalemic-induced changes.

B. **Intracellular shifting** of potassium occurs relatively rapidly.
   1. **Bicarbonate** distributes potassium into cells within 15–30
      minutes, lasting 1–2 hours.
   2. **Insulin** and **albuterol** begin to act over 15–30 minutes, last-
      ing from 4–6 and 2–4 hours, respectively.
C. **Potassium removal** can be accomplished in several ways.
   1. **Loop diuretics** (e.g., 40–160 mg of furosemide either PO or
      IV)
   2. **Sodium polystyrene sulfonate (Kayexalate)** is an ion-
      exchange binding resin that administers a sodium load in ex-
      change for binding potassium.
      a. Consider giving 15–30 g PO or up to 60 g PR.
      b. Its onset is over a few hours.
   3. **Hemodialysis and peritoneal dialysis** result in the extracor-
      poreal removal of potassium. As much as 300 mEq of potas-
      sium can be removed during each treatment.

References
Perazella MA. Drug-induced hyperkalemia: old culprits and new offenders. Am J Med 2000;109(4):307–314.
Rastergar A, Soleimani M. Hypokalaemia and hyperkalaemia. Postgrad Med 2001;77 (914):759–764.
Slovis C, Jenkins R. ABC of clinical electrocardiography: conditions not primarily affecting the heart. [Erratum appears in BMJ 2002;325(7358):259]. BMJ 2002;324 (7349):1320–1323.

47. Hypertension

I INTRODUCTION

A. Definition. Patients who consistently have **systolic blood pressure > 140 mm Hg** or **diastolic blood pressure > 90 mm Hg** are considered to be hypertensive. Certain subgroups of patients are at greater risk for complications of hypertension and are considered "hypertensive" at lower cutoffs (i.e., diabetic patients with blood pressure greater than 130/85 mm Hg).

B. Hypertension is an extremely **common disorder** in both outpatients and hospitalized patients. In general, hypertension in inpatients is a major concern primarily when patients present with hypertensive urgencies or emergencies.

II CAUSES OF SECONDARY HYPERTENSION. Although 95% of hypertensive patients have essential (primary) hypertension, causes of secondary hypertension must be considered in patients with characteristic signs or symptoms, onset of hypertension at a very young or old age, or when the blood pressure is refractory to medical therapy. The causes of secondary hypertension can be remembered using the following memory aid:

Causes of Secondary Hypertension

One anatomic cause
Two renal causes
Three adrenal causes
Four CENTs
Calcium (hypercalcemia)
Ethanol abuse or Estrogen use
Neurologic disease
Thyrotoxicosis

A. One anatomic cause. Aortic coarctation, a congenital disorder characterized by aortic constriction at the origin of the left subclavian artery, usually presents in children or young adults and can lead to hypertension.

B. Two renal causes

1. **Intrinsic renal disease.** Almost any parenchymal kidney disorder can lead to hypertension, usually as a result of in-

creased intravascular volume, increased endothelial reactivity, and/or increased activity of the renin-angiotensin-aldosterone system.

2. **Renal artery stenosis,** a relatively common cause of secondary hypertension, is usually caused by fibromuscular dysplasia in young women (very infrequent) and atherosclerosis in older patients (much more common). The stenosis leads to decreased renal blood flow, which leads to increased renin release and hypertension.

H O T Always consider renal artery stenosis as the cause of hypertension when a patient shows a dramatic increase in serum creatinine after starting angiotensin-converting enzyme (ACE)
K E Y inhibitor therapy.

C. Three adrenal causes

1. **Primary hyperaldosteronism,** an uncommon cause of secondary hypertension, is caused by an aldosterone-secreting adenoma or bilateral adrenal hyperplasia.

H O T

Primary hyperaldosteronism should be suspected if a hypertensive patient is hypokalemic and not taking diuretics.

K E Y

---

2. **Cushing's syndrome.** Excess glucocorticosteroids (as a result of any cause) will often cause the patient to be hypertensive. Usually the other clinical manifestations of glucocorticoid excess will be present to aid in making the diagnosis.

3. **Pheochromocytoma** is a rare norepinephrine- and epinephrine-secreting tumor that may be malignant and can also lead to headaches and glucose intolerance. It is most commonly—but not always—located near the adrenals.

D. Four CENTs

1. **Calcium.** Hypercalcemia is an uncommon cause of hypertension but should be considered in those who have underlying diseases apt to lead to hypercalcemia (see Chapter 77).

2. **Ethanol abuse** or **estrogen use.** The most common causes of secondary hypertension are the use of alcohol and oral contraceptives. Pregnancy can also lead to hypertension.

3. **Neurologic disease.** Any process that leads to increased intracranial pressure can lead to the triad of hypertension,

bradycardia, and irregular respiration (known as Cushing's triad).

4. Thyrotoxicosis. Patients with hyperthyroidism can also be hypertensive.

III HYPERTENSIVE CRISES: URGENCIES AND EMERGENCIES

A. Hypertensive urgencies are situations in which the patient has systolic blood pressure > 220 mm Hg or diastolic blood pressure > 120 mm Hg and no evidence of end-organ damage. Urgencies are usually treated with **oral antihypertensive agents** (e.g., labetalol, clonidine, or captopril) in the emergency department. After blood pressure is lowered to an acceptable level, these patients can usually be discharged but warrant very close follow-up.

HOT KEY

Sublingual nifedipine should be avoided in almost all patients.

B. Hypertensive emergencies are those situations in which elevated blood pressure leads to end-organ damage.
   1. Examples. The following situations qualify as hypertensive emergencies:
   a. Hypertensive encephalopathy (altered mental status)[1]
   b. Intracranial hemorrhage
   c. Aortic dissection
   d. Myocardial infarction
   e. Unstable angina
   f. Hypertensive nephropathy (progressive acute renal failure with proteinuria and hematuria)
   2. Treatment for hypertensive emergencies usually requires admission to the intensive care unit (ICU) and the administration of **parenteral antihypertensives** (e.g., nitroglycerin, nitroprusside, labetalol). Typically, blood pressures should not be lowered by more than 25% over the first 1–2 days (i.e., not lower than 170/110 mm Hg) to minimize organ hypoperfusion.

---

[1]Malignant hypertension is an outdated term that implies hypertension associated with encephalopathy (or neuropathy) and accompanied by papilledema. It is a form of hypertensive emergency.

References

Beevers G, Lip GY, O'Brien E. ABC of hypertension: the pathophysiology of hypertension. BMJ 2001;322(7291):912–916.

Garg J, Messerli AW, Bakris GL. Evaluation and treatment of patients with systemic hypertension. Circulation 2002;105(21):2458–2461.

Nally JV, Barton DP. Contemporary approach to diagnosis and evaluation of renovascular hypertension. Urol Clin North Am 2001;28(4):781–791.

Phillips RA, Greenblatt J, Krakoff LR. Hypertensive emergencies: diagnosis and management. Progr Cardiovasc Dis 2002;45(1):33–48.

PART VI

INFECTIOUS DISEASES

48. Approach to Fever

I   INTRODUCTION

A. Normal body temperature. Body temperature varies throughout the day. The nadir is usually in the early morning, and temperature peaks at 4–6 PM. This is the circadian temperature rhythm. The normal oral temperature is 36°C-37.4°C (average = 36.7°C).

   1. In adults 18–40 years of age, the upper limit of normal temperature should be considered 37.2°C at 6 AM and 37.7°C overall.

   2. The average rectal temperature is 0.5°C higher, and the average axillary temperature is 0.5°C lower than the oral temperature.

> **HOT KEY**
>
> Think of the three temperatures (axillary, oral, and rectal) in alphabetical order to remember which is lowest and which is highest: A < O < R.

B. Fever reflects an upward shift in the body's temperature set point triggered by release of pyrogens. Hyperthermia reflects the body's inability to lower temperature by the usual mechanisms because of overheating or other mechanisms.

C. Causes of fever. Fever may be a manifestation of infection, malignancy, connective tissue disorders, drug reactions, central nervous system (CNS) disorders, inflammatory diseases, or other diseases.

II   APPROACH TO THE PATIENT.

In many cases, the etiology of the fever is clinically obvious; other times, fever can be the initial manifestation of an elusive illness. This chapter provides a way to approach patients with recent onset of fever from an obscure source. If the fever persists for weeks without a diagnosis, a fever of unknown origin (FUO) may be present (see Chapter 51).

> Remember:
> • Patients who are elderly, immunocompromised, or taking steroids or nonsteroidal anti-inflammatory drugs (NSAIDs) may not mount a fever, even in the presence of a severe infection.
> • The degree of fever is of little predictive value in assessing the severity of an underlying illness in a given patient.
> • Hypothermia may signal the presence of an overwhelming infection and should therefore be evaluated as thoroughly as hyperthermia.
>
> HOT
> KEY

A. Patient history

1. **Immune status.** Is the patient immunocompromised [e.g., as a result of leukemia, chemotherapy, steroid use, human immunodeficiency virus (HIV) infection, liver disease]?

2. **Medical history.** Patients with a known illness may have a fever caused by their underlying illness (e.g., tumor fever from lymphoma or a fever from a lupus flare); however, this is a diagnosis of exclusion, and infectious causes must be ruled out. Also, some illnesses predispose patients to certain infectious complications (abdominal abscess as a complication of Crohn's disease, endocarditis in a patient with an aortic valve replacement).

3. **Medication history.** What prescription or over-the-counter drugs is the patient taking? The medication history is aimed at discovering drugs that cause immunosuppression (e.g., steroids) and those that may result in drug fever (e.g., neuroleptics, anticholinergics, anesthetics, antibiotics).

4. **Social history.** What is the patient's travel history? Is there a history of injected drug use or other HIV risk factors? What is the patient's sexual history? Does the patient have pets or frequent animal contact? What are his or her occupation and hobbies? This information may lead to expanding the differential diagnosis to include diseases common in the developing world, HIV-related infections, sexually transmitted disease, tick-borne illnesses, endemic fungal disease, infectious complications such as endocarditis that are common in those using injected drugs, and so on.

> HOT
>
> Fever should be presumed to be secondary to an infection until proven otherwise, because infections cause the majority of fevers and can be life-threatening.
>
> KEY

B. Top-to-bottom approach. One way of determining the cause of a fever is to start at the patient's head and work your way down. Characteristic signs and symptoms (shown in parentheses) may increase your suspicion for the following disorders:

1. **Meningitis** (headaches, neck stiffness, photophobia)
2. **Sinusitis** (sinus tenderness)
3. **Otitis** (ear pain, diminished hearing)
4. **Pharyngitis** (sore throat, lymphadenopathy)
5. **Pneumonia** (cough, pleurisy, dyspnea)
6. **Endocarditis** (recent dental or other procedure, back pain, new skin lesions)
7. **Abdominal processes** (pain, change in bowel habits, nausea, vomiting)
8. **Urinary tract infection (UTI)** or **pyelonephritis** (dysuria, frequency, suprapubic or costovertebral angle tenderness)
9. **Pelvic infection** (discharge, dysuria)
10. **Prostatitis** (lower abdominal pain, tender prostate)
11. **Perirectal abscess** (pain, tenderness, swelling)
12. **Cellulitis** (erythema, pain, swelling)
13. **Joint infections** (pain, warmth, swelling)
14. **Local intravenous catheter site infection** (pain, pus)

HOT

KEY

In patients exposed to antibiotics and presenting with diarrhea, always consider *Clostridium difficile* colitis.

C. Physical examination. A complete physical examination is critical and should cover all the areas mentioned in the review of systems.

HOT

KEY

Easily overlooked portions of the physical include: a complete skin examination, a dental examination, careful evaluation of the joints particularly the hips, a rectal and perirectal evaluation, and a pelvic examination. Each may provide critical clues that lead to the correct diagnosis.

D. Laboratory studies. The history and physical examination may provide enough information to make a diagnosis. Quite commonly, however, you may remain unsure about the etiology of the fever. The following laboratory tests will help you assess the likelihood of an infection and may also help to localize the source.

1. **Complete blood count (CBC) with platelets**
    a. **Neutropenia** with fever is a medical emergency and requires hospitalization and broad-spectrum antibiotics.

  b. A **leftward shifted white blood cell (WBC) count** often implies significant bacterial infection.

  c. A **low WBC count** may be just as worrisome as a high one; the WBC count may not be elevated in alcoholics, the elderly, HIV-infected patients, and other immunocompromised patients in the presence of a serious infection. Overwhelming infection can cause bone marrow suppression and a reduced WBC, which may be manifest before the presence of hemodynamic compromise. Many indolent infections may not be associated with elevations in the WBC. On the other hand, African-American patients normally have WBC counts slightly below the given "normal" range.

2. Electrolytes with blood urea nitrogen (BUN) and **creatinine.** The presence of an anion gap acidosis may indicate sepsis.

3. Prothrombin time (PT) and **partial thromboplastin time (PTT).** Abnormal coagulation studies may indicate disseminated intravascular coagulation (DIC), which may accompany serious infection.

4. Liver tests (e.g., bilirubin, alkaline phosphatase, and transaminase levels) help evaluate the possibility of hepatobiliary disease (e.g., cholecystitis, ascending cholangitis, liver abscess, hepatitis).

5. Amylase levels may be helpful if pancreatitis is suspected.

6. Urinalysis should always be done to evaluate the possibility of UTI.

7. Urine pregnancy test. A pregnancy test should be considered in all women of childbearing age.

8. Cultures

  a. Blood cultures provide the gold standard for diagnosing bacteremia. A minimum of two sets of blood cultures should be drawn. Depending on the organism, determining if a single positive blood culture represents true infection or skin contamination can be difficult. Patients at higher risk for endocarditis, such as those with prosthetic valves or a history of injected drug use, should always have blood cultures drawn.

HOT ▶ **KEY** Persistently positive blood cultures or multiple positive sets of cultures suggest an intravascular infection such as endocarditis, infectious aortitis, septic thrombophlebitis, or a vascular graft infection.

---

  b. Urine culture with a urinalysis should be obtained; however, bacteriuria in the absence of pyuria is unlikely to be the cause of fever.

c. **Sputum evaluation** may be useful for patients with respiratory tract symptoms.

d. **Throat culture** may be useful in patients with pharyngitis.

e. **Cerebrospinal fluid (CSF) analysis** and **culture** is necessary in patients with meningeal symptoms or signs, altered mental status, or HIV infection and an unexplained fever.

f. **Body fluid analysis** and **culture.** Patients with a fever accompanied by ascites, a pleural or joint effusion, or any other type of fluid collection need a diagnostic tap.

HOT KEY

Patients that present with fever and rash should have a skin biopsy unless the diagnosis is straightforward.

E. Radiographs

1. **Chest.** Posterior-anterior (PA) and lateral views should be taken on all patients with unexplained fever.

2. **Abdomen.** Flat and upright views are useful when the patient has a fever and abdominal pain. Make sure to look for air-fluid levels, bowel distention, kidney stones, and free air.

F. Ancillary studies. At this point, you have systematically ruled out most of the possible infections from head to toe. If a diagnosis still has not been made, you need to consider the **easiest place for an infection to hide—the abdomen and pelvis.**

1. **Computed tomography (CT).** A CT scan is the best radiographic test in this situation. It provides a thorough evaluation of the intra-abdominal organs and is more sensitive than ultrasound for detecting occult abscesses.

2. **Ultrasound.** Abdominal ultrasound is often inadequate for ruling out intra-abdominal abscesses and other pathology, but may be better than a CT scan for evaluating the gallbladder and bile ducts (e.g., for cholecystitis or ascending cholangitis).

3. **Other tests** (e.g., **bone marrow biopsy, liver biopsy, indium** or **PET scans, bone scans**) may be obtained if the cause of the fever is still in question (see Chapter 51).

III **TREATMENT.** If a potentially dangerous infection is suspected, or close follow-up is uncertain, admission to the hospital is warranted. Patients who are elderly, immunocompromised, or have other organ system disease may also require admission.

A. General measures

1. **Fluids** need to be administered to keep up with increased insensible losses.

2. **Discontinuing medications** that may be responsible for a fever can be both diagnostic and therapeutic.
B. **Empiric antibiotic therapy**
   1. Nontoxic patients who are otherwise stable can be closely watched without antibiotics until a diagnosis is made.
   2. Patients hospitalized for fever and neutropenia, meningitis, or who are critically ill should be treated empirically pending culture results.
   3. A low threshold for giving empiric antibiotics should also be used for patients who are immunocompromised, including those with HIV infection, diabetes, alcoholism, or liver or renal disease, and patients who are asplenic or taking steroids or immunosuppressants.
C. **Antipyretic therapy**
   1. **Acetaminophen** (325–650 mg every 4 hours as needed) is given initially to provide symptomatic relief. It should preferentially be administered in response to fever rather than around-the-clock so the temperature curve can be monitored.
   2. **Indomethacin** (25–50 mg every 8 hours) and cold sponge baths may be useful for persistent fevers.
   3. **Evaporative cooling** is often used for patients with a temperature greater than 41°C. In this technique, the patient is sprayed with cool water while fans move ambient air across the body. Cooling blankets can be utilized as well.

References
Cunha BA. Fever in the critical care unit. Crit Care Clin 1998;14:1–14.
Pizzo PA. Current concepts: fever in immunocompromised patients. N Engl J Med 1999;341:893–900.
Suh KN, Kozarsky PE, Keystone JS. Evaluation of fever in the returned traveler. Med Clin North Am 1999;83:997–1017.

49. Approach to Microbiology

OVERVIEW OF MICROBIOLOGY. The simplest way to approach microbiology is to divide the organisms into **six major categories** (based on Gram stain, morphology, and aerobic requirements) and consider the most important diseases each organism can cause.

A. **Gram-positive cocci**
  1. *Streptococcus*
      a. **Group A** streptococci cause "strep throat," scarlet fever, rheumatic fever, erysipelas, cellulitis, and pneumonia.
      b. **Group B** streptococci cause mainly perinatal infections and a variety of infections in adults [e.g., urinary tract infection (UTI), sepsis].
      c. *S. pneumoniae* causes pneumonia (usually lobar), bacteremia, meningitis, and endocarditis.
      d. **Viridans** streptococci are the most common cause of bacterial endocarditis.
      e. *S. milleri* originates from the gastrointestinal (GI) tract and causes abscesses, including pulmonary and central nervous system abscesses.
  2. *Enterococcus* causes UTIs, intra-abdominal infections, endocarditis, and nosocomial infections. Infections caused by *Enterococcus* can be difficult to treat.
  3. *Staphylococcus*
      a. *S. aureus* (coagulase-positive) causes skin infections, toxic shock syndrome, endocarditis, intravascular line infections, osteomyelitis, septic arthritis, pneumonia, and nosocomial infections. *S. aureus* is a virulent organism that has a propensity to cause "metastatic" infections.
      b. *S. epidermidis* (coagulase-negative) causes intravascular line infections and prosthetic valve endocarditis.
      c. *S. saprophyticus* (coagulase-negative) causes UTIs.

B. **Gram-positive rods**
  1. *Clostridium* (anaerobic) can cause tetanus, botulism, food poisoning, antibiotic-associated colitis, cellulitis and skin infections, gas gangrene, abscesses, and septicemia.
  2. *Bacillus* can cause cutaneous and pulmonary anthrax (woolsorter's disease, recently an agent of bioterrorism). Most cases in the United States are cutaneous; pulmonary anthrax is usually fatal. *B. cereus* is a common cause of diarrhea.

3. ***Nocardia*** usually causes pulmonary disease that may disseminate (in immunocompromised hosts), leading to brain abscesses and subcutaneous nodules. *Nocardia* species are weakly acid-fast.

4. ***Actinomyces*** (anaerobic) causes cervicofacial infections (following dental infection or trauma), chronic pneumonia, abdominal infections (which may be confused with Crohn's disease), and pelvic inflammatory disease (PID) associated with the use of an intrauterine contraceptive device (IUD).

5. ***Listeria monocytogenes*** causes sporadic cases of meningitis and bacteremia as well as food-borne outbreaks in elderly or immunocompromised adults.

6. ***Erysipelothrix*** causes three types of human illness: erysipeloid (a localized skin lesion); a diffuse skin eruption accompanied by systemic illness; and bacteremia (usually associated with endocarditis). *Erysipelothrix* is acquired through skin abrasions following contact with infected swine, fish, turkeys, ducks, and sheep.

7. ***Corynebacterium***
   a. ***C. diphtheriae*** causes cutaneous, nasopharyngeal, and oropharyngeal infections. Infections of the respiratory tract are characterized by a thick, gray membrane over the pharynx and tonsils.
   b. ***C. jeikeium*** (group JK) causes sepsis, primarily in hospitalized, neutropenic cancer patients who are receiving multiple antibiotics and have some type of skin disruption.
   c. **"Diphtheroids"** are common, nonpathogenic skin contaminants.

Gram-Positive Rods ("**CL**umsy **BA**cteria **NO**rmally **AC**t **LI**ke **ER**ror-prone **CO**rnballs")

Clostridium
Bacillus
Nocardia
Actinomycosis
Listeria monocytogenes
Erysipelothrix
Corynebacterium

C. **Gram-negative cocci**
   1. ***Neisseria***
      a. ***N. meningitidis*** causes meningitis (in children and young adults), meningococcemia (30%-50% of patients have meningococcemia without meningitis), and sinusitis.

b. *N. gonorrhoeae* commonly causes urethritis (in both men and women) and endocervicitis, which may progress to PID or disseminated gonococcal infection (DGI). *N. gonorrhoeae* also causes pharyngitis and conjunctivitis.

2. *Moraxella catarrhalis* causes sinusitis, bronchitis, and pneumonia; however, it is often difficult to distinguish colonization from actual infection.

D. Gram-negative rods comprise the largest category of pathogenic organisms. Infections can involve many different systems, including the genitourinary, hepatobiliary, GI, and respiratory systems. Sepsis involving gram-negative rods is a major cause of mortality, especially for neutropenic or otherwise immunocompromised patients. A partial list of pathogens in this category follows.

1. *Escherichia coli* causes the majority of UTIs and can cause intra-abdominal and biliary infections—all of which may lead to sepsis.

2. *Klebsiella* causes the same diseases as *E. coli* as well as sinusitis and pneumonia (especially in alcoholics).

3. *Pseudomonas* is a destructive organism that can lead to sepsis following a variety of illnesses (e.g., skin, ear, sinus, eye, urinary tract, or lung infections). *Pseudomonas* infection is often nosocomial and usually occurs in the setting of local tissue damage or impaired host defenses.

4. *Haemophilus influenzae* causes pneumonia, bacteremia (especially in patients who have undergone splenectomy), cellulitis, otitis media, epiglottitis, sinusitis, chronic bronchitis, and meningitis (although less commonly now because of the availability of an effective vaccine).

5. *Bordetella pertussis* causes whooping cough (primarily in children) and prolonged bronchitis in adults.

6. *Brucella* causes an insidious febrile illness characterized by easy fatigability, headache, cervical and axillary lymphadenopathy, hepatosplenomegaly, and lymphocytosis. Acquisition of brucellosis is usually via animal contact or following ingestion of contaminated milk.

7. *Francisella tularensis* causes tularemia, a multisystemic disorder (fever, headache, lymphadenopathy, prostration) usually acquired via rabbit or tick contact.

8. *Yersinia pestis* causes plague and is acquired via flea or rodent bites.

9. *Salmonella, Shigella, Campylobacter, Yersinia enterocolitica,* and *Vibrio* species can all cause infectious diarrhea.

E. Anaerobes. The anaerobes *Actinomyces* and *Clostridium* are discussed with the gram-positive rods. *Bacteroides fragilis, B. (Prevotella) melaninogenicus, Peptostreptococcus,* and *Fusobacterium* are also anaerobes.

1. In general, anaerobes are implicated (either alone or in combination) in gingivitis, sinusitis, otitis, abscesses (dental, brain, lung, intra-abdominal), aspiration pneumonia, empyema, skin and soft tissue infections, and pelvic infections.
2. As a rule of thumb, treatment of an abscess primarily depends on drainage and only secondarily depends on antibiotics.

F. Miscellaneous organisms

1. ***Rickettsia.*** Infections include Rocky Mountain spotted fever, murine (endemic) typhus fever, louse-borne (epidemic) typhus fever, and Q fever.
2. ***Mycoplasma pneumoniae*** is the most common cause of pneumonia ("walking pneumonia") in young adults.
3. ***Chlamydiae.*** Infections include chlamydia (the most common sexually transmitted disease in the United States), lymphogranuloma venereum (LGV), trachoma, conjunctivitis, psittacosis, and pneumonia (in young adults).

II ANTIMICROBIAL THERAPY. The best way to learn about antibiotics is to know the organisms that each antibiotic (or class of antibiotics) covers well and which organisms are missed. This information can be found in many antimicrobial guides.

III APPROACH TO THE PATIENT

A. List approximately three of the most common or potentially lethal organisms that can cause the illness with which you are confronted.
B. Select an antibiotic that covers the organisms that are most likely responsible for the infection, making sure to consider cost, convenience, and coverage of potentially life-threatening pathogens.

> **HOT** **KEY** If a patient is very ill, elegant antibiotic combinations are less important than broad coverage to protect against a potentially lethal organism.

References

Bernaldo de Quiros JC, Moreno S, Cercenado E, et al. Group A streptococcal bacteremia. A 10-year prospective study. Medicine 1997;76(4):238–248.

Catterall JR. Streptococcus pneumoniae. Thorax 1999;54(10):929–937.

Lowy FD. *Staphylococcus aureus* infections. N Engl J Med 1998;339(8):520–532.

Opal SM, Cohen J. Clinical gram-positive sepsis: does it fundamentally differ from gram-negative bacterial sepsis? Crit Care Med 1999;27(8):1608–1616.

50. Fever and Rash

I **INTRODUCTION.** Like chest pain, the symptom complex of fever and rash may represent an acute, life-threatening disease or a benign condition.

II **SEVEN KILLER CAUSES OF FEVER AND RASH.** Although there are many causes of fever and rash, you must first consider the diseases that may kill the patient within hours. A SMARTTT physician can easily remember these seven killer causes:

Seven Killer Causes of Fever and Rash ("SMARTTT")

Sepsis
Meningococcemia
Acute endocarditis
Rocky Mountain spotted fever
Toxic erythemas
Toxic epidermal necrolysis (TEN)
Travel-related infections

A. Sepsis. Fever accompanied by a generalized erythematous rash may signal impending sepsis (usually caused by gram-negative organisms).

B. Meningococcemia. Patients usually appear acutely ill. A petechial rash develops in most patients.

HOT

KEY

Disseminated gonococcal infection (DGI) is a less dangerous *Neisseria* infection that may also produce fever and rash. DGI often presents with palpable purpuric pustules and may be associated with fever, tenosynovitis, polyarthralgias, or septic arthritis.

C. Acute endocarditis should be considered in all patients with fever and a petechial rash. A careful cardiac examination is always necessary.

D. Rocky Mountain spotted fever. After 2–6 days of a flu-like febrile illness, a macular rash usually appears over the ankles or wrists. The rash spreads centrally and may evolve into a petechial rash.

E. **Toxic erythemas** include **toxic shock syndrome (TSS), staphylococcal scalded skin syndrome (SSSS), scarlet fever,** and **scarlatiniform eruptions.**

HOT KEY Common features of toxic erythemas include fever and an erythematous rash that is most significant in the flexural folds and later desquamates; mucocutaneous involvement occurs frequently.

---

1. **TSS** results in a diffuse erythematous rash that blanches easily; desquamation occurs after 1–2 weeks (see Chapter 90). Both *Staphylococcus aureus* and *Streptococcus pyogenes* can cause TSS.
2. **SSSS** results in generalized erythema and desquamation.
3. **Scarlet fever** follows *S. pyogenes* pharyngitis. Although it may not be immediately life-threatening, scarlet fever should always be considered when the patient presents with toxic erythema. Scarlatiniform eruptions resemble the rash of scarlet fever and are usually caused by *S. aureus.*

F. **Toxic epidermal necrolysis (TEN)** is caused by a reaction to **drugs.** It is a "SNAP" to remember the drugs that commonly cause TEN:

Drugs That Commonly Cause TEN ("SNAP")

Sulfonamides
Nonsteroidal anti-inflammatory drugs (NSAIDs)
Allopurinol
Phenytoin

TEN results in large areas of erythema and desquamation and may be clinically indistinguishable from SSSS.

G. **Travel-related infections.** Fever and rash in a recent traveler should alert you to the possibility of a potentially life-threatening viral illness. Most of these dangerous viruses are acquired in Latin America, Africa, or Asia.
1. **Hemorrhagic fevers** are the most worrisome and include Ebola, Lassa, and Hanta virus infection. These disorders are often characterized by petechiae or purpura as well as other types of bleeding, and are associated with a high mortality rate.

III APPROACH TO THE PATIENT

A. Rule out the seven killer causes of fever and rash. In general, you will be able to rule out these life-threatening causes of fever and rash by paying attention to the patient history and the clinical manifestations of disease, including the rash.

1. **Patient history.** Always remember to obtain a **medication** and **travel history.** A negative drug and travel history usually rules out **TEN** and **hemorrhagic fever** as potential etiologies.

2. **Clinical manifestations**

   a. **Ill appearance.** Patients with **meningococcemia, Rocky Mountain spotted fever,** or **sepsis** usually appear systemically ill.

   b. **Cardiac murmur. Acute endocarditis** is usually accompanied by a cardiac murmur (see Chapter 54).

   c. **Rash**

      (1) **Desquamating rashes** often signal **toxic erythema** or **TEN.**

      (2) **Petechial rashes** should always alert you to the possibility of meningococcemia, Rocky Mountain spotted fever, or endocarditis.

3. **Helpful data**

   a. Laboratory evaluation to assess other organ systems may be necessary when toxic shock is still a consideration (e.g., in a patient who appears ill or has low blood pressure).

   b. Most of the toxic erythemas (with the exception of SSSS) can usually be ruled out on clinical grounds; however, a skin biopsy is always indicated to differentiate **SSSS** from **TEN.** A split epidermis (i.e., intraepidermal separation) is found in SSSS, whereas total epidermal separation (i.e., subepidermal separation) is seen in TEN.

B. Address other diagnostic possibilities

1. **Types of lesions.** One way to establish a concise differential diagnosis of a fever and rash is to first determine the type of primary lesion (Table 50–1).

2. **Differential diagnoses.** Some common etiologies for each primary lesion associated with a fever are provided below.

   a. **Macules** and **papules** (or a **maculopapular rash**)

      (1) **Drug reactions** commonly present with a pruritic, confluent eruption over the trunk that usually occurs within 1 week of starting a new medication. Fever is usually absent.

      (2) **Viral infections** [e.g., measles and other childhood viral exanthems, infectious mononucleosis, primary human immunodeficiency virus (HIV)] usually result in rashes that are nonpruritic. Fever and other viral symptoms are often present.

TABLE 50-1: Types of Cutaneous Lesions	
Lesion	**Description**
Macules	Discolored, flat lesions
Papules	Raised lesions; < 0.5 cm in diameter
Vesicles	Lesions filled with clear fluid; < 0.5 cm in diameter
Bullae	Large vesicles (i.e., > 0.5 cm in diameter)
Pustules	Pus-filled vesicles
Nodules	Raised lesions > 0.5 cm in diameter and depth
Plaques	Raised lesions > 0.5 cm in diameter, but without depth
Purpura	Purple, nonblanchable lesion
Petechiae	Purpuric lesions < 3 mm in diameter
Ecchymoses	Purpuric lesions > 3 mm in diameter

(3) **Toxic erythemas** are usually accentuated in the flexural folds, are not pruritic, and may have mucous membrane involvement.

(4) **Connective tissue diseases** [e.g., systemic lupus erythematosus (SLE), Still's disease] often present with rash in association with other characteristic symptoms (e.g., arthralgias).

(5) **Bacterial infections** are less likely causes.

    (a) **Lyme disease** may cause erythema chronicum migrans.

    (b) **Secondary syphilis** most often results in scaling papules that are present on the palms and soles.

    (c) **Typhoid fever** can cause "rose spots," which are usually seen as an individual papule on the trunk that fades with pressure.

b. Vesicles and **bullae** (see mnemonic on next page)

c. Pustules (see mnemonic on next page)

d. Nodules and **plaques**

    (1) **Nonpainful**

        (a) **Fungal infections**

        (b) **Lymphoma**

    (2) **Painful**

        (a) **Erythema nodosum** presents with tender nodules on the lower legs. It is often associated with another

Differential Diagnoses for Vesicles and Bullae
Accompanied by Fever ("VESICLES")

Viral infections (e.g., varicella-zoster, herpes simplex,
Coxsackie)
Erythema multiforme
SSSS
Impetigo (bullous)
Contact dermatitis
LESs likely etiologies (e.g., porphyria cutanea tarda, bul-
lous pemphigoid, pemphigus vulgaris, dermatitis her-
petiformis)

Differential Diagnoses for Pustules Accompanied by
Fever ("Very Full of PUS")

Viral infections (e.g., varicella-zoster, herpes simplex)
Fungal infections (e.g., candidiasis)
Pustular psoriasis
Urethritis-related (i.e., DGI)
Syphilis

illness (e.g., tuberculosis, coccidioidomycosis, sarcoid, poststreptococcal infection) or pregnancy.

(b) Sweet's syndrome should be suspected in patients
with fever, neutrophilia, and red-brown lesions
(usually on the head and upper extremities). The
syndrome may be associated with leukemias (usually acute myelogenous leukemia), lymphomas,
myelodysplasia, or other malignancies. Infiltration
of neutrophils into the dermis is seen on biopsy.

e. Purpura

(1) Palpable purpura is pathognomonic for **vasculitis** (see
Chapter 76).

(2) Nonpalpable purpura. Petechiae usually indicate a
bleeding disorder (e.g., thrombocytopenia), and ecchymoses often result from vessel fragility (e.g., actinic
purpura); however, overlap does exist [e.g., necrotic
ecchymoses may occur with disseminated intravascular coagulation (DIC)].

> **HOT**
> ▶
> **KEY**
>
> Purpuric lesions in a patient with fever may be the harbinger of a life-threatening illness. Hemorrhagic fever, meningococcemia, Rocky Mountain spotted fever, endocarditis, sepsis, and vasculitis all need to be considered carefully and ruled out.

References

Cunha BA. Rash and fever in the critical care unit. Crit Care Clin 1998;14:35–53.

Schlossberg D. Fever and rash. Infect Dis Clin North Am 1996;10:101–110.

51. Fever of Unknown Origin (FUO)

I **INTRODUCTION.** Fever of unknown origin (FUO) is defined as a temperature greater than 38.3°C for more than 3 weeks that eludes diagnosis even after 1 week of in-hospital evaluation. More recent authors have suggested that the duration of time in the hospital be modified to include patients whose illness remains undiagnosed after at least 3 outpatient visits or 3 days in the hospital. These definitions were designed to exclude common undiagnosed viral syndromes and to identify a homogenous population to describe in studies. This definition is arbitrary, and the following approach should be used in patients in whom the etiology of fever is obscure despite an initial work-up.

II **COMMON CAUSES OF FUO** (Table 51-1)

A. Although the percentage of FUOs due to infectious etiologies is declining, infections still account for the majority of FUOs.
   1. **Bacterial infections**
      a. **Intra-abdominal abscesses** (e.g., in the liver, spleen, or kidney) are especially common causes of FUO.
      b. **Osteomyelitis** and **sinusitis** are other localized infections that may elude initial diagnosis.
      c. **Bacteremias** from endocarditis, salmonellosis (typhoid fever), and brucellosis commonly cause FUO. Intravascular graft infections present with bacteremia and can be very difficult to diagnose.
      d. **Mycobacterial infections**
         (1) Tuberculosis is a common cause of FUO and is likely the most common cause worldwide. Human immunodeficiency virus (HIV)-infected patients have a higher rate of extrapulmonary tuberculosis.
         (2) *Mycobacterium avium* **complex infections** is the leading cause in the United States of FUO in patients with acquired immune deficiency syndrome (AIDS). CD4 counts are typically < 50 in this setting.
      e. **Spirochetal infections. Secondary syphilis, leptospirosis,** and **Lyme disease** should be considered.
      f. **Rickettsial infections** include the typhus group (epidemic, endemic, and scrub typhus), the spotted fever group

TABLE 51-1: Common Causes of Fever of Unknown Origin (FUO)	
° Disease Category	Examples
Infectious	Bacterial, mycobacterial, viral, fungal, parasitic, spirochetal, rickettsial
Neoplastic	Lymphomas, leukemias, hepatic cancer, renal cancer, atrial myxoma
Connective tissue disorders	Systemic lupus erythematosus (SLE), rheumatoid arthritis, Still's disease, vasculitides
Miscellaneous	Inflammatory bowel disease, granulomatous hepatitis

(Rocky Mountain spotted fever, rickettsialpox, and tick fever), and other similar illnesses (Q fever, trench fever, and ehrlichiosis).

2. **Viral infections**
   a. **Cytomegalovirus (CMV) infection** is a common cause of FUO. Acute CMV infection in immunocompetent patients often presents without localizing signs.
   b. **Epstein-Barr virus infection** causes mononucleosis (especially in adolescents and young adults).
3. **Fungal infections**
   a. **Histoplasmosis** and **coccidioidomycosis** can cause FUO in immunocompetent or immunocompromised patients.
   b. **Candidiasis** and **aspergillosis** are opportunistic fungal infections that may cause FUO.
4. **Parasitic infections. Amebiasis, malaria,** and **toxoplasmosis** may cause FUO and are common causes of FUO in developing countries.

B. **Neoplasms.** Lymphomas, leukemias, hepatic and renal cancers, and atrial myxomas are often associated with febrile syndromes. Concurrent infection should always be ruled out.
C. **Connective tissue disorders.** Systemic lupus erythematosus (SLE), rheumatoid arthritis, Still's disease, giant cell arteritis, and the vasculitides (see Chapter 76) can all cause FUO.
D. **Other causes.** Inflammatory bowel disease, sarcoidosis, and granulomatous hepatitis may cause prolonged fever. Factitious fever and drug fever should also be considered.

III **APPROACH TO THE PATIENT.** Because the cause of an FUO is elusive (by definition), there is a tendency to try to "net the diagnosis" by ordering every test under the sun. Proceeding in a logical, stepwise fashion will decrease the number of tests your patient must undergo, the cost of the total work-up, and the incidence of false-positive results. Before delving into an extensive evaluation, rule out factitious (patient-induced) fever by observing the elevated temperature reading yourself.

A. Go where the money is! The best bet for making a diagnosis is pursuing any symptoms, signs, or abnormal laboratory test results that present along with the fever. Make sure to always go down the list of possibilities from head to toe as outlined in Chapter 48. For example:

1. **Persistent headaches with a normal cerebrospinal fluid analysis.** A computed tomography (CT) scan or magnetic resonance imaging (MRI) may be indicated to rule out an intracranial abscess or sinusitis.

2. **Cardiac murmurs** associated **with negative blood cultures** may be evaluated with echocardiography (transthoracic or transesophageal).

3. **Hemoptysis** or **chronic cough** in the presence of an unremarkable chest radiograph may be further evaluated with a chest CT scan or bronchoscopy.

4. **Hematuria** may prompt an intravenous pyelogram or ultrasound to evaluate the possibility of renal carcinoma.

5. **Lymphadenopathy** may be evaluated by biopsy.

6. **Bone pain** can be pursued with radiographs and a bone scan.

7. **Cytopenias** can be evaluated by bone marrow biopsy.

HOT KEY

In HIV-infected patients, you can use the **CD4 count** to help predict the disease processes a patient is likely to have (see Chapter 55). Mycobacterium avium complex infections and CMV infections are common causes of FUO in AIDS patients with low CD4 counts (less than 100 cells/μl).

B. Diagnostic studies
   1. **Initial considerations**
      a. **Abdominal and pelvic CT scan.** There is no better place for an infection (e.g., an abscess) or malignancy (e.g., liver or renal carcinoma) to hide than in the abdomen or pelvis; therefore, performing this test early in the diagnostic work-up may be valuable.
      b. **Chest CT.** Although occult pulmonary infection is less common than occult abdominal abscess, unexpected findings (including infiltrates, cavitation, and lymphadenopathy) may lead to the diagnosis.

c. Screens for tuberculosis, Epstein-Barr virus, and **syphilis** may be performed with a purified protein derivative (PPD) test, a heterophil antibody test, and a serum Venereal Disease Research Laboratory (VDRL) test, respectively.

d. Rheumatologic work-up. An antinuclear antibody (ANA) assay, rheumatoid factor assay, and an erythrocyte sedimentation rate (ESR) are often requested early in the evaluation. Any rashes that are purpuric should be biopsied to rule out vasculitis (see Chapter 76).

e. Other tests may be ordered based on epidemiologic exposures. For example:

(1) Thick and thin blood smears examined every 8 hours for 2–3 days are appropriate if the patient has traveled to areas where malaria is endemic.

HOT

KEY

Fever in a traveler should be considered malaria until proven otherwise.

---

(2) Stool for culture or **ova and parasite (O&P) examination** is also useful in patients with an appropriate travel history.

(3) Amebic titers can help evaluate chronic intestinal amebiasis in patients with a remote travel history because O&P stool examination is usually negative in patients with chronic disease.

(4) Toxoplasmosis titers are approximately 85% sensitive for end-organ toxoplasmosis.

(5) Specific serologies or **cultures** for brucellosis, leptospirosis, Lyme disease, Rocky Mountain spotted fever, and other spirochetal and rickettsial diseases may be sent, depending on the geographic region, exposures to animals or the outdoors, and the clinical presentation.

(6) *Mycobacterium avium* **complex** blood cultures may be performed in HIV-positive patients with low CD4 counts.

2. Secondary considerations

a. Radionuclide studies

(1) Gallium scans, indium-labeled white blood cell (WBC) scans, and PET scans are often used when no etiology has been found. These tests are limited by low specificity.

(2) Bone scans may be performed to rule out osteomyelitis and primary or metastatic malignancies of bone.

b. Invasive tests

    (1) Bone marrow biopsies are generally of low diagnostic yield, but are low-risk and are often performed when the diagnosis is still in question.

    (2) Liver biopsies have a higher yield in patients with abnormal liver tests.

    (3) Endoscopy (upper and lower) should be performed earlier in the work-up if there are any gastrointestinal symptoms, signs, or suggestive laboratory abnormalities (e.g., a positive fecal occult blood test, iron deficiency anemia).

    (4) Temporal artery biopsy may be revealing in elderly patients with FUO, even in the absence of localizing symptoms.

    (5) Bronchoscopy should be performed in patients with suggestive abnormalities on chest radiograph, chest CT, or by symptoms. In HIV-infected patients, bronchoscopy should be pursued as part of the standard work-up of FUO even in the asymptomatic patient.

    (6) Exploratory laparotomy in the absence of abnormal findings on imaging studies no longer plays a significant role in the evaluation of FUO.

References

Armstrong WS, Katz JT, Kazanjian PH. Human immunodeficiency virus-associated fever of unknown origin: a study of 70 patients in the United States and review. Clin Infect Dis 1999;28:341–345.

Cunha BA. Fever of unknown origin. Infect Dis Clin North Am 1996;10:111–127.

Hirschmann JV. Fever of unknown origin in adults. Clin Infect Dis 1997;24:291–300

Petersdorf RO, Beeson PB. Fever of unexplained origin: report on 100 cases. Medicine (Baltimore) 1961;40:1–30. (classic article)

52. Skin and Soft Tissue Infections

I. INTRODUCTION

A. The **severity** of skin and soft tissue infections **can vary from insignificant to life-threatening** and is determined by both the causative organism and the depth of tissue involvement.

B. **Cellulitis** and **animal bites** are common reasons for emergency department visits and hospital stays.

C. **Pyomyositis** and **necrotizing fasciitis** are two clinical entities that may be difficult to distinguish from cellulitis but require different therapies. Necrotizing fasciitis is associated with a high mortality.

II. CELLULITIS

A. Definition. Cellulitis is an **infection of the dermal and subcutaneous tissues,** including the deep dermis and fat.

B. Clinical manifestations. Patients are often febrile and complain of pain at the affected site. On physical examination, erythema, warmth, tenderness, and edema are notable.

C. Microbiology. The most common etiologic agents are *Staphylococcus aureus* and **streptococcal species,** most commonly group A streptococcus. In specific settings, other organisms may cause cellulitis, including gram-negative bacilli and anaerobes.

D. Approach to the patient. Several historical features may provide important clues about the etiology of disease and may lead the physician to broaden empiric therapy or to watch for serious manifestations.

  1. Has any trauma occurred in the involved area? Injections (diabetics requiring insulin, intravenous drug users) and skin tears can provide routes of entry for bacteria.

  2. Has the involved area been exposed to soil or fresh or salt water? Soil exposure may increase the risk of anaerobes or gram-negative infections. Water exposure increases the risk of infection with organisms such as *Aeromonas hydrophila* or *Vibrio vulnificus.*

  3. Does the patient have any comorbid conditions? Underlying diabetes or neoplasm may increase the risk of group B streptococcal infection. Patients with cirrhosis are at increased risk of *V. vulnificus* infection after salt water exposure or eating raw shellfish.

4. **Is the cellulitis adjacent to a surgical wound or a diabetic foot ulcer?** Both these circumstances increase the risk of infection with gram-negative organisms or resistant gram-positive organisms (e.g., methicillin-resistant *S. aureus*).

5. **Did the cellulitis start in an area of an animal bite** (see III)?

6. **Does the patient's pain seem out of proportion to the examination? Is the area of cellulitis spreading over minutes to hours? Is there crepitus, or are there bullous lesions?** A positive answer to any of these questions should lead the physician to consider more serious diagnoses that require more aggressive intervention (see V).

7. **Is the border of the lesion raised and well-demarcated? Is the involved area significantly edematous and indurated?** The presence of these findings likely indicate **erysipelas,** which is actually a more superficial infection than cellulitis. Erysipelas is almost always caused by group A streptococci.

E. **Treatment**
1. **In the absence of several of the risk factors** discussed in II D (e.g., animal bite, surgical wound, presence of underlying diabetes mellitus or malignancy, contamination of the site with soil or environmental water), narrow coverage with an agent that covers streptococcal and staphylococcal species is preferred. Reasonable intravenous choices include nafcillin or cefazolin; good oral choices include cephalexin or dicloxacillin.

2. **If cellulitis is associated with a surgical wound,** vancomycin may be a more appropriate initial choice. Gram-negative coverage should be tailored to the appropriate organisms based on historical exposures.

III ANIMAL BITES

A. **Epidemiology.** Animal bites are a common reason for emergency department visits. Patients often present acutely, within hours of the bite, or later after cellulitis or deeper infections have developed.

B. **Microbiology.** Infections due to bites from dogs and cats most often are caused by *S. aureus,* streptococcal species, gram-positive anaerobes, and *Pasteurella multocida*. Less common organisms include *Capnocytophaga canimorsus,* which causes fulminant disease in patients with liver disease or splenectomy; *Francisella tularensis* (tularemia); and rabies virus.

C. **Approach to the patient**
1. **Determine the history of the bite**

a. **What type of animal was it? Was the bite unprovoked?** The first responsibility of the treating physician is to determine whether the patient needs **rabies prophylaxis.** Rabies is uncommon in the United States, but it is fatal without appropriate prophylaxis. Bats and raccoons are known to harbor the rabies virus. Domesticated dogs are not a common source of the virus, but an unprovoked attack should lead to observation of the animal and consideration of prophylaxis.

b. **How rapidly have symptoms developed after the bite?** Rapidly progressive cellulitis should lead to consideration of *P. multocida* infection.

c. **Was the bite a cat bite and was it near a joint?** Cat bites can leave deep puncture wounds, which appear unimpressive but can inoculate organisms deep into a joint or tendon sheath, leading to septic arthritis, osteomyelitis, or tenosynovitis. Examination should be performed carefully to consider these complications, and patients with cat bites should be followed closely and treated aggressively.

2. **Culture the wound** if possible.

D. **Treatment.** In non-penicillin-allergic patients, the **treatment of choice is ampicillin/sulbactam** or **amoxacillin/clavulanate.** Ciprofloxacin plus clindamycin may be considered in the penicillin-allergic patient.

IV PYOMYOSITIS

A. **Definition.** Pyomyositis is a bacterial infection of the muscle, which can mimic cellulitis.

B. **Epidemiology.** In the United States, pyomyositis occurs most often in immunocompromised patients (patients with diabetes or cirrhosis, individuals taking corticosteroids) and those with local trauma (intravenous drug users).

C. **Microbiology.** The most common etiology is *S. aureus.* Streptococci and gram-negative bacilli are much less common.

D. **Approach to the patient.** Typically, the onset is subacute. Pyomyositis progresses to a febrile illness with pain, erythema, and fluctuance at the involved site.

1. Pyomyositis should be considered in the differential diagnosis in patients with the following conditions:
   a. Risk factors (e.g., patients receiving systemic corticosteroids, presence of diabetes mellitus or cirrhosis, intravenous drug use HIV infection)
   b. Slowly resolving cellulitis despite usual treatment
   c. "Cellulitis" in a less typical location (e.g., thigh) or with more induration or fluctuance than expected

2. Magnetic resonance imaging (MRI) or computed tomography (CT) of the affected area can aid in diagnosis.

E. Treatment. Adequate therapy requires both antistaphylococcal antimicrobial therapy (e.g., nafcillin) and adequate drainage (e.g., percutaneous aspiration or open surgical drainage).

V NECROTIZING FASCIITIS

> **HOT** Necrotizing fasciitis is a **true clinical emergency** and has a mortality rate of 30%. Differentiation of necrotizing fasciitis from cellulitis in the early stages requires an astute clinician and **KEY** close follow-up.

A. Definition. Necrotizing fasciitis is a necrotizing cellulitis that involves the superficial fascia and subcutaneous tissues.

B. Epidemiology. Patients at increased risk include those with diabetes or alcoholism, with immunosuppressed status, or with peripheral vascular disease.

C. Clinical manifestations
   1. There is often a **preexisting history of trauma,** including recent surgery, but the insult may be minor (e.g., a small cut or site of injection).
   2. The **most common involved areas** are the **extremities, perineum,** and **abdominal wall.**
   3. **Spread of infection is rapid.** The initial stages are notable for **pain out of proportion to the examination,** with minimal or absent skin changes. Over hours to days, **loss of sensation can occur** due to tissue ischemia and nerve destruction. Erythema, edema, cyanosis, and bullous formation may develop. **Crepitus** (subcutaneous gas) is an ominous sign. Patients are ill-appearing, with high fevers, and become hemodynamically unstable.

D. Microbiology. Two primary types of necrotizing fasciitis have been described. The first is **polymicrobial** and may involve gram-positive and gram-negative organisms, including anaerobes. The second is caused by **group A streptococci.**

E. Approach to the patient
   1. **Diagnosis of this condition in the early stages is difficult.** Serial clinical examinations are necessary in patients who appear to have cellulitis with atypical features (**too much pain, too high a fever, bullous lesions, hemodynamic instability**) and in those with **underlying immunosuppressive conditions** (diabetes, alcohol abuse, end-stage renal disease) or **recent trauma.** Marking the involved area with a pen is helpful to gauge progression over time.
   2. **CT or MRI may be helpful** but should be reserved for stable patients. The diagnosis should be confirmed in the operating room in acutely ill patients.

HOT KEY

If a diagnosis of necrotizing fasciitis is seriously being considered, it is never too early to ask for a surgical evaluation.

F. Treatment. Adequate therapy combines urgent **surgical debridement with antimicrobial therapy.** Blood cultures and surgical wound cultures can help guide therapy. Antimicrobial therapy should be broad and include anaerobic coverage until the etiologic organisms are identified. Many clinicians favor including clindamycin in the regimen because its mechanism (protein synthesis inhibition) leads to inhibition of bacterial toxin synthesis.

References

Bisno AL, Stevens DL. Streptococcal infections of skin and soft tissues. N Engl J Med 1996;334:240–245.

Christin L, Sarosi GA. Pyomyositis in North America: case reports and review. Clin Infect Dis 1992;15:668–677.

Green RJ, Dafoe DC, Raffin TA. Necrotizing fasciitis. Chest 1996;110:219–229.

53. Acute Rheumatic Fever

I INTRODUCTION

A. Definition. Acute rheumatic fever is a systemic, immune-mediated disorder that occurs as a **sequela** to **group A streptococcal pharyngeal infection.** (Skin infections are not associated with rheumatic fever.)

B. Epidemiology. Acute rheumatic fever most commonly occurs in school-age children, 1–5 weeks (mean, 19 days) after an acute throat infection.

1. Acute rheumatic fever rarely occurs in patients younger than 5 years of age or older than 40 years of age.
2. It is uncommon in the United States but can be seen in recent immigrants.

C. Rheumatic fever **"bites the heart and licks the joints"** [i.e., chronic arthritis is not a sequela of rheumatic fever, but valve disease and congestive heart failure (CHF) can be]. The incidence of valve involvement varies depending on the valve.

1. The **mitral valve** is affected in the **majority** of cases.
2. The **aortic valve** is affected in **less than half** of cases (but almost never as the sole valve).
3. The **tricuspid** and **pulmonary valves** are affected in **less than 5%** of cases, usually in association with mitral valve involvement.

II DIAGNOSIS

A. Jones criteria. Diagnosis of rheumatic fever is based on evidence of a preceding streptococcal pharyngitis [e.g., a positive anti-streptolysin O (ASO) titer or culture], plus two major Jones criteria or one major and two minor Jones criteria.

1. **Major**
   a. **Arthritis.** The arthritis takes the form of a migratory polyarthritis that tends to involve the large joints sequentially; however, adults may have only single joint involvement. Arthritis resolves spontaneously within 1 month, and there are no residual joint deformities.
   b. **Heart involvement.** Evidence of carditis includes pericarditis, myocarditis, cardiomegaly, congestive heart failure, and mitral or aortic regurgitation.
   c. **Nodules.** Small, firm, nontender subcutaneous nodules occur over areas of bony prominence and over tendons. Nodules are rarely seen in adults.

d. **Erythema marginatum** is the classic rash seen in less than 10% of cases. It is erythematous and nonpruritic. Individual lesions are evanescent with a serpiginous border.

e. **Sydenham's chorea (St. Vitus' dance)**—the most diagnostic of the major criteria—is characterized by involuntary choreoathetoid movements of the face, hands, and feet.

Major Jones Criteria ("J♥NES")

Joints (arthritis)
♥ **I**nvolvement
Nodules
Erythema marginatum
Sydenham's chorea

2. **Minor**
   a. **Prolongation of the PR interval** on the electrocardiogram (ECG)
   b. **Increased erythrocyte sedimentation rate (ESR) and/or C-reactive protein (CRP)**
   c. **Fever**
   d. **Polyarthralgias**
   e. **Supporting evidence of antecedent group A streptococcal infection** including either a positive throat culture or rapid antigen test or an elevated or rising streptococcal antibody titer

B. **Clinical presentation.** Rheumatic fever usually presents in one of three ways:
   1. **Insidious carditis**
   2. **Acute-onset polyarthritis**
   3. **Chorea** (least common)

III TREATMENT

A. **Bed rest.** The patient should be confined to bed until the fever, tachycardia, and ECG changes resolve.

B. **High-dose salicylates** will rapidly decrease fever and joint swelling, but do not affect the natural course of the illness. If salicylates do not provide symptomatic relief, steroids should be considered.

C. **Antibiotics**
   1. **Prophylactic** antibiotics are recommended to prevent further streptococcal infections. The preferred regimen remains IM penicillin every 4 weeks and should be continued

for a minimum of 5 years after the last episode *and* until the patient is in his or her mid-20s.

References

Bisno AL. Group A streptococcal infections and acute rheumatic fever. N Engl J Med 1991;325:783–793.

Stollerman GH. Rheumatic fever. Lancet 1997;349:935–942.

Thatai D, Turi ZG. Current guidelines for the treatment of patients with rheumatic fever. Drugs 1999;57:545–555.

54. Infective Endocarditis

I INTRODUCTION

A. Once uniformly fatal, infective endocarditis (IE) continues to cause significant morbidity and mortality in the post-antibiotic era. Early diagnosis by an astute clinician and proper therapy can improve outcomes substantially.

B. Before the availability of effective antibiotics, IE was classified as acute or subacute based on the organism and the clinical course. Today these distinctions are less meaningful.

C. Certain subgroups of patients are at increased risk of IE development and should be evaluated carefully for evidence of disease. They include (1) persons with valvular abnormalities, including congenital bicuspid aortic valves and those with a history of rheumatic fever, (2) patients with prosthetic valves, and (3) intravenous drug users.

II CAUSES OF INFECTIVE ENDOCARDITIS

A. Streptococci. Viridans streptococci (*Streptococcus salivarius, Streptococcus sanguis, Streptococcus mitis/mitior,* and *Streptococcus milleri*) remain the most common cause of IE. However, in recent years, staphylococcal species are increasing in importance. Other streptococcal species including **enterococci,** *S. bovis* (nonenterococcal group D streptococci), and occasionally *S. pneumoniae* are important causes of IE as well.

B. Staphylococci. IE caused by *Staphylococcus aureus* and *Staphylococcus epidermidis* has increased in frequency and now is nearly as common as viridans streptococcal endocarditis. *S. aureus* is the most frequent cause of IE in those with a history of intravenous drug use and is an important cause of nosocomial endocarditis. *S. epidermidis* is the most common bacteria isolated in cases of prosthetic valve endocarditis.

C. Gram-negative bacteria can cause endocarditis, usually in association with genitourinary or gastrointestinal procedures, surgery, or intravascular catheters.

D. Fungi. Fungal endocarditis has a poorer prognosis than bacterial IE and is associated with injection drug use, long-term antimicrobial therapy, and chronic hyperalimentation therapy. Candida spp. account for the majority of cases of fungal IE.

E. Culture-negative endocarditis is most frequently encountered in patients who have received prior antibiotics leading to sterile blood cultures. Certain organisms may be difficult to detect in routine culture systems, however. These include:

1. **HACEK group organisms.** *Haemophilus, Actinobacillus, Cardiobacterium, Eikenella,* and *Kingella* are gram-negative organisms that often grow slowly over weeks; therefore, ask the laboratory to save the blood cultures for a prolonged period if culture-negative endocarditis is suspected.
2. **Nutritionally variant streptococcal species (now known as Abiotrophia spp.)** require specific media supplementation for growth.
3. **Fungi.** Large vegetations are often found in patients with endocarditis associated with fungal infection. An intravascular source is frequently noted (e.g., an indwelling intravenous catheter). Candida species are easily isolated in routine cultures; however, Aspergillus is almost never recovered from cultures. Other rare fungal causes of IE, including *Histoplasma capsulatum,* may require special fungal cultures (lysiscentrifugation system).
4. **Legionella, Brucella species, Coxiella burnetii** (Q fever), *Bartonella henselae* (cat scratch disease), and **chlamydia species** (including *Chlamydia psittaci*) are rare causes of culture-negative endocarditis.

III **CLINICAL MANIFESTATIONS OF INFECTIVE ENDO-CARDITIS.** The clinical manifestations of endocarditis are variable, but most closely depend on which organism is involved and whether the patient has left-sided (aortic or mitral) or right-sided (usually tricuspid) disease.

A. **Fever** occurs in almost all patients; however, elderly patients, patients with congestive heart failure or renal failure, and patients taking steroids or nonsteroidal anti-inflammatory drugs (NSAIDs) may be afebrile. Other systemic symptoms such as **anorexia** and **malaise** are common.
B. **Murmurs.** Although a cardiac murmur is a classic sign of endocarditis, a murmur may be absent in as many as 15% of patients, and a new or changing murmur is present in only 3–5% and 5–10% of patients, respectively.
C. **Low back pain, arthralgias,** and **myalgias** are very common and may be the patient's presenting symptoms.
D. **Splenomegaly** may be seen in one-quarter to one-half of patients.
E. **Classic findings,** including **Osler's nodes, Janeway lesions, Roth spots** (retinal hemorrhages), **petechiae of the palate or conjunctivae,** and **subungual splinter hemorrhages** are often not found, probably because of early treatment of disease in the antimicrobial era.

HOT KEY Although Osler's nodes are typically violaceous nodules located on the pads of the fingers or toes and Janeway lesions are typically erythematous and found on the palms or soles, the predominant distinction between the two is that **Osler's nodes are painful,** whereas **Janeway lesions are painless.**

IV COMPLICATIONS OF INFECTIVE ENDOCARDITIS

A. **Congestive heart failure (CHF).** Pulmonary edema and hypotension may occur with significant left-sided (aortic and mitral) valve dysfunction, whereas peripheral edema may result from right-sided (tricuspid) disease.

B. **Myocardial abscess formation** can lead to bundle branch block (aortic valve abscesses) or heart block (mitral valve abscesses). Perivalvular abscesses are common in patients with prosthetic valve endocarditis.

C. **Emboli.** Left-sided endocarditis may result in visceral infarcts, including splenic, hepatic, renal, central nervous system, and mesenteric infarcts as well as cutaneous infarcts. Right-sided endocarditis may cause septic pulmonary emboli with pulmonary infarction, abscess formation, or both.

D. **Hematogenous seeding** of other sites may occur, including bone (vertebral osteomyelitis), joint (septic arthritis), and other vessels (mycotic aneurysms).

V APPROACH TO THE PATIENT

A. **Patient history**
1. IE is a diagnosis that is often missed; therefore, always make sure to include endocarditis in the "head to toe" approach to fever (see Chapter 48).
2. Be sure to ask the patient about risk factors for endocarditis (i.e., IVDU, known valvular disease, recent procedures or surgery).

B. **Physical examination.** In addition to performing a complete physical examination, pay special attention to the:
1. **Funduscopic examination** (to search for Roth spots)
2. **Cardiovascular examination** (to detect murmurs or evidence of CHF)
3. **Skin and mucous membrane examination** (to search for Osler's nodes, Janeway lesions, splinter hemorrhages, and conjunctival or palatal petechiae)
4. **Bone and joint examination** (to detect septic joints or osteomyelitis)

C. **Laboratory studies.** Patients who have an unexplained fever, a low clinical probability of endocarditis, and are conscientious concerning follow-up can sometimes be evaluated as outpatients. Patients with fever and a prosthetic valve, history of intravenous drug use, or examination findings concerning for endocarditis and no obvious alternative source of infection are almost always admitted to rule out endocarditis.

1. **Blood cultures** are the **gold standard** for diagnosis. **A minimum of two sets** of aerobic and anaerobic cultures are usually obtained; however, three sets may increase the sensitivity to greater than 90%.

   a. Different venous sites are usually used to avoid confounding skin contamination.

   b. Cultures should always be taken before initiating empiric antibacterial therapy.

2. **Urinalysis.** Abnormal urinalysis findings are common in endocarditis. Hematuria or proteinuria are common; red blood cell casts suggestive of glomerulonephritis should be sought.

3. **Echocardiography.** Because the duration of therapy may differ depending on which side of the heart (left or right) is involved, echocardiography is often performed to define which valve is infected and to identify complications of disease such as myocardial abscesses. Transthoracic echocardiography is often performed first, followed by transesophageal echocardiography in cases in which the diagnosis is still in question; however, the cost-effectiveness of this approach is unclear.

   a. **Transthoracic echocardiography (TTE),** with a sensitivity of approximately 60%, is not sensitive enough to rule out endocarditis. In addition, TTE is notoriously poor for ruling out mitral valve disease and evaluating prosthetic valves.

   b. **Transesophageal echocardiography (TEE)** increases the sensitivity to approximately 95% and is significantly better for evaluating the mitral valve.

VI TREATMENT

A. **Empiric therapy.** Empiric therapy should be initiated only when the patient appears unstable or acutely ill. Patients with stable symptoms for days to weeks should be watched carefully while not taking antibiotics until a causative agent is discovered. Ill patients should receive vancomycin and gentamicin pending cultures. Penicillin and gentamicin is an appropriate empiric regimen in patients suspected of having viridans streptococcal endocarditis, but often these patients are not acutely ill and the diagnosis can be made with blood culture data before urgently starting therapy.

**HOT
KEY**

The benefits of added gentamicin include the following:
- Synergy against *S. aureus*, which decreases the duration of bacteremia
- Broader coverage against gram-negative and multi-organism infections, an important advantage in intravenous drug users.

1. **Suspected prosthetic valve endocarditis** may be treated with vancomycin, rifampin, and an aminoglycoside. This regimen will cover methicillin-resistant *S. epidermidis* (a common offender) while treating possible enterococcal infection as well.

B. Organism-specific therapy. The duration of therapy may vary depending on the causative organism, the severity of the illness, and whether disease is right- or left-sided.

1. **Streptococcal viridans infections** are usually treated with penicillin or ceftriaxone with or without an aminoglycoside. Therapy most commonly lasts for 4 weeks.

2. **Enterococcal infections** usually require prolonged combination therapy and are often treated with ampicillin or vancomycin and an aminoglycoside for 4–6 weeks.

3. **Staphylococcal infections**
   a. **Methicillin-sensitive *S. aureus* (MSSA) infections** may be treated with nafcillin or oxacillin.
   b. **Methicillin-resistant *S. aureus* (MRSA) infections** may be treated with vancomycin.
   c. **Prosthetic valve staphylococcal infections** should be treated with combination therapy with rifampin and 2 weeks of an aminoglycoside in addition to the above agents when possible.

C. Surgery. Valve replacement is often indicated when:

1. Fungal infection is strongly suspected
2. A prosthetic valve is infected
3. Complications have developed (e.g., myocardial abscess, acute valvular dysfunction with refractory CHF)
4. Uncontrolled infection (inability to clear blood cultures)
5. The patient has experienced more than one embolic event

VII FOLLOW-UP

A. Frequent examinations are essential. Listen carefully for a new or changing murmur, look closely for embolic phenomena, and watch for widening of the pulse pressure (which should alert you to possible aortic regurgitation).

1. **Bilateral disease.** Although intravenous drug users more commonly have right-sided disease, they may also have left-

sided or bilateral endocarditis. You should therefore continue to assess possible left-sided involvement.
2. **Persistent fever.** Defervescence occurs within 1 week in 72% of patients. Prolonged fevers is an important prognostic sign. Drug reactions are the most common cause of persistent or recurrent fever, but myocardial and metastatic abscess formation should always be considered.
B. **Electrocardiograms (ECGs).** Lengthening of the PR interval or a new bundle branch block should prompt an echocardiogram to evaluate possible myocardial abscess formation (TEE is more sensitive). An ECG should be obtained on admission and often on a frequent basis thereafter.

References
Bayer AS. Infective endocarditis. Clin Infect Dis 1993;17:313–320.
Hermans PE. The clinical manifestations of infective endocarditis. Mayo Clin Proc 1982;57:15–21.
Wilson WR, Karchmer AW, Dajani AS, et al. Antibiotic treatment of adults with infective endocarditis due to streptococci, enterococci, staphylococci and HACEK microorganisms. JAMA 1995;274:1706–1713.

55. CD4 Counts and Complications of HIV Infection

I **INTRODUCTION** In human immunodeficiency virus (HIV)-positive patients, a physician must consider many different possible diagnoses when the patient presents with a new symptom. These diagnoses include causes of disease present in nonimmunocompromised patients as well as those opportunistic infections and malignancies that present more frequently in patients with HIV. Furthermore, HIV-infected patients may present with protean symptoms such as fever and weight loss instead of classic manifestations of disease that may be produced by a vigorous inflammatory response. The list of possible diagnoses can often be simplified because patients infected with HIV acquire opportunistic infections and malignancies at relatively predictable CD4 counts. Therefore, a recent CD4 count may help you exclude etiologies of disease more likely at greater degrees of immunosuppression. Remember, however, that patients with very low CD4 counts may get any of the conditions noted as occurring at any higher CD4 count.

HOT **KEY** Remember that a CD4 count obtained during an acute illness may be falsely low or falsely high. It is therefore best to use the most recent CD4 count before the development of acute illness if available.

II **DIFFERENTIAL DIAGNOSES ACCORDING TO CD4 COUNT.** CD4 counts should only be used as a general guide because there is a great deal of variability among patients. Common diseases that occur as the CD4 count falls are discussed here.

A. **CD4 count > 200 cells/μl**
  1. **Bacterial infection.** Pneumococcal pneumonias are common.
  2. **Pulmonary tuberculosis.** Both primary tuberculosis and reactivation disease can be seen at relatively high CD4 counts. As CD4 counts drop below 200 cells/μl, less common manifestations such as extrapulmonary tuberculosis and miliary

tuberculosis are encountered more frequently. Extrapulmonary sites may include the central nervous system (CNS), peritoneum, lymph nodes, pleura, and bone and joints.
3. **Lymphoma.** B-cell lymphomas are more common in HIV-infected patients at any CD4 count, and diagnosis of B-cell lymphoma in any individual should prompt HIV testing even in the absence of known risk factors. In patients with CD4 counts in this range, lymphomas are systemic, not the primary CNS lymphomas that occur with lower counts.
4. **Kaposi's sarcoma.** Patients may have pulmonary and gastrointestinal involvement as well as the typical cutaneous lesions.
5. **Herpes zoster.** Herpes zoster may present with a multidermatomal or single dermatome distribution.
6. **Candidiasis**
   a. **Oral and vaginal candidiasis** and **esophagitis** are very common.
   b. **Disseminated disease** is more likely in patients with neutropenia or intravascular catheters, or in those taking broad-spectrum antibiotics.
B. **CD4 count < 200 cells/μl**
   1. *Pneumocystis carinii* **pneumonia** (see Chapter 56)
   2. *Cryptococcus* **infection** is a common cause of meningitis.
   3. **Coccidioidomycosis** may be manifested as pneumonia, meningitis, or skin and soft tissue infection.
   4. **Histoplasmosis** can cause pulmonary disease or disseminate with pulmonary, hepatic, bone marrow, and CNS involvement as well as fungemia.
   5. **Extrapulmonary or miliary tuberculosis.** See A 2 above.
   6. **Progressive multifocal leukoencephalopathy (PML).** Caused by JC virus, PML can lead to focal neurologic deficits (see Chapter 58).
C. **CD4 count < 100 cells/μl**
   1. **Toxoplasmosis** often manifests with CNS disease (see Chapter 58)
   2. **Cryptococcosis** most commonly causes meningitis, but patients may have pulmonary or cutaneous disease as well.
   3. **Candida esophagitis.** Although other manifestations of candidiasis may present at higher CD4 counts, esophagitis tends to be seen in patients with more impaired immunity.
D. **CD4 count < 50 cells/μl**
   1. **Disseminated *Mycobacterium avium* complex (MAC) infection** usually causes fever, cytopenias, and cachexia.
   2. **Cytomegalovirus (CMV) infection.** Retinitis, esophagitis, colitis, AIDS cholangiopathy, and polyradiculopathy may all be seen with CMV infection.
   3. **Primary CNS lymphoma** (see Chapter 58)

Reference

http://hopkins-aids.edu. This website is maintained by Johns Hopkins University and includes a PDF version of their book, "The Abbreviated Guide to Medical Management of HIV Infection" by John G Bartlett, MD. This and the full version ("Medical Management of HIV Infection") are valuable and up-to-date resources about HIV infection.

56. Pulmonary Disease in HIV-Infected Patients

I **INTRODUCTION.** At least two-thirds of patients with HIV have symptomatic pulmonary disease at some time during their lives. One way to approach respiratory complaints in HIV-infected patients is to:

A. Consider the organisms that can cause disease based on the patient's **CD4 count** (see Chapter 55).

B. Narrow the list of possible diagnoses by considering the appearance of the **chest radiograph** (Table 56-1). These patterns are not mutually exclusive, and each pattern can be caused by many disorders. When it comes to HIV disease, there are few absolute truths—use Table 56-1 as a starting point and modify it based on your clinical experience.

C. Further narrow the list based on the **clinical picture, laboratory data,** and results of **diagnostic testing.**

II **DIFFERENTIAL DIAGNOSIS OF PULMONARY INFILTRATES IN HIV**

A. Bacterial. Bacterial pathogens remain the most likely cause of pneumonia in HIV-infected patients. Pneumonia due to *Streptococcus pneumoniae* is most common. Remember that *Haemophilus influenzae,* gram-negative bacilli (including Pseudomonas, particularly in late-stage HIV), Legionella species, and Nocardia can also be seen.

B. Mycobacterial. Tuberculosis and nontuberculous mycobacteria such as *M. kansasii* are not uncommon. *Mycobacterium avium* complex frequently colonizes sputum but is rarely viewed as a pathogen.

C. Fungal. Cryptococcosis, histoplasmosis, and aspergillosis all may present with pulmonary manifestations in HIV-infected patients.

D. Viral. The respiratory viruses including influenza, adenovirus, and respiratory syncytial virus must be remembered. A nasal swab for antigen testing can provide evidence of infection.

E. *Pneumocystis carinii.* See III.

F. Noninfectious. Both lymphoma and Kaposi's sarcoma may cause pulmonary disease.

TABLE 56-1: Radiographic Patterns in HIV-Associated Pulmonary Disease

Radiographic Pattern	Common Disease
Normal	Pneumocystis Carinii pneumonia (PCP)
Diffuse interstitial infiltrates	PCP
	Disseminated fungal infection
	Tuberculosis
	Kaposi's sarcoma*
	Congestive heart failure (CHF)
	Viral and atypical pneumonia
Focal consolidation	Bacterial pneumonia
	Kaposi's sarcoma
	Tuberculosis
Pleural effusion	Tuberculosis
	Lymphoma
	Bacterial pneumonia
	Kaposi's sarcoma
	CHF
	Disseminated fungal infection

*Usually patchy infiltrates.

III APPROACH TO THE HIV-INFECTED PATIENT WITH POSSIBLE PCP Whenever a patient with HIV disease presents with respiratory complaints, the diagnosis of *Pneumocystis carinii* pneumonia (PCP) should always be considered because *P. carinii* is an extremely common pathogen.

A. The following questions are important to ask when considering PCP as a possible diagnosis:
   1. What is the **CD4 count**? The CD4 count will indicate the patient's risk for PCP; those with CD4 counts > 200 cells/μl are at much less risk.
   2. Is the patient receiving **PCP prophylaxis**? Compliant patients taking trimethoprim-sulfamethoxole or dapsone are less likely to have PCP.
   3. What is the **clinical scenario**? Patients with PCP usually present with a subacute onset of shortness of breath (especially on exertion) that is associated with fever, fatigue, weight loss, and a dry cough. Community-acquired pneumonia, on the other hand, usually presents with the acute onset

of a productive cough, fever, and evidence of consolidation on lung examination.

4. Does the physical examination reveal **evidence of a different disorder (e.g., tuberculosis, lymphoma, or Kaposi's sarcoma)?**

5. Does the chest radiograph reveal **diffuse interstitial infiltrates?** Diffuse interstitial infiltrates are the classic finding; patients may, however, present with minimal changes or atypical findings (e.g., pleural effusions, pneumothorax).

HOT KEY The radiographic appearance of the lung fields often looks much worse than predicted by auscultation in patients with PCP; however, a normal chest radiograph does not exclude PCP.

---

6. What is the patient's **alveolar-to-arterial (A-a) gradient?** The blood gas report allows definition of the degree of hypoxemia as well as evaluation for the necessity of steroid therapy in patients with PCP. (Patients with an A-a gradient > 35 usually benefit when treated with corticosteroids.)

HOT KEY Oxygen saturation monitoring can be very useful. Patients who exhibit dramatic desaturation on ambulation may have PCP.

---

7. Is the **sputum purulent?** Finding *P. carinii* organisms is extremely difficult in purulent sputum. On the other hand, culturing sputum for routine pathogens and AFB organisms may be diagnostic.

B. **There are many ways to evaluate patients for the possibility of PCP.** The algorithm in Figure 56–1 is one approach; it should be modified based on the sensitivity and specificity of the various tests available at your institution.

C. **Treatment.** First-line therapy for PCP in nonallergic patients is intravenous trimethoprim-sulfamethoxazole 5 mg/kg IV every 8 hours. If the A-a gradient is > 35, corticosteroids (e.g., prednisone) should be added. The usual dose is 40 mg twice daily for 5 days followed by 40 mg once daily for 5 days, then a taper to zero over the ensuing 11 days. Treatment of PCP should be continued for 21 days. Patients may be switched to oral therapy once defervescence occurs and the patient is no longer hypoxic on ambulation at room air. Stable, reliable patients who are not initially hypoxic may receive their entire course of therapy orally. TMP-

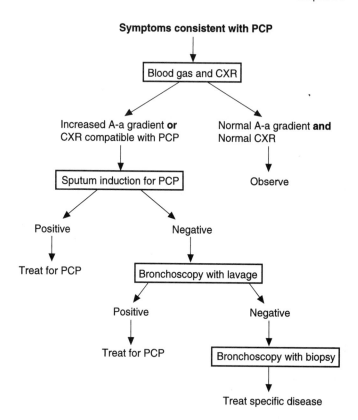

FIGURE 56-1. Algorithm for the assessment of patients with suspected *Pneumocystis carinii* pneumonia (*PCP*). *A-a gradient* = alveolar-to-arterial gradient; *CXR* = chest radiograph.

SMX 2 DS tablets orally 3 times/day is recommended. Options for TMP-SMX-intolerant patients include intravenous pentamidine, dapsone plus trimethoprim, or clindamycin plus primaquine.

References

Bartlett JG. Pneumonia in the patient with HIV infection. Infect Dis Clin North Am 1998;12:807–820.

Meduri GU, Stein DS. Pulmonary manifestations of acquired immunodeficiency syndrome. Clin Infect Dis 1992;14:98–113.

Seminars in Respiratory Infections. 1998;13. (Issue devoted to *Pneumocystis carinii* pneumonia; articles on diagnosis, treatment, and prophylaxis.)

57. Gastrointestinal Manifestations of HIV Disease

I **INTRODUCTION.** More than 50% of HIV-infected patients develop a gastrointestinal illness during the course of their disease. Esophagitis, enterocolitis, and hepatobiliary disease are commonly seen.

II **ESOPHAGITIS** usually presents with dysphagia, odynophagia, or a substernal sensation of pain or burning.

A. **Causes of HIV-related esophagitis.** Common causes include the following:
   1. **Infectious**
      a. *Candida*
      b. Cytomegalovirus (CMV)
      c. Herpes simplex virus (HSV)
   2. **Noninfectious**
      a. Aphthous ulcers
      b. Pill-induced
B. **Approach to the patient**
   1. **Empiric antifungal therapy.** Patients with symptoms of esophagitis and oral thrush are usually treated empirically for candidal esophagitis. **Fluconazole** (often 200 mg orally once daily) may be administered for 2–3 weeks. A rapid improvement in symptoms is expected. Failure to improve should lead to further testing.
   2. **Upper endoscopy** is usually indicated for patients without oral thrush and for those who are unresponsive to empiric antifungal therapy. Abnormal areas on endoscopy should be biopsied and sent for pathology as well as viral and fungal cultures. Viral and fungal esophagitis can coexist. Aphthous ulcers are an important consideration in those with negative cultures and pathology.
C. **Treatment**
   1. **Fungal esophagitis**
      a. **Fluconazole** is usually the first-line treatment, unless fluconazole-resistant Candida is suspected. **Intravenous amphotericin** (0.1–0.3 mg/kg/day) may be necessary in pa-

tients with resistant species. Itraconazole and amphotericin solution are also options.
  b. **Maintenance therapy** may be given as one-half of the
     treatment dose (e.g., fluconazole 100 mg once daily).
  2. **Viral esophagitis**
     a. **CMV esophagitis** is usually treated with **ganciclovir** (often
        5 mg/kg intravenously twice daily for 2–3 weeks). The
        maintenance dose is often 5 mg/kg intravenously daily.
        New oral agents (valganciclovir) also have a role in main-
        tenance therapy.
     b. **HSV esophagitis** is usually treated with **acyclovir.** Intra-
        venous therapy may be necessary in patients who are un-
        able to swallow and in those who are very ill (e.g., in pa-
        tients with esophageal bleeding or fevers).
  3. **Noninfectious esophagitis including aphthous ulcers** may be
     treated with **steroids** (often prednisone, 40 mg orally daily
     for 2 weeks followed by a taper) or **thalidomide.**

III **ENTEROCOLITIS.** More than 50% of HIV-positive patients
develop diarrhea at some time during their illness.
  A. **Causes of HIV-related enterocolitis**
     1. **Opportunistic infection**
        a. **Bacteria.** *Salmonella, Shigella, Yersinia, Escherichia coli,*
           and *Campylobacter* are common causes of acute diarrhea
           in HIV-positive patients. *Clostridium difficile* is an im-
           portant consideration even in patients without recent ex-
           posure to antibiotics.
        b. **Protozoa.** Commonly implicated organisms include *Ent-*
           amoeba histolytica, Giardia lamblia, Cryptosporidium,
           Microsporidia, and *Isospora belli.*
        c. **Viruses.** **CMV** and **adenovirus** are common causes of en-
           terocolitis in HIV-infected patients.
        d. *Mycobacterium avium* **complex (MAC)** can cause diar-
           rhea; however, stool is frequently colonized with this or-
           ganism in the absence of disease.
     2. **AIDS-associated enteropathy** is a diagnosis of exclusion. It
        is not known whether this entity is directly caused by HIV
        itself.
  B. **Approach to the patient**
     1. **Laboratory studies**
        a. **Fecal white blood cell (WBC) count.** A fecal WBC should
           be performed.
        b. **Stool culture** should be performed to rule out bacterial
           infection.
        c. **Stool ova and parasites (O&P).** Three samples are gener-

ally sent to increase the yield. The evaluation for Cryptosporidium and Microsporida is enhanced by an **acid-fast stain** and a **modified trichrome stain,** respectively.

d. Enzyme-linked immunosorbent assay (ELISA) for *C. difficile* **toxin.** *C. difficile* may be a commonly missed diagnosis.

e. Routine blood cultures for Salmonella should be considered. In patients with CD4 counts < 50 cells/μl, mycobacterial blood cultures for **MAC** should be obtained.

2. Endoscopy is often necessary when symptoms continue and no etiology has been identified.

   a. CMV is a very common pathogen that is often missed by the initial screening studies.

   b. Colonoscopy with biopsy (followed by upper endoscopy with small bowel biopsy if colonoscopy findings are normal) should be performed.

C. Treatment

1. Specific therapy depends on the causative organism. Most bacterial causes of enterocolitis are fluoroquinolone susceptible but increasing resistance is being reported, particularly with Campylobacter. Oral metronidazole is first-line for *C. difficile* and Giardia. Isospora responds to trimethoprim-sulfamethoxazole. Amebiasis can be treated with metronidazole plus paromomycin. Cryptosporidium and Microsporidium are challenging to treat and tend to respond poorly, although paromomycin and fumagillin or albendazole may be effective, respectively.

IV **HEPATOBILIARY DISEASE.** Abnormal transaminases, alkaline phosphatase, and bilirubin are common among HIV-infected patients. These abnormalities may be clinically insignificant and asymptomatic, but may be the initial indication of opportunistic infections and neoplastic disease or dangerous drug toxicity.

A. Causes of HIV-related hepatic parenchymal disease

1. Viruses, including **hepatitis B, hepatitis C,** and **CMV**

2. *Mycobacterium avium* **complex and less commonly,** *Mycobacterium tuberculosis* **infection**

3. Fungal infections including **histoplasmosis**

4. Malignancy including **lymphoma, Kaposi's sarcoma, and hepatocellular carcinoma**

5. Medications

   (a) Sulfa drugs, isoniazid, rifampin, and **fluconazole** are well known causes of hepatitis.

   (b) All **antiretroviral medications** have been associated with transaminase elevations. Of these, the most serious is hepatitis due to **nevirapine** (a non-nucleoside reverse transcriptase inhibitor) which can lead to fulminant hepatic failure.

(c) **Nucleoside reverse transcriptase inhibitors** can cause hepatic steatosis in association with lactic acidosis leading to a transaminitis. If not recognized early, the lactic acidosis may be fatal.

6. Peliosis hepatis from ***Bartonella henselae*** or ***B. quintana***

B. **Causes of HIV-associated obstructive biliary tract disease**
   1. **Sclerosing cholangitis** (i.e., **AIDS cholangiopathy**) often presents with right upper quadrant pain accompanied by significant elevation in alkaline phosphatase level that is out of proportion to transaminase elevations. Infection with CMV, MAC, *Cryptosporidium,* or *Microsporidium spp.* may be involved in the pathogenesis.
   2. Remember that the protease inhibitor **indinavir** can cause an asymptomatic unconjugated hyperbilirubinemia.

C. **Approach to the patient**
   1. **Patient history.** A medication history should be obtained to search for potentially hepatotoxic medications. Pain should be carefully characterized, including location and relationship to food.
   2. **Physical examination.** As always, a careful physical examination should be performed, looking for cutaneous and other manifestations of disease such as drug rash, skin lesions suggestive of Kaposi's sarcoma or fungal infection, and lymphadenopathy.

HOT ▶ **KEY**

After obtaining the history, performing the examination, and obtaining initial liver chemistries, think about whether the patient is presenting predominantly with obstructive or infiltrative disease (elevations of alkaline phosphatase out of proportion to transaminases) or hepatitis (transaminases elevated out of proportion to alkaline phosphatase) and whether the process is acute or chronic. This can help direct the remainder of your work-up. As a rough guideline, drugs and viral hepatitis tend to present with hepatitis, whereas many of the other listed etiologies are more likely to show an alkaline phosphatase predominant pattern.

---

3. **Laboratory studies**
   a. **Liver studies** (AST, ALT, alkaline phosphatase, fractionated bilirubin)
   b. **Hepatitis A, B,** and **C serologies** should be obtained.

    c. **Blood cultures** for *Mycobacterium avium* **complex, fungi, and Bartonella species** may be ordered.

    d. If hepatic steatosis with lactic acidosis is a consideration, obtain a **serum lactate** level.

    e. A **urine histoplasmosis antigen** may be diagnostic of disseminated histoplasmosis.

    f. **Serum quantitative CMV** studies should be obtained (pp65 antigenemia, CMV DNA by PCR or Digene assay).

    g. **Stool studies** for Cryptosporidia, Microsporidia

4. **Imaging studies.** Although initial evaluation may uncover a potential etiology, it is often unclear whether that disease is an incidental finding or the cause of the hepatobiliary process. Imaging studies are often performed to rule out other disorders (e.g., lymphoma).

    a. **Ultrasound** may be especially useful for evaluating the bile ducts and is therefore often chosen for patients suspected of having biliary obstruction.

    b. **Computed tomography (CT).** A CT scan provides better resolution of the liver parenchyma and is useful for patients suspected of having parenchymal disease.

    c. **Endoscopic retrograde cholangiopancreatography (ERCP)** may be used for the diagnosis and treatment of sclerosing cholangitis. In this disease, intraluminal irregularities of the bile ducts are often accompanied by distal narrowing of the common bile duct (i.e., papillary stenosis). Biliary brushings for culture and cytology can be obtained during the procedure.

5. **Liver biopsy** may be considered for patients with a negative evaluation and persistent symptoms.

D. **Treatment** depends on the cause. In patients with sclerosing cholangitis, **papillary sphincterotomy** may provide symptomatic benefit.

References

Cappell MS. Hepatobiliary manifestations of the acquired immune deficiency syndrome. Am J Gastroenterol 1991;86:1–15.

Cello JP. Acquired immunodeficiency syndrome cholangiopathy: spectrum of disease. Am J Med 1989;86:539–546.

Smith PD. Gastrointestinal infections in AIDS. Ann Intern Med 1992;166:63–77.

Tanowitz HB, Simon D, Weiss LM, et al. Gastrointestinal manifestations. Med Clin North Am 1996;80:1395–1414.

58. Neurologic Manifestations of HIV Disease

I **INTRODUCTION.** HIV-infected patients frequently develop neurologic disorders, which can be divided into five clinical categories: meningitis, space-occupying lesions, encephalopathy, myelopathy, and peripheral neuropathy.

II **MENINGITIS**

A. **Causes of meningitis.** The following are common causes of meningitis in HIV-positive patients.
  1. **Bacteria** (see Chapter 88)
  2. **Viruses. Herpes simplex virus (HSV) and cytomegalovirus (CMV)** may cause aseptic meningitis and encephalitis. **HIV** itself may cause a slight cerebrospinal fluid (CSF) pleocytosis and elevated CSF protein even without clinical meningitis.
  3. **Fungi.** Cryptococcal meningitis is common, often presenting as fever and headache without neck stiffness or photophobia. A lumbar puncture with no pleocytosis does not rule out cryptococcal meningitis. When this infection is in the differential diagnosis, an opening pressure should always be obtained.
  4. **Spirochetes.** The incidence of central nervous system (CNS) syphilis is increased in HIV-infected patients.
  5. **Mycobacteria.** Tuberculosis is the most common mycobacterial cause of CNS disease in HIV-positive patients.
  6. **Malignancy.** Lymphomatous meningitis is the most common malignant etiology.
B. **Approach to the patient.** In general, the approach to an HIV-positive patient with suspected meningitis is the same as that for other patients (see Chapter 88 V). However, the increased likelihood of certain etiologies leads to a few specific considerations for HIV-infected patients with possible meningitis.
  1. A serum or CSF **cryptococcal antigen (CRAG) titer** should be obtained in HIV-infected patients who are being evaluated for possible meningitis. The serum CRAG is more sensitive than the CSF CRAG, but the sensitivities of each may exceed 90%.
  2. A CSF **Venereal Disease Research Laboratory (VDRL) test** is often performed to evaluate the possibility of neurosyphilis.

3. The presence of an unexplained CSF lymphocytic pleocytosis or evidence of a basilar meningitis (e.g., meningitis with cranial nerve findings) usually raises suspicion of meningitis related to tuberculosis, other endemic fungal infections, or lymphoma.

    a. CSF analysis. Multiple CSF samples should be sent for cytology, fungal, and acid-fast bacillus staining and culture.

    b. A **tuberculin purified protein derivative (PPD) skin test** may be performed to evaluate exposure to tuberculosis; however, a negative test does not exclude the diagnosis.

    c. Magnetic resonance imaging (MRI) is often useful to look for basilar meningitis; a biopsy of the brain or meninges is sometimes necessary for definitive diagnosis.

C. Treatment depends on the cause.

    1. Bacteria. Treatment of routine bacterial meningitis is not different from that in an immunocompetent patient.

    2. Viruses. HSV and CMV are treated with acyclovir and ganciclovir as first-line agents, respectively. See Section IV for details on therapy of disease caused by JC virus.

    3. Fungi. Combination therapy with Amphotericin B (0.7 mg/kg/d) and 5-flucytosine (25 mg/kg po q6 hr) is recommended for initial treatment of cryptococcal meningitis. After 14 days, if the CSF is sterile, these drugs are discontinued and fluconazole (400 mg/day) is initiated orally. After 3 months, the dose may be reduced for maintenance therapy to 200 mg/day. The duration of this therapy depends on the patient's CD4 count and HIV viral load over time but may be lifelong.

    4. Spirochetes. Intravenous penicillin G for 14 days is recommended for patients with CNS syphilis.

    5. Mycobacteria. Standard regimens for tuberculosis are used for CNS tuberculosis, but the duration of therapy is extended and corticosteroids may be beneficial.

    6. Malignancy. HIV infection is not a contraindication to chemotherapy or radiation therapy, and the appropriate treatment of the underlying malignancy should be pursued.

III **SPACE-OCCUPYING LESIONS** may present as headaches, seizures, focal sensory or motor deficits, visual field defects, or altered mental status.

A. Causes of space-occupying lesions. Although all the following causes should be considered in a patient who presents with signs and symptoms of a space-occupying lesion, the first two are the most common in HIV-positive patients.

    1. Toxoplasmosis

    2. Primary CNS lymphoma

3. **Bacterial abscess**
4. **Cryptococcoma**
5. **Histoplasmoma**
6. **Tuberculoma**
7. **Nocardiosis**
B. **Approach to the patient**
1. **Imaging studies.** A **computed tomography (CT)** or **MRI scan** is often useful for evaluating suspected CNS disease in HIV-infected patients.
   a. **CT scan.** Many space-occupying lesions are better seen with contrast enhancement, which should be used in the absence of contraindications.
   b. **MRI** is generally a more sensitive test and may reveal multiple lesions when only a single lesion is seen on CT scan.
2. **Laboratory studies**
   a. A **serum CRAG titer** is frequently ordered.
   b. **Blood cultures** and a **PPD test** may also be obtained, depending on the clinical situation.
   c. **Toxoplasmosis IgG titers.** A *Toxoplasma gondii* IgM titer has limited utility because nearly all cases of toxoplasmosis in HIV-infected patients are due to reactivated disease. Determining whether a patient has been exposed to *T. gondii* in the past (e.g., a positive Toxoplasmosis IgG serology) can help determine if the patient is at risk of reactivation. Individuals receiving prophylaxis for toxoplasmosis are also at decreased risk of developing CNS disease. Daily trimethoprim-sulfamethoxazole is the first-line prophylaxis regimen for patients with CD4 counts < 100 cells/μl.
   d. **CD4 counts.** The patient's risk of disease depends on the degree of immunosuppression. Bacterial abscess, tuberculoma, and lymphoma can be seen at relatively high CD4 counts, whereas cryptococcomas and toxoplasmosis more commonly occur in patients with CD4 counts < 100 cells/μl.

HOT KEY

Lumbar punctures are rarely useful for evaluating space-occupying lesions in HIV-infected patients and are contraindicated in patients with mass effect or posterior fossa lesions.

---

3. **Stereotactic brain biopsy.** This procedure should be performed early in the diagnostic work-up if the patient does not have a high likelihood of CNS toxoplasmosis, including:
   a. Those with negative Toxoplasma IgG serologies
   b. Those with an increased risk for processes other than tox-

oplasmosis (e.g., intravenous drug users, who have an increased risk of brain abscess)
  c. Those with single lesions on MRI (because finding a single lesion makes toxoplasmosis less likely)
  d. Those with progressive neurologic deficits or mass effect on imaging (because appropriate treatment is needed immediately)
  e. Those who do not have regression of the space-occupying lesion or lesions after 2 weeks of empiric toxoplasmosis therapy
 C. **Treatment** depends on the cause. In individuals believed to be at high risk for toxoplasmosis, empiric therapy is often given for 2 weeks, followed by repeat imaging to evaluate for response. Standard therapy is sulfadiazine (or high-dose clindamycin) combined with pyrimethamine.

IV ENCEPHALOPATHY

 A. Any alteration in mental status requires a thorough evaluation to rule out reversible causes (see Chapter 82). An **imaging study** (preferably an MRI) and **spinal fluid analysis** are necessary to rule out infectious or malignant processes. **Neuropsychiatric testing** is frequently performed to help rule out depression.
 B. **Progressive multifocal leukoencephalopathy** (PML) due to JC virus is a common cause of cognitive impairment and focal neurologic deficits in patients with late-stage HIV infection. Imaging studies reveal patchy periventricular and/or subcortical white matter lesions best seen on MRI. A PCR for JC virus may be positive even in the absence of a CSF pleocytosis. No definitive therapy exists. Highly active antiretroviral therapy (HAART) may improve symptoms, and limited data suggest a possible benefit with cidofovir.
 C. Many patients are ultimately diagnosed as having **AIDS dementia complex,** an illness that occurs late in the course of HIV infection and is often characterized by memory deficits, gait difficulty, behavioral changes including depression, and psychomotor slowing. CT scanning may reveal brain atrophy. MRI findings include symmetric subcortical white matter lesions with high intensity on T2-weighted images. Significant improvement has been seen in some patients after initiating successful HAART therapy.

V MYELOPATHY

usually presents with progressive lower extremity weakness that may be accompanied by bladder or bowel incontinence. Evidence of upper motor neuron disease with spastic paraparesis and hyperreflexia are usually noted unless peripheral neuropathy is also present.

A. Causes of myelopathy. Spinal cord disease often results from infection, external compression injury (i.e., cord compression), or miscellaneous insults.

1. **Infection.** Viruses (CMV, HSV, and HIV), fungi (*Cryptococcus*), spirochetes (*Treponema pallidum*), and parasites (*Toxoplasma*) can infect the spinal cord, leading to myelopathy.

2. **Cord compression** may result from epidural abscesses (e.g., from bacterial infection or tuberculosis) or from malignancy (e.g., CNS lymphoma).

3. **Miscellaneous causes**
   a. **Vascular insults** (e.g., vasculitis)
   b. **Vitamin B_{12} deficiency**
   c. **HIV-related vacuolar myelopathy** is a diagnosis of exclusion and usually occurs late in the course of HIV infection. Motor weakness and decreased proprioception often reflect preferential loss of myelin from the lateral and dorsal columns, respectively. Examination reveals a spastic paraparesis with lower extremity hyperreflexia. There is no proven therapy.

B. Approach to the patient

1. **Imaging studies. MRI** of the involved area of spinal cord helps to rule out spinal cord compression.

2. **Laboratory studies**
   a. **Spinal fluid analysis** with PCR for CMV and HSV, **CRAG titers** (serum, CSF, or both), and a **CSF VDRL** should be obtained.
   b. **Culture** and **serology for CMV** may be useful to evaluate the possibility of **CMV polyradiculopathy** (see VI A).
   c. A **vitamin B_{12}** level should be obtained.

VI PERIPHERAL NEUROPATHY is common in patients with AIDS.

A. Causes of peripheral neuropathy. All causes of peripheral neuropathy should be considered (see Chapter 83); however, common causes and patterns of peripheral neuropathy in patients with AIDS are given here.

1. **Polyneuropathy**
   a. **Distal symmetric peripheral neuropathies** are the most commonly seen peripheral neuropathies in HIV-infected patients. Typically, patients present with painful dysesthesias. The etiologies are many but common causes include antiretroviral medications (most commonly didanosine, zalcitabine, and stavudine) or HIV itself. The latter is seen in late stage disease. In cases in which medication is the suspected cause, therapy should be changed (when possible) to agents not associated with neuropathy. **Symp-**

tomatic therapy with tricyclic antidepressants or gabapentin may be helpful.

  b. Predominantly motor neuropathies

    (1) CMV polyradiculopathy may cause progressive lower extremity weakness associated with a CSF neutrophilic pleocytosis (in the absence of bacterial infection). Therapy with **ganciclovir** may result in clinical improvement.

    (2) An **inflammatory demyelinating polyneuropathy** may result in severe motor weakness and significantly depressed nerve conduction velocities. The clinical scenario resembles that of the more acute Guillain-Barré syndrome. **Plasmapheresis** is often used as treatment.

  2. Mononeuritis multiplex is much less common than polyneuropathy. Although HIV itself is an etiology, other infections (e.g., CMV, VZV) and malignancies (e.g., lymphoma) should be ruled out.

B. Approach to the patient. Other potentially reversible causes of peripheral neuropathy should be considered (see Chapter 83).

References

Simpson DM, Tagliati M. Neurologic manifestations of HIV infection. Ann Intern Med 1994;121:769–785.

Thorner A, Katz J. Progressive multifocal leukoencephalopathy. Curr Infect Dis Rep 2001;3:352–359.

Weisberg LA. Neurologic abnormalities in human immunodeficiency virus infection. South Med J 2001;94:266–275.

PART VII

HEMATOLOGY/ONCOLOGY

59. Pancytopenia

I **INTRODUCTION** Pancytopenia is defined as a decrease in all blood cell lines.

II **CLINICAL MANIFESTATIONS OF PANCYTOPENIA**

A. Pancytopenia usually presents with signs and symptoms that are related to a decrease in each cell line.
  1. **Anemia** can result in increased fatigue, shortness of breath, lightheadedness, and pallor.
  2. **Thrombocytopenia**
     a. Patients with platelet counts greater than 90,000 cells/μl have normal bleeding times (unless platelet function is abnormal) and are usually asymptomatic.
     b. Easy bruisability may be noted as the platelet count approaches 50,000 cells/μl.
     c. Counts below 20,000 cells/μl can be associated with petechiae, mucosal bleeding, and spontaneous internal bleeds.
  3. **Neutropenia** predisposes patients to bacterial infections, but patients usually present with symptoms related to anemia or thrombocytopenia first. The risk of infection increases substantially once the neutrophil count falls below 500 cells/μl.
B. Disease-specific symptoms (e.g., neurologic symptoms in vitamin B_{12} deficiency, cachexia in malignancy) may also be present.

HOT **KEY** Pancytopenia is a great reminder that even mild, nonspecific symptoms can be the harbinger of a serious illness. You should therefore consider getting a complete blood count (CBC) on all patients with a prolonged or recurring illness.

III **CAUSES OF PANCYTOPENIA.** Many textbooks attempt to differentiate causes of decreased production from those of increased destruction. For pancytopenia, this distinction is not very useful because both processes are often involved. The mnemonic "PANCYTO" can help you remember the most common causes of pancytopenia.

Common Causes of Pancytopenia ("PANCYTO")

Paroxysmal nocturnal hemoglobinuria (PNH)
Aplastic anemia
Neoplasms and Near neoplasms
Consumption
Vitamin deficiencies (the "V" looks like a "Y")
Toxins, drugs, and radiation therapy
Overwhelming infections

A. PNH is a disorder of stem cells that results in an increased sensitivity for complement-mediated cell lysis. PNH can clinically manifest as chronic intravascular hemolysis, a hypercoagulable state, and/or bone marrow aplasia.

B. Aplastic anemia is one of the misnomers in medicine because it involves a disorder of stem cells and therefore affects all cell lines. An immune mechanism is probable. Exposures and disorders associated with aplastic anemia are listed below; many cases of aplastic anemia have no identifiable association.

  1. Fanconi's anemia is an autosomal recessive disease that usually appears in childhood and is often associated with other congenital abnormalities (e.g., cardiac and renal malformations, hypoplastic thumbs, hyperpigmented skin).

  2. Drugs and **toxins.** Chemotherapeutic agents, chloramphenicol, sulfa drugs, gold, ionizing radiation, benzene, and various other drugs have been associated with aplastic anemia.

  3. Infections. Hepatitis (especially hepatitis C and possibly hepatitis G), Epstein-Barr virus infection, parvovirus B19 infection, and other viral infections have been associated with aplastic anemia.

  4. Immune disorders such as systemic lupus erythematosus may be associated with aplastic anemia.

  5. Idiopathic. The cause remains unclear in a large number of patients. In these cases, the leading hypothesis is that damage from unrecognized causes leads to a host immune response causing aplastic anemia.

C. Neoplasms (e.g., **leukemia, metastatic malignancies**) and **near neoplasms** (i.e., **myelodysplasia**) can cause pancytopenia.

D. Consumption
  1. **Hypersplenism** (see Chapter 31), regardless of the cause, can result in pancytopenia.
  2. **Immune-mediated destruction** usually results in decreases of one or two cell lines but can also cause pancytopenia.
E. Vitamin deficiencies (e.g., vitamin B_{12} and folate deficiencies) should always be considered in patients with pancytopenia.
F. Toxins, drugs, and **radiation therapy.** For example, ethanol use may result in pancytopenia.
G. Overwhelming infections. Sepsis, tuberculosis, or fungal infection can cause pancytopenia. HIV infection can also result in pancytopenia, from the infection itself, superimposed infections, or medications used to treat the infection.

IV APPROACH TO THE PATIENT

HOT

KEY

Pancytopenia should be considered leukemia until proven otherwise.

A. Patient history. Inquire about medications, exposures, and human immunodeficiency virus (HIV) risk factors. Perform a review of systems, asking the patient about cachexia and other symptoms of an occult malignancy.
B. Physical examination. Carefully examine the spleen and lymph nodes. The presence of splenomegaly increases the likelihood of malignancy and essentially rules out aplastic anemia.
C. Laboratory studies. Although a bone marrow biopsy is usually indicated and diagnostic, there are some potential clues to the diagnosis that can be obtained on a routine peripheral blood smear. Other tests may also be indicated in certain patients.
  1. **Peripheral blood smear**
     a. **Megaloblastosis** increases the likelihood of vitamin B_{12} or folate deficiency.
     b. **Blasts** implicate a possible leukemia.
     c. **Leukoerythroblastic smear.** A leukoerythroblastic smear, which reveals **early (nucleated) red blood cells (RBCs)** and **early white blood cells (WBCs)** (i.e., bands, metamyelocytes, myelocytes), implies marrow invasion by malignancy, fibrosis, or infection. **Teardrop cells** (i.e., RBCs shaped like a teardrop from being "squeezed" out of the bone marrow) are frequently seen with leukoerythroblastosis.
     d. **Pelger-Huet anomaly** (i.e., neutrophils with bilobed nuclei) is seen in patients with myelodysplasia (see Chapter 70).

2. **Vitamin B$_{12}$** and **folate** levels are often obtained.
3. **HIV test.** An HIV test should be performed in patients with risk factors.
4. **PNH workup.** PNH results in intravascular hemolysis that can cause iron deficiency from urinary losses; therefore, PNH should be ruled out in all patients with pancytopenia and suspected iron deficiency [e.g., when the mean corpuscular volume (MCV) is low]. The **sucrose lysis test** and the **Ham test** assess the susceptibility of RBCs to lysis and are both sensitive and specific for PNH.

D. **Bone marrow biopsy.** Because a "dry tap" may occur (i.e., one in which bone marrow aspirate is unobtainable as a result of aplasia, fibrosis, or malignancy), a core biopsy is essential to determine the etiology of pancytopenia. Patients with HIV and pancytopenia often still undergo bone marrow biopsy to rule out a contributing infection or malignancy.

1. **Increased cellularity** suggests peripheral destruction (hypersplenism, PNH, immune-mediated disorders) or ineffective erythropoiesis (myelodysplasia). Of note, PNH and myelodysplasia may also display decreased cellularity.
2. **Decreased cellularity** is the more common finding and may implicate aplastic anemia.
3. **Cytogenetic analysis** may help make the diagnosis of myelodysplastic syndrome or a malignant process.
4. **Other findings.** Evidence of malignancy, infection, or myelodysplasia may also be found.

V TREATMENT

A. **General treatment** is aimed at preventing the complications associated with a decrease in each cell line.

1. **Packed RBC transfusions** are usually given to maintain the hematocrit above 30% in symptomatic patients and older patients with known or suspected coronary artery disease. Younger patients may tolerate a much lower hematocrit. For each unit of packed RBCs transfused, the hemoglobin is expected to rise by 1 g/dl and the hematocrit by 3%.
2. **Platelet transfusions** may be necessary (see Chapter 60).
3. **Infection prevention and treatment**
   a. **Granulocyte-macrophage colony-stimulating factor (GM-CSF)** is sometimes used to increase neutrophil counts.
   b. **Neutropenic precautions** (e.g., **handwashing, minimizing injections, avoiding unpeeled fruit and fresh flowers**). The risk from neutropenia is highest when the patient's absolute neutrophil count is less than 500 cells/μl. Neutropenic precautions should be used for these patients. Pro-

phylactic antibiotics in the absence of signs or symptoms of infection are not recommended.

   c. Broad-spectrum antibiotics should be used for patients with fever and neutropenia, which should be treated as a medical emergency.

B. Specific treatment is aimed at the underlying illness. Specific treatments for most of the causes of pancytopenia are found in the relevant chapters. Therapies for PNH and aplastic anemia will be briefly discussed here.

   1. PNH carries approximately a 40% lifetime risk of thrombosis. (The mechanism is unclear.) Bleeding from thrombocytopenia can also occur; approximately 50% of patients with PNH die of one of these two complications. Spontaneous remission may occur in approximately 15% of patients.

   a. Chronic anticoagulation therapy is indicated for all patients with a history of thrombosis and should also be considered prophylactically for patients without severe thrombocytopenia.

   b. Bone marrow transplantation may be curative for a small group of eligible, young patients.

   2. Aplastic anemia

   a. Removal of potential etiologies (e.g., medications) is always important.

   b. Pharmacologic therapy

   (1) Antithymocyte globulin (ATG) is usually the first-line pharmacologic treatment.

   (2) Immunosuppressive agents (e.g., cyclosporine) are also used in conjunction with ATG.

   (3) Androgens are sometimes useful for patients with mild aplasia but are generally not effective in patients with more severe disease.

   c. Bone marrow transplantation may cure 80% of the young, eligible patients selected. Because transfusions may increase the risk of rejection, transplant candidates should only receive transfusions when it is absolutely necessary, and transfusions from potential donors should never be given.

   d. Spontaneous recovery is uncommon and usually is seen only in mild or moderate cases.

References

Hillmen P, Lewis SM, Bessler M, et al. Natural history of paroxysmal nocturnal hemoglobinuria. N Engl J Med 1995;333:1253–1259.

Rayson D, Kang EM, Inwards DJ. 27-year-old woman with pancytopenia. Mayo Clin Proc 1995;70(2):185–188.

Young NS, Maciejewski J. The pathophysiology of acquired aplastic anemia. N Engl J Med 1997;336:1365–1372.

60. Thrombocytopenia

I **INTRODUCTION.** Thrombocytopenia, a common disorder in hospitalized patients, is defined as a **platelet count < 150,000 cells/µl.**

II **CLINICAL MANIFESTATIONS OF THROMBOCYTOPENIA.** Signs and symptoms are related to the degree of thrombocytopenia (in the absence of concomitant disorders of coagulation or platelet dysfunction).

A. **Platelet count 50,000–90,000 cells/µl.** Clinical manifestations are usually absent.

B. **Platelet count 20,000–50,000 cells/µl.** Patients may report easy bruisability, but spontaneous bleeding is usually not seen.

C. **Platelet count < 20,000 cells/µl.** Patients are at increased risk for spontaneous bleeding (e.g., petechiae, gastrointestinal bleeding).

III **CAUSES OF THROMBOCYTOPENIA.** It is easiest to remember the causes of thrombocytopenia if you classify them according to the underlying mechanism: decreased production, splenic sequestration, or increased destruction (Figure 60–1).

A. **Decreased production.** Because diseases of the bone marrow are involved, there is often a decrease in other cell lines as well. The causes of decreased platelet production are almost identical to those of pancytopenia. (see chapter 59)

1. **PNH** is more commonly associated with increased destruction, but may also be associated with a production defect.

2. **Aplasia. Aplastic anemia** causes pancytopenia; rare congenital diseases that result in isolated decreased megakaryocytic proliferation include **congenital amegakaryocytic hypoplasia** and **thrombocytopenia and absent radii** (the **TAR syndrome**).

3. **Neoplasms** and **near neoplasms** include **leukemia, metastatic malignancies,** and **myelodysplasia.**

4. **Vitamin deficiencies,** including **vitamin B$_{12}$** and **folate deficiency,** are rare causes of isolated thrombocytopenia.

5. **Toxins, drugs,** and **radiation therapy. Ethanol, thiazide diuretics, estrogens,** and **chemotherapeutic agents** can cause thrombocytopenia.

FIGURE 60-1. Causes of thrombocytopenia. *MAHA* = microangiopathic hemolytic anemia; *PNH* = paroxysmal nocturnal hemoglobinuria.

6. **Overwhelming infections,** including sepsis, tuberculosis, fungal infection, and human immunodeficiency virus (HIV) disease, can cause thrombocytopenia.

B. **Increased splenic sequestration** can result from **hypersplenism** of any cause, leading to thrombocytopenia.

C. **Increased destruction** is probably the most common cause of isolated thrombocytopenia. Disorders that cause increased destruction of platelets can be classified as nonimmunologic or immunologic.

1. **Nonimmunologic**

   a. **Microangiopathic hemolytic anemia (MAHA)** may cause platelet destruction as a result of shearing in small vessels (see Chapter 62).

   b. **PNH** predisposes all cell lines to complement-mediated lysis and is therefore a rare cause of isolated thrombocytopenia.

2. **Immunologic.** Destruction may be related to autoimmune phenomena [e.g., **immune thrombocytopenic purpura (ITP)** or **rheumatologic disease**], alloimmune phenomena (e.g.,

post-transfusion reaction), or drug-dependent antibodies from **medications.**

IV APPROACH TO THE PATIENT

A. **Exclude pseudothrombocytopenia.** Pseudothrombocytopenia is an artifact of platelet clumping in the test tube in EDTA-anticoagulated blood. Examining the peripheral blood smear may alert you to the problem, and sending a heparinized specimen will confirm your suspicion.

B. **Try to determine the cause of thrombocytopenia.**
 1. **Patient history.** Pay particular attention to the patient's medications. Risk factors for HIV or a history of substance abuse (e.g., alcohol) also deserve attention. A review of systems and asking about "B symptoms" (i.e., fevers, night sweats, and weight loss) may help reveal an occult malignancy. A bleeding history including questions about menstrual bleeding, surgical complications, and prior transfusions may help elucidate the chronicity of the problem.
 2. **Physical examination.** A complete physical examination is always necessary.
    a. Examination of the **spleen** is of particular importance (see Chapter 31 IV).
    b. A detailed skin examination for petechiae, purpura, and ecchymoses should be performed.
    c. In addition, a thorough examination for **lymphadenopathy** should be performed (see Chapter 68 II).
 3. **Laboratory studies**
    a. **Peripheral blood smear.** A peripheral blood smear is often helpful.
       (1) **Large platelets.** This finding implies increased destruction and early release from the bone marrow. ITP is classically associated with finding large platelets on the peripheral blood smear. These large platelets are young and hyperfunctional. As a result, patients with ITP may not have as high of an incidence of bleeding relative to their platelet count.
       (2) **Schistocytes.** The finding of fragmented red blood cells (RBCs) implies microangiopathic hemolytic anemia.
       (3) **Other abnormalities** that may offer clues are discussed in Chapter 59 IV C 1.
    b. **Prothrombin time (PT), partial thromboplastin time (PTT),** and **lactate dehydrogenase (LDH)** may be used to evaluate the possibility of a MAHA. **Blood urea nitrogen (BUN)** and **creatinine levels** should be obtained when hemolytic-uremic syndrome/thrombotic thrombocytopenic purpura (HUS/TTP) is a consideration.

    c. Serologic studies. Antinuclear antibody (ANA), HIV, and other specific viral serologies are useful for evaluating the possibility of immunologic destruction associated with systemic lupus erythematosus (SLE) or infections with HIV or another virus.

        (1) An HIV test is especially necessary in patients with HIV risk factors.

        (2) Epstein-Barr virus, cytomegalovirus (CMV), hepatitis, and toxoplasmosis serologies are most useful when the patient has systemic symptoms, lymphadenopathy, or splenomegaly on examination.

    d. Vitamin B_{12} and **folate levels** and **tests for PNH** are sometimes performed but are usually not helpful, because these disorders are rarely associated with isolated thrombocytopenia.

    e. Anti-platelet antibody testing is not necessary to make the diagnosis of ITP and is therefore usually not performed.

4. Bone marrow biopsy is performed in many patients with thrombocytopenia. If the cause of thrombocytopenia is readily identifiable (e.g., thiazide diuretic therapy), a trial of removing the possible inciting agent may be both diagnostic and therapeutic and may obviate the need for a bone marrow biopsy. Pertinent findings on bone marrow biopsy include the following:

    a. Decreased megakaryocytes are diagnostic of one of the production problems. Evidence of the specific cause of the decreased production may also be found (e.g., malignancy, infection).

    b. Increased megakaryocytes are found when increased destruction or sequestration is the mechanism of thrombocytopenia. Increased megakaryocytes on bone marrow biopsy without other identifiable causes of increased destruction or sequestration are usually diagnostic for ITP.

    c. Evidence for myelodysplasia can also be seen on bone marrow biopsy (see Chapter 70).

V TREATMENT

A. General treatment

1. Discontinue medications that may cause thrombocytopenia.

    a. The platelet count will usually return to normal in 7–10 days.

    b. Heparin-induced thrombocytopenia and thrombosis (HITT) is a disorder in which immune-mediated thrombocytopenia and, paradoxically, systemic thrombosis coexist. Increasing the heparin dose in these patients is contraindicated; the only therapy is heparin withdrawal. If systemic anticoagulation is required, other agents such as danaparoid (a heparinoid), recombinant hirudin, or argatroban (direct thrombin inhibitors) may be used until warfarin levels are therapeutic.

2. Platelet transfusions. Unnecessary platelet transfusions should be avoided because they may induce immune resistance; if this complication occurs, human leukocyte antigen (HLA)-matched platelets can be administered.

   a. Platelet transfusions are usually not indicated for patients with platelet counts > 20,000 cells/μl and no evidence of bleeding.

HOT KEY

In general, platelet transfusions in asymptomatic patients with TTP should be avoided, because transfusions may worsen the patient's condition.

---

   b. Indications. Platelet transfusions are indicated in the following situations:

     (1) Before surgery. The platelet count is usually maintained above 50,000 cells/μl when surgery is to be performed, although in patients with ITP, this may be both impossible and unnecessary. When neurosurgery is to be performed, the platelet count is usually maintained above 90,000 cells/μl in an attempt to normalize the bleeding time.

     (2) In a patient with active bleeding

       (a) Severe bleeding. The platelet count is always maintained above 50,000 cells/μl and is sometimes increased to 90,000–100,000 cells/μl.

       (b) Mild bleeding or **petechiae.** The platelet count should be maintained above 20,000 cells/μl.

     (3) To prevent spontaneous bleeding. The platelet count is usually kept above 10,000–20,000 cells/μl, depending on physician preference.

B. Specific treatments for **ITP** (including HIV-associated ITP) are discussed here; specific treatments for other causes are discussed in relevant chapters.

   1. Observation is often appropriate for patients with platelet counts > 20,000 cells/μl and no evidence of bleeding. Children frequently have an acute form of ITP that is usually related to a viral illness and resolves spontaneously over 3–6 months. In adults, ITP usually follows a chronic course.

   2. Pharmacologic therapy

     a. Steroids will benefit approximately two thirds of patients, leading to an increase in platelet count in approximately 3 weeks.

b. Intravenous gammaglobulin or **anti-D** (a component of intravenous gammaglobulin) often increases the platelet count faster than steroids; it is therefore useful for patients who are actively bleeding and those with extremely low counts in the "window" before steroids take effect.

c. Immunosuppressive agents can be used for patients with ITP associated with SLE or other connective tissue disorders. The most commonly used agents include cyclophosphamide, azathioprine, vincristine, or vinblastine.

d. Danazol is sometimes useful for patients with refractory ITP.

e. Zidovudine may be useful in patients with HIV-associated ITP.

f. Rituximab, a monoclonal antibody directed against a B cell antigen (CD20), shows some promise for treating patients who have failed to respond to other modalities.

3. Splenectomy is reserved for patients in whom steroid therapy fails or for those who experience relapse after a steroid taper.

References

Cines DB, Blanchette VS. Immune thrombocytopenic purpura. N Engl J Med 2002; 346:995–1008.

Elalamy I, Lecrubier C, Horellou MH, Conard J, Samama MM. Heparin-induced thrombocytopenia: laboratory diagnosis and management. Ann Med 2000;32 (Suppl 1):60–67.

Stasi R, Pagano A, Stipa E, Amadori S. Rituximab chimeric anti-CD20 monoclonal antibody treatment for adults with chronic idiopathic thrombocytopenic purpura. Blood 2001;98:952–957.

61. Thrombocytosis

I **INTRODUCTION.** Thrombocytosis is defined as a **platelet count > 450,000 cells/μl.**

II **CLINICAL MANIFESTATIONS OF THROMBOCYTOSIS**

A. Primary. If thrombocytosis is caused by a myeloproliferative disorder, the platelets are frequently abnormal and the patient may be prone to both bleeding and clotting events.

B. Secondary. If thrombocytosis is secondary to another disorder (reactive), even patients with extremely high platelet counts (e.g., > 1,000,000 cells/μl) are usually asymptomatic.

III **CAUSES OF THROMBOCYTOSIS**

A. Primary causes. Any of the four **myeloproliferative disorders** can increase the platelet count through clonal proliferation of the stem cells (see Chapter 70).

B. Secondary causes. Reactive thrombocytosis is the most common cause of thrombocytosis.
   1. **Malignancies**
   2. **Infections** and **inflammatory disorders** (e.g., Crohn's disease)
   3. **Connective tissue disorders**
   4. **Iron deficiency anemia**
   5. **Splenectomy**

IV **APPROACH TO THE PATIENT**

A. Patient history
   1. A history of **gastrointestinal bleeding** may imply possible iron deficiency.
   2. **Fevers, night sweats,** or **weight loss** may implicate malignancy or chronic infection (e.g., tuberculosis). A complete review of systems should be performed to help identify the presence of an occult malignancy or infection.
   3. A history of recent **splenectomy** may provide a simple explanation for thrombocytosis.
   4. Patients should be questioned regarding potential symptoms related to thrombocytosis including thrombosis, bleeding complications, and vasomotor symptoms of headache, visual symptoms, and **erythromelalgia** (burning pain of extremities associated with warmth and redness). Presence of these

symptoms would point more toward a primary cause of thrombocytosis.

B. Physical examination. Perform a thorough physical examination, including pelvic and rectal examinations. Pay special attention to the spleen and lymph nodes because enlargement may signal malignancy or infection.

C. Laboratory studies can further narrow the differential diagnosis.

   1. Serum ferritin. The serum ferritin level will help evaluate the possibility of iron deficiency anemia and is especially important in patients with a history of gastrointestinal bleeding, guaiac-positive stools, or a low mean corpuscular volume (MCV).

   2. Hematocrit and white blood cell (WBC) count. The hematocrit and WBC count are often elevated in patients with myeloproliferative disorders, although essential thrombocytosis may result in an isolated elevation of the platelet count.

   3. Peripheral smear. Rarely, automated hematology counters may count small fragmented RBCs as platelets and report an elevated count. This spurious diagnosis of thrombocytosis can be found by evaluating the peripheral smear. Howell-Jolly bodies, target cells, or abnormally shaped cells on smear may suggest a post-splenectomy state as a cause of thrombocytosis.

   4. Other tests may be performed if reactive thrombocytosis is suspected [e.g., a purified protein derivative (PPD) test for possible tuberculosis, a computed tomography (CT) scan for suspected intraabdominal malignancy]. If a reactive cause is ruled out, a bone marrow biopsy may be necessary to look for a primary cause.

V TREATMENT

A. Primary causes. Myeloproliferative disorders may predispose the patient to both bleeding and thrombosis as a result of abnormal platelet function. Immediate platelet apheresis should be considered in patients with acute thromboses and a platelet count > 800,000 cells/UL. Hydroxyurea or anagrelide can be used for longer-term management of patients with significant thrombocytosis or thromboses.

B. Secondary causes. Most causes of reactive thrombocytosis do not require treatment to lower the platelet count. The platelet count usually returns to normal following treatment of the underlying disorder. Patients with reactive thrombocytosis rarely have associated thromboses, so anticoagulant therapy is usually not warranted.

References

Gilbert HS. Diagnosis and treatment of thrombocythemia in myeloproliferative disorders. Oncology 2001;15:989–996.

Murphy S, Peterson P, Iland H, Laszlo J. Experience of the Polycythemia Vera Study Group with essential thrombocythemia: a final report on diagnostic criteria, survival, and leukemic transition by treatment. Semin Hematol 1997;34:29–39.

Tefferi A, Solberg LA. Silverstein MN. A clinical update in polycythemia vera and essential thrombocythemia. Am J Med 2000;109:141–149.

62. Anemia

I INTRODUCTION. Anemia is a common disorder among hospitalized patients.

A. Definition. Anemia is defined as a **decrease in the volume of red blood cells (RBCs) as reflected by the hematocrit.** Anemia is a manifestation of disease, not a disease in and of itself.

B. Normal values are both gender- and age-dependent.
1. In men, a hematocrit < 40% is considered anemic.
2. In women, a hematocrit < 37% is considered anemic.

C. Clinical manifestations of anemia. Patients with anemia may be asymptomatic or complain of **fatigue, dyspnea on exertion,** or **exertional angina.** Signs and symptoms of the underlying disorder may also be present.

D. Classification. Anemia is classified as **microcytic, normocytic,** or **macrocytic** using the **mean corpuscular volume (MCV)** as a basis.
1. The **normal MCV is 80–100 μm^3.**
2. If more than one disorder is present, the MCV may be an average of the different populations of RBCs, producing a normal MCV. In mixed disorders, the **red cell distribution width (RDW)** will be increased.

II MICROCYTIC ANEMIA (MCV < 80 μm^3)

A. Causes of microcytic anemia
1. **Iron deficiency** is a very common cause of microcytic anemia and is important to diagnose because it may be indicative of an underlying gastrointestinal malignancy.
2. **Thalassemia** ranges in severity. Patients with alpha or beta thalassemia minor may even present with microcytosis without anemia.
3. **Anemia of chronic disease (ACD)** is associated with inflammatory diseases (e.g., rheumatoid arthritis, serious infection, carcinoma).
4. **Sideroblastic anemias** are a heterogenous group of disorders that have in common various defects in the porphyrin pathway that lead to an increase in cellular iron uptake. Congenital sideroblastic anemia causes microcytosis, whereas other etiologies may lead to a variable MCV. Causes of sideroblastic anemia include:
   a. Heredity
   b. Drugs and **toxins** [e.g., Lead, Isoniazid, Ethanol (LIE)]

    c. Malignancy (e.g., leukemia, lymphoma, myelofibrosis, multiple myeloma, solid tumor)

    d. Collagen vascular disease (e.g., rheumatoid arthritis)

B. Approach to the patient. It is important to differentiate iron deficiency from the other causes of microcytic anemia.

  1. Iron deficiency versus thalassemia. Iron deficiency can be distinguished from thalassemia using the **thalassemia index** (i.e., the **MCV divided by the RBC count**). A thalassemia index < 13 suggests thalassemia; one > 13 suggests iron deficiency.

  2. Iron deficiency versus other etiologies

    a. Determine the probability that a patient has iron deficiency. The pretest probability is based on clinical factors. By estimating the pretest probability and using likelihood ratios for a given ferritin level (Table 62-1), you can estimate the posttest probability (see Chapter 2 III C 1).

    b. Laboratory studies

      (1) Serum ferritin. This test may be less helpful in patients with liver disease. Like most tests, ferritin is most useful when the pretest probability is approximately 50%.

        (a) If the serum ferritin is < 15 μg/L, it practically guarantees that the patient has iron deficiency.

        (b) Similarly, a value > 100 μg/L essentially rules out the diagnosis.

      (2) Serum transferrin is occasionally helpful because it is usually elevated in iron deficiency and decreased in ACD, probably because transferrin is a protein.

    c. Bone marrow biopsy remains the gold standard test to diagnose iron deficiency.

TABLE 62-1: Serum Ferritin Values and Corresponding Likelihood Ratios

Serum Ferritin (μ/L)	Likelihood Ratio
> 100	0.1
25–100	Not helpful
15–24	10
< 15	50

Based on data from Guyatt GH, Oxman AD, Ali M, Willan A, McIlroy W, Patterson C. Laboratory diagnosis of iron-deficiency anemia: an overview. J Gen Intern Med 1992;7(2):145–153.

C. Treatment

   1. Iron deficiency anemia therapy involves treating the underlying cause of blood loss and replacing lost iron. Oral iron is most commonly used; side effects include constipation, abdominal discomfort, and black discoloration of stools. Rarely, patients have difficulties absorbing iron and can be given iron intravenously. With therapy, reticulocytosis should occur within a few days and the hemoglobin should rise in 1–2 months.

HOT KEY

If iron deficiency is diagnosed, endoscopy of the upper and lower gastrointestinal tract may need to be performed because of the possibility of an underlying gastrointestinal malignancy.

   2. Thalassemia treatment varies with disease severity. Patients can require no treatment, deferoxamine (iron chelation therapy) for iron overload, or intermittent transfusions. Severe disease can be treated successfully with bone marrow transplantation.

III MACROCYTIC ANEMIA (MCV > 100 μm³)

A. Megaloblastic anemias are caused by various defects in DNA synthesis that lead to hematologic abnormalities. Causes of megaloblastic anemia include:
   1. Vitamin B_{12} deficiency
   2. Folate deficiency
   3. Drugs (e.g., methotrexate, azathioprine)
   4. Miscellaneous (e.g., Lesch-Nyhan syndrome, thiamine-responsive or pyridoxine-responsive anemias)

HOT KEY

The finding of hypersegmented polymorphonuclear neutrophils (PMNs) on the peripheral blood smear strongly suggests megaloblastic anemia.

B. Chronic liver disease causes a macrocytosis as a result of ineffective erythropoiesis.

C. Alcoholism produces erythrocyte membrane abnormalities, leading to macrocytic anemia.

D. Hypothyroidism causes macrocytic anemia via an unclear mechanism.

E. Reticulocytosis. An MCV greater than 110 μm³ is usually not due to reticulocytosis alone.

F. Myelodysplasia. There are five myelodysplastic syndromes (see Chapter 70).

HOT KEY

Practically all HIV-infected patients taking zidovudine will have an elevated MCV; therefore, this finding can aid in gauging compliance with medications.

IV NORMOCYTIC ANEMIA. An **absolute reticulocyte count** is the initial test to order in a patient with normocytic anemia, because the absolute reticulocyte count allows the anemia to be classified as **proliferative** or **hypoproliferative** (Figure 62–1).

A. Proliferative normocytic anemia is characterized by erythrocyte loss.
 1. Hemolysis. Clues that hemolysis may be present include elevated lactate dehydrogenase (LDH) and increased total bilirubin levels. If hemolysis is a concern, the **peripheral smear** must be examined. The cause of hemolytic anemia can be determined based on the morphology of the erythrocytes (e.g., schistocytes, sickle cells). Two important causes of hemolysis include autoimmune hemolytic anemia (AIHA) and microangiopathic hemolytic anemia (MAHA).
  a. AIHA is caused by antibodies to RBCs. IgG autoantibodies are termed warm antibodies, and IgM autoantibodies are termed cold antibodies. Underlying etiologies include collagen vascular disorders, malignancy, infection (e.g., *Mycoplasma* and mononucleosis), drugs, or idiopathic causes.
  b. MAHA is characterized by intravascular shearing of RBCs, which leads to schistocyte formation. A few of the important causes of MAHA are listed here.
   (1) Disseminated intravascular coagulation (DIC). In acute DIC, the major concern is bleeding, whereas in chronic DIC, thrombosis is more of a problem.

Causes of DIC ("MOIST")

Malignancy
Obstetric complications
Infection
Shock
Trauma

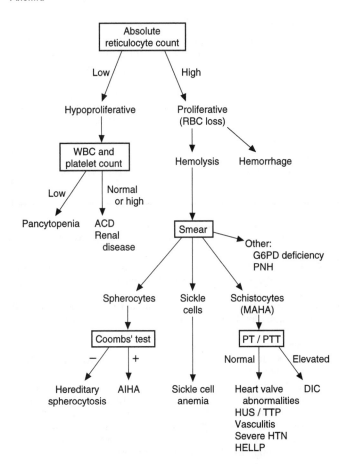

FIGURE 62-1. Determining the cause of normocytic anemia. *ACD* = anemia of chronic disease; *AIHA* = autoimmune hemolytic anemia; *DIC* = disseminated intravascular coagulation; *G6PD* = glucose-6-phosphate dehydrogenase; *HELLP* = Hemolysis, Elevated Liver enzymes, and Low Platelet count syndrome; *HTN* = hypertension; *HUS/TTP* = hemolytic-uremic syndrome/thrombotic thrombocytopenic purpura; *MAHA* = microangiopathic hemolytic anemia; *PNH* = paroxysmal nocturnal hemoglobinuria; *PT* = prothrombin time; *PTT* = partial thromboplastin time; *RBC* = red blood cell; *WBC* = white blood cell.

(2) Hemolytic-uremic syndrome (HUS)/thrombotic thrombocytopenic purpura (TTP). The triad of HUS is hemolysis, uremia, and thrombocytopenia. TTP is hemolytic-uremic syndrome plus fever and neurologic changes. In general, if uremia is the primary disorder, the disease is referred to as HUS. If the central nervous system (CNS) manifestations are more significant, then TTP is the appropriate term.

HOT KEY — An LDH level less than 1000 U/l makes HUS/TTP very unlikely.

(3) Heart valve abnormalities
(4) Hemangiomas (e.g., Kasabach Merritt syndrome)
(5) Malignant hypertension
2. Hemorrhage. If hemorrhage is suspected, the source of the blood loss (e.g., the gastrointestinal tract) must be determined.
B. Nonproliferative normocytic anemia. Low white blood cell (WBC) and **platelet counts** indicate pancytopenia, whereas normal or high counts usually indicate ACD or renal disease.
C. Therapy
    1. AIHA. In idiopathic cases, primary treatment includes steroids and/or splenectomy.
    2. MAHA treatment should be aimed at correcting the underlying disorder if possible. Immediate therapy for TTP is critical and includes plasmapheresis and possibly steroids.
    3. Anemia of chronic disease or renal disease. If anemia is profound enough to require intermittent transfusions, a trial of recombinant erythropoietin can be given.

References
Elliott MA, Nichols WL. Thrombotic thrombocytopenic purpura and hemolytic uremic syndrome. Mayo Clin Proc 2001;76(11):1154-1162.
Fisch P, Handgretinger R, Schaefer HE. Pure red cell aplasia. Br J Haematol 2000; 111(4):1010–1022.
Goodnough LT, Monk TG, Andriole GL. Erythropoietin therapy. N Engl J Med 1997;336:933–938.
Olivieri NF. The beta-thalassemias. N Engl J Med 1999;341:99–109.
Packman CH. The spherocytic haemolytic anaemias. Br J Haematol 2001;112(4): 888–899.

63. Polycythemia

I **INTRODUCTION.** A hematocrit greater than 54% in men or 51% in women constitutes polycythemia (or erythrocytosis).

A. **Absolute polycythemia** is characterized by an increase in red blood cell (RBC) mass.

B. **Relative polycythemia** is characterized by a decrease in plasma volume.

II **CLINICAL MANIFESTATIONS OF POLYCYTHEMIA**

A. Patients are often asymptomatic if the hematocrit is lower than 60%. Higher hematocrits may cause vaso-occlusive episodes resulting in headaches, blurry vision, dizziness, strokes, cardiac ischemia, and peripheral thromboses. A "ruddy" cyanosis may be found on physical examination.

B. Symptoms specific to polycythemia vera are described in Chapter 70.

III **CAUSES OF POLYCYTHEMIA.** Polycythemia may be a secondary, physiologic response to another disorder (e.g., chronic hypoxia), or it may herald a primary, more malignant disorder (e.g., polycythemia vera or an erythropoietin-secreting tumor).

A. **Absolute polycythemia.** There are five common causes of absolute polycythemia. Remember, "Hypoxia Can Cause Polycythemia Every Time."

Causes of Absolute Polycythemia ("Hypoxia Can Cause Polycythemia Every Time")

Hypoxia (chronic)
Carboxyhemoglobinemia
Cushing's syndrome or **C**orticosteroids
Polycythemia vera
Erythropoietin-secreting **T**umors or post-renal **T**ransplant

---

    1. Hypoxia. Chronic hypoxia, as a result of cardiopulmonary disease or high altitude, can lead to polycythemia.

2. **Carboxyhemoglobinemia** or **methemoglobinemia.** Carboxy-hemoglobin, methemoglobin, and other high-affinity variants cause a leftward shift of the hemoglobin dissociation curve, decreased oxygen delivery to the tissues, and a compensatory polycythemia. Smoking is a common cause of carboxyhemoglobinemia.

3. **Cushing's syndrome** or **corticosteroid therapy.** Corticosteroids have an erythropoietic effect, which can lead to polycythemia.

4. **Polycythemia vera** causes polycythemia by clonal proliferation of stem cells independent of erythropoietin.

5. **Erythropoietin-secreting tumors** are primarily renal cell carcinomas, hemangioblastomas (of the cerebellum), uterine fibroids, or hepatocellular carcinomas.

6. **Post-renal transplant.** Due to unclear mechanisms, erythrocytosis can occur in up to 15% of patients after a renal transplant.

B. **Relative polycythemia.** There are two main causes of relative polycythemia.

1. **Dehydration** (e.g., from vomiting, diarrhea, excessive sweating, or diuretics) can deplete plasma volume, leading to a relative polycythemia.

2. **Stress erythrocytosis (Gaisböck's polycythemia)** actually results from contraction of the plasma volume and is therefore a misnomer. This benign disorder is seen most often in hypertensive, obese men.

IV APPROACH TO THE PATIENT

A. **Rule out hypoxia and carboxyhemoglobinemia.** These are common, relatively easy to evaluate causes of polycythemia. If abnormalities significant enough to result in polycythemia are found, the need for additional work-up may be eliminated. An **arterial blood gas with carboxyhemoglobin level** is necessary for all patients who smoke and is more accurate than oxygen saturation measurements. The methemoglobin level can also be checked if there is clinical suspicion.

B. **Look at the patient's hematocrit**

1. **Greater than 60% in men or 55% in women**

   a. A hematocrit greater than 60% in men or 55% in women essentially rules out steroid excess, which usually causes a mild polycythemia. Furthermore, because an elevated RBC mass is found in 99% of these patients, decreased plasma volume is unlikely, and an RBC mass study is usually not necessary.

   b. A hematocrit greater than 60% in men or 55% in women usually reduces the list of possible diagnoses to either polycythemia vera (more common) or an erythropoietin-secreting tumor (less common). The following criteria may be used to help diagnose polycythemia vera. In patients without a definitive diagnosis, the possibility of an erythropoietin-secreting tumor should be considered.

(1) **Polycythemia vera (PCV)**

   (a) Polycythemia associated with splenomegaly, thrombocytosis, and a normal oxygen saturation is diagnostic for PCV.

   (b) A history of bleeding or thrombotic complications points toward PCV.

   (c) An increased leukocyte alkaline phosphatase (LAP) score, concomitant iron deficiency anemia, and/or increased vitamin B_{12} level offer additional evidence for polycythemia vera (see Chapter 70).

   (d) A decreased erythropoietin level is also useful (almost all patients with polycythemia vera have a level less than 20 mU/ml).

(2) **Erythropoietin-secreting tumors**

   (a) An abdominal computed tomography (CT) scan may help rule out renal pathology (including cancer) and hepatic malignancies.

   (b) Brain imaging [preferably with magnetic resonance imaging (MRI)] may be performed if there is any clinical suspicion of a cerebellar lesion.

2. **Hematocrit less than 60% in men or 55% in women.** An **RBC mass study** should be performed to rule out **decreased plasma volume,** which is responsible for polycythemia in approximately 50% of cases. In general, secondary causes will account for far more cases than polycythemia vera.

 TREATMENT is aimed at the underlying disorder. Stress erythrocytosis requires no treatment. General therapeutic measures include the following.

A. **Oxygen therapy** is useful in patients with an arterial oxygen tension (PaO_2) lower than 60 mm Hg.

B. **Smoking cessation** is encouraged (especially in patients with carboxyhemoglobinemia).

C. **Hydration** is recommended for patients with evidence of dehydration.

D. An **ACE inhibitor** is used to treat post-renal transplant polycythemia.

E. **Phlebotomy** to lower the hematocrit is usually only indicated for patients with polycythemia vera (see Chapter 70).

References
Montanaro D, Groupuzzo M, Boscutti G, Risaliti A, Bresadola F, Mioni G. Long-term
    therapy for postrenal transplant erythrocytosis with ACE inhibitors: efficacy,
    safety and action mechanisms. Clin Nephrol 2000;53:47–51.
Pearson TC, Messinezy M. Investigation of patients with polycythaemia. Postgrad
    Med 1996;72:519–524.
Spivak JL. The optimal management of polycythaemia vera. Br J Haematol 2002;
    116:243–254.

64. Leukocytosis

I   INTRODUCTION

A. The **circulating pool of white blood cells** (WBCs, leukocytes) consists of:
1. Neutrophils
2. Lymphocytes
3. Monocytes
4. Eosinophils
5. Basophils

B. **Definitions**
1. **Leukocytosis.** In leukocytosis, the total WBC count **exceeds 11,000 cells/mm³ (11 × 10⁹/L).**
2. **Leukemoid reaction.** A leukemoid reaction occurs when the leukocyte count **exceeds 30,000 cells/mm³** and there is no evidence of immature WBCs or nucleated red blood cells (RBCs) on the peripheral smear. This process reflects a healthy bone marrow that is reacting to some type of stress (e.g., trauma, inflammation, infection, malignancy).
3. **Leukoerythroblastosis.** This term is used when there is evidence of immature WBCs and nucleated RBCs on the peripheral smear, regardless of the total WBC count. Leukoerythroblastosis usually implies bone marrow infiltration.

C. Because each cell type can be increased in response to various stimuli, determining the predominant cell type in patients with leukocytosis may offer some insight into the cause.

II   NEUTROPHILIA   is defined as a neutrophil count that **exceeds 7500 cells/mm³.**

A. **Causes of neutrophilia.** Neutrophilia can be caused by many of the major disease categories discussed in Chapter 1 (Table 64-1).

B. **Approach to the patient.** When evaluating patients with neutrophilia, the most important initial consideration should be **infection.** If this and other benign disorders are excluded, a search for malignancy (which may include a bone marrow biopsy) is usually warranted. Acutely infected or injured patients have elevated levels of endogenous glucocorticoids, which in turn will lead to low levels of eosinophils and basophils. The presence of eosinophils and basophils in acutely ill patients usually indicates one of the following:

TABLE 64-1: Common Causes of Neutrophilia	
Category of Disease	**Specific Causes**
Hematologic	Hemolytic anemia, splenectomy
Pregnancy-related	Pregnancy-induced neutrophilia
Drugs/toxins	Corticosteroids, lithium, mercury, ethylene glycol
Metabolic/endocrine	Hyperthyroidism, ketoacidosis
Inflammatory	Rheumatoid arthritis, vasculitis, gout
Infectious	Bacteria, viruses, fungi, parasites
Neoplastic	Myeloproliferative disorders, myelo-dysplastic syndromes, gastrointestinal or renal malignancy, melanoma, Hodgkin's disease
Trauma	Insects bites, jellyfish stings, crush injuries, electric shock

1. Concomitant adrenal insufficiency
2. Granulocyte-macrophage colony-stimulating factor (GM-CSF)-secreting tumor
3. Hematologic malignancy

III **LYMPHOCYTOSIS** is defined as a lymphocyte count that exceeds 5000 cells/mm^3.

A. **Causes of lymphocytosis** (Table 64-2). The severity of lymphocytosis may indicate possible causes.
B. **Approach to the patient**
  1. The first step in evaluating a patient with lymphocytosis is to look for leukoerythroblastosis on the peripheral smear. If leukoerythroblastosis is present, bone marrow biopsy is necessary.
  2. In patients without evidence of **leukoerythroblastosis,** a benign cause should be sought. If none of these causes can be reasonably diagnosed, the patient should have a bone marrow biopsy to exclude neoplasm.

IV **MONOCYTOSIS** is defined as a monocyte count that **exceeds 500 cells/mm^3.**

A. **Causes of monocytosis** (Table 64-3). Monocytes are very important, not only in the killing of **obligate intracellular parasites**

TABLE 64-2: Common Causes of Lymphocytosis

Type of Lymphocytosis	Specific Causes
Mild to moderate (5000–15,000/mm³)	Viral illness (mononucleosis, hepatitis) Secondary to other infections (e.g., tuberculosis, toxoplasmosis, syphilis) Malignancy (e.g., Hodgkin's disease early CLL)
Severe (> 15,000/mm³)	Mononucleosis Hepatitis Pertussis Late CLL ALL

ALL = acute lymphocytic leukemia; CLL = chronic lymphocytic leukemia.

(e.g., fungi, parasites, yeast), but also in **granulomatous inflammation.**

B. Approach to the patient. If the levels of monocytes are extremely high, a hematologic malignancy should be strongly suspected.

TABLE 64-3: Common Causes of Monocytosis

Category of Disease	Specific Cause
Infectious	Tuberculosis, endocarditis, brucellosis, syphilis, fungal or protozoal infections, listeriosis
Neoplastic	Hodgkin's disease, leukemia, carcinoma
Inflammatory	Inflammatory bowel disease, sarcoidosis

V BASOPHILIA is defined as a basophil count that **exceeds 100 cells/mm³.**

A. Causes of basophilia. Basophilia is an uncommon phenomena. It can be caused by myeloproliferative disorders especially chronic myelogenous leukemia, hypothyroidism, post-splenectomy, pregnancy, and allergic, infectious, or neoplastic phenomena.

B. Approach to the patient. If no clear underlying etiology is found, a bone marrow biopsy should be considered to look for a myeloproliferative disorder.

References
Abramson N, Melton B. Leukocytosis: basics of clinical assessment. Am Fam Phys 2000;62:2053–2060.
Vignola AM, Gjomarkaj M, Arnoux B, Bousquet J. Monocytes. J Allergy Clin Immunol 1998;101:149–152.

65. Eosinophilia

I INTRODUCTION

A. **Eosinophils, a type of white blood cell (WBC), normally dwell in tissues. Eosinophils:**
   1. Play a major role in defending the body against multicellular, helminthic parasites
   2. Elaborate mediators that promote mucus secretion and alter vascular permeability in allergic diseases
   3. Induce mast cells and basophils to release allergic mediators
B. **Eosinophil count.** The normal range of eosinophils in the blood is 0–450 cells/mm^3 (0%–4%). Counts are highest in the very early morning hours (e.g., 4 AM).
   1. **Eosinopenia** is commonly seen in bacterial and viral infections and with exogenous corticosteroid use.
   2. **Eosinophilia** is associated with many diseases (see II).

II CAUSES OF EOSINOPHILIA

A. **Pulmonary diseases.** Many primary lung disorders can lead to eosinophilia, including Löffler's syndrome and eosinophilic pneumonia.
B. **Helminthic infections**
   1. **Filariasis**
   2. **Ascariasis**
   3. **Schistosomiasis**
   4. **Strongyloidiasis**

HOT KEY Disseminated strongyloides sometimes does not cause eosinophilia because of the superimposed bacterial infection that may accompany parasitic dissemination.

---

   5. **Trichinosis**
C. **Other infections**
   1. **Allergic bronchopulmonary aspergillosis**

HOT KEY Invasive aspergillosis does not cause eosinophilia.

Causes of Eosinophilia

PHILIA   CAN

ACT   FAST

Pulmonary disease
Helminthic infections
  Filariasis
  Ascariasis
  Schistosomiasis or Strongyloides infection
  Trichinosis
Infections, other
  Allergic bronchopulmonary aspergillosis
  Coccidioidomycosis
  Tuberculosis (especially chronic)
L-Tryptophan
Immunologic disorders
Addison's disease

Cutaneous disorders
Allergic disorders
Neoplasms

2. Coccidioidomycosis

3. Tuberculosis, especially chronic tuberculosis

D. Contaminated L-tryptophan can cause eosinophilia-myalgia syndrome.

E. Immunologic disorders [e.g., vasculitis (especially Churg-Strauss syndrome), severe rheumatoid arthritis, eosinophilic fasciitis]

F. Addison's disease

G. Cutaneous disorders (e.g., bullous pemphigoid, scabies, eosinophilic cellulitis)

H. Allergic disorders (e.g., asthma, allergic rhinitis, atopic dermatitis, drug reactions, acute urticaria)

I. Neoplasms. Solid tumors, lymphoma, and leukemia can lead to eosinophilia.

References
Brigden ML. A practical workup for eosinophilia. You can investigate the most likely causes right in your office. Postgrad Med 1999;105:193–194, 199–202, 207–210.
Rothenberg ME. Eosinophilia. N Engl J Med 1998;338:1592–1600.
Wolfe MS. Eosinophilia in the returning traveler. Med Clin North Am 1999;83:1019–1032.

66. Bleeding Disorders

I **INTRODUCTION.** A predisposition to bleeding can result from **problems with platelets** (either number or function) or **problems with coagulation** (factor deficiency or factor inhibitors).

II **CLINICAL MANIFESTATIONS OF BLEEDING DISORDERS**

A. **Recurrent bleeding** since childhood or a family history of bleeding suggests an **inherited problem.**

B. **Mucocutaneous petechiae** or ecchymoses are usually indicative of **platelet problems.**

C. **Spontaneous deep bleeding** into hematomas or joints (hemarthroses) or **delayed bleeding** after surgery or trauma is suggestive of **coagulation problems.**

III **APPROACH TO THE PATIENT.** Figure 66-1 summarizes the general approach to a patient with a bleeding disorder.

A. **Platelet count.** The platelet count must be < 90,000 cells/μl to prolong the bleeding time. Therefore, mildly decreased counts are not responsible for clinical bleeding, and a concurrent problem of platelet function or coagulation should be considered.

B. **Prothrombin time (PT)/partial thromboplastin time (PTT).** There are three types of PT/PTT abnormalities: increased PT/normal PTT, increased PT/increased PTT, or normal PT/increased PTT.

1. **Increased PT/normal PTT**
   a. **Differential diagnosis**
      (1) **Early disseminated intravascular coagulation (DIC)**
      (2) **Liver disease**
      (3) **Warfarin therapy**
      (4) **Vitamin K deficiency**
      (5) **Factor VII deficiency** (isolated factor VII deficiency is a rare cause of an elevated PT/normal PTT)
   b. **Recommended work-up**
      (1) **Patient history.** Ask about medications and note factors that may predispose a patient to vitamin K deficiency (e.g., malnutrition, pancreatic insufficiency, recent antibiotic use).
      (2) **DIC panel (D-dimers, fibrinogen) and peripheral smear.** Evidence for DIC may include a low fibrino-

FIGURE 66-1. Approach to the patient with a bleeding disorder. *DIC* = disseminated intravascular coagulation; *PT* = prothrombin time; *PTT* = partial thromboplastin time; *vWD* = von Willebrand's disease.

gen level (< 150 mg/dl), elevated D-dimers, or schistocytes on the peripheral blood smear. D-Dimers can also be elevated in cirrhosis or with clinical bleeding, and hypofibrinogenemia may also occur with severe liver dysfunction; therefore, the presence of schistocytes may be the only distinguishing feature for DIC in a patient with concomitant liver failure.

(3) **Liver tests** (bilirubin, albumin, and transaminase levels) are often obtained.

(4) **Factor VII level.** A factor VII level is rarely necessary but can be obtained if the cause of the increased PT is still unknown.

2. **Increased PT/increased PTT**

a. **Differential diagnosis.** The differential diagnosis for this abnormality is generally the same as for an isolated elevated PT, but the conditions are more severe.[1]

(1) **Severe DIC**

(2) **Severe liver disease**

(3) **Warfarin overdose**

(4) **Severe vitamin K deficiency**

(5) **Factor II, V, or X deficiency** (extremely rare causes of an elevated PT/PTT)

b. **Recommended work-up.** The recommended evaluation is the same as that for increased PT/normal PTT, except that on the extremely rare occasion of a completely negative work-up, different factor levels need to be tested.

3. **Normal PT/increased PTT**

a. **Differential diagnosis.** After excluding the obvious cause (i.e., heparin therapy), you need to consider three possibilities.

(1) **Coagulation factor deficiency**

(2) **Coagulation factor inhibitor**

(3) **Antiphospholipid antibodies (including lupus anticoagulant and anticardiolipin antibody)**

b. **Recommended work-up**

(1) **Patient history.** The patient history can provide valuable information. If the patient has a history of bleeding, a factor deficiency or a factor inhibitor is likely. If the patient has a history of clotting, an antiphospholipid syndrome is implicated.

(2) **50:50 mixing study.** Only 30% factor activity is needed to have a normal PTT. By mixing the patient's

---

[1]Heparin therapy can also cause an elevated PT/PTT, but the PT is usually only mildly increased.

blood with an equal amount of blood with a normal PTT, enough factor will be provided to correct any factor deficiency (if that is the problem).

    (a) **If the PTT corrects** (and stays corrected on later testing) a **factor deficiency** is diagnosed. The most common factor deficiencies are factor VIII (**hemophilia A**), factor IX (**hemophilia B**), and factor XI deficiencies; therefore, **factor VIII, IX, and XI levels should be drawn first.**

    (b) **If the PTT does not correct** with mixing, an **antiphospholipid antibody** or a **factor inhibitor** is present. Laboratory tests for lupus anticoagulant and anticardiolipin antibody should be sent. A dilute Russell's viper venom time (see III D 1) can also be sent to evaluate the presence of an antiphospholipid antibody.

    (c) **If the PTT initially corrects but prolongs on later testing**, a **factor inhibitor** is probably present. Initially, there is enough factor present to normalize the PTT, but the inhibitor "eats up" the factor until the level decreases to below 30%, prolonging the PTT. **Factor VIII inhibitor is most common** and should be checked first.

C. Bleeding time. If the platelet count and PT/PTT are normal, the next step in the work-up of a patient with a suspected bleeding disorder is to obtain a bleeding time.

  1. If the bleeding time is prolonged with a platelet count > 90,000 cells/μl, platelet dysfunction is implicated.

    a. Acquired platelet dysfunction

      (1) Differential diagnosis. Acquired platelet disorders are usually systemic.

        (a) Severe renal disease (i.e., uremia)

        (b) Severe liver disease

        (c) Malignancy. Myeloproliferative disorders, multiple myeloma, and Waldenstrom's macroglobulinemia (from paraproteinemias) can all lead to platelet dysfunction.

        (d) Autoantibodies [e.g., caused by β lactam antibiotic therapy or idiopathic thrombocytopenic purpura (ITP)] can coat platelets and increase the bleeding time even with a normal platelet count.

        (e) DIC. The fibrin split products produced in DIC inhibit platelet function.

        (f) Acquired storage pool disease. Cardiopulmonary bypass surgery or vasculitis can cause platelets to release all their granules, resulting in dysfunctional platelets.

(g) **Aspirin** irreversibly inhibits platelet function for the life of the platelet (7–10 days); other non-steroidal anti-inflammatory drugs (NSAIDs) reversibly inhibit platelet function and the effect is more transient.

(h) **Clopidogrel** is increasingly used for cardiovascular disease and works by inhibiting platelet aggregation.

HOT KEY

Bleeding time may be prolonged with aspirin or NSAIDs but will only become abnormal if another underlying cause of platelet dysfunction is present.

---

(2) **Recommended work-up**

(a) **Patient history.** A medication history (including all over-the-counter drugs) should always be obtained. Immune-mediated platelet dysfunction may be suspected with the use of certain medications, a history of ITP, or with mild thrombocytopenia accompanied by obvious platelet dysfunction (prolonged bleeding time). Acquired storage pool disease is suspected if the clinical setting is appropriate.

(b) **Complete blood count (CBC) with differential.** A CBC with differential will help evaluate the possibility of a myeloproliferative disorder (see Chapter 70).

(c) **DIC panel.** A DIC panel can help evaluate the possibility of DIC.

(d) **Liver tests** and a **blood urea nitrogen (BUN) level** will help exclude liver and renal disease, respectively.

(e) **Protein electrophoresis** may be used to evaluate the presence of a paraproteinemia (see Chapter 72).

b. **Inherited platelet dysfunction.** Platelets need to first adhere to the endothelium during injury, and then to aggregate by binding fibrinogen.

(1) **Differential diagnosis.** The first two disorders involve problems with platelet adherence, and the second two involve problems with platelet aggregation.

(a) **von Willebrand's disease (vWD).** von Willebrand's factor (vWF) is elaborated by megakaryocytes and endothelial cells and circulates in the plasma in multimers of varying size bound to factor VIII (which vWF stabilizes). vWF binds to the glycoprotein Ib receptor on platelets and helps platelets adhere to endothelium.

  (i) In **type I vWD** (80% of cases), the amount of vWF is decreased.

  (ii) In **type III vWD**, vWF is completely lacking.

  (iii) In **type II vWD**, there is a qualitative decrease in vWF activity. In **type IIa vWD**, the qualitative defect results from a decrease in the large multimers of vWF, the active forms in platelet adhesion. In **type IIb vWD**, there is also a decrease in the large multimers of vWF; however, type IIb vWD differs from type IIa vWD in that the decrease is caused by abnormal vWF adherence to platelets.

  (b) **Bernard-Soulier syndrome** results from a loss in the platelet receptor for vWF (glycoprotein Ib).

  (c) **Glanzmann's thrombasthenia** results from the loss of the IIb–IIIa glycoprotein platelet receptor, which leads to decreased fibrinogen binding and, therefore, defective platelet aggregation.

  (d) **Storage pool disease** is caused by defective release of platelet granules [especially adenosine diphosphate (ADP)], which results in decreased platelet aggregation.

(2) **Recommended work-up**

  (a) **Patient history.** vWD is an autosomal dominant disorder, and Bernard-Soulier syndrome and Glanzmann's thrombasthenia are autosomal recessive disorders; therefore, obtaining the family history is important.

  (b) **vWD panel.** Screen for vWD first because vWD is the most common inherited disorder of platelet function. A vWD panel includes the following tests:

  (i) **Ristocetin cofactor activity.** The patient's plasma is mixed with normal platelets and ristocetin. Ristocetin should cause plasma vWF to bind to the platelet surface (via the glycoprotein Ib receptor), resulting in platelet aggregation. The absence of platelet aggregation implies a quantitative or qualitative decrease in vWF.

  (ii) **Factor VIII antigen** is another way to assess the vWF level.

  (iii) **Factor VIII activity** may be decreased with a decrease in vWF level and may cause a prolonged PTT.

HOT KEY Type I vWD often shows a parallel decrease in all parts of the panel, whereas type III vWD demonstrates no activity in any part of the panel. In type II vWD, there will be decreased ristocetin cofactor activity out of proportion to the decreased factor VIII antigen level.

    (c) Ristocetin aggregation test. The patient's plasma and platelets are mixed with ristocetin. **Bernard-Soulier syndrome** is diagnosed by a normal vWD panel but an abnormal ristocetin aggregation test.

    (d) Platelet aggregometry is used to diagnose **Glanzmann's thrombasthenia** and storage pool diseases.

        (i) In storage pool diseases, platelets will not aggregate with low doses of ADP, but higher doses will result in aggregation.

        (ii) In Glanzmann's thrombasthenia, neither low nor high doses of ADP will induce aggregation because the necessary IIb-IIIa receptor is missing.

2. If the bleeding time is not prolonged in a patient with a normal PT/PTT and platelet count, but there is still clinical suspicion of a bleeding diathesis, a few rare disorders still need to be considered. All these involve a defect in cross-linking of fibrin.

    a. Differential diagnosis

        (1) Factor XIII ("fibrin-stabilizing factor") deficiency

        (2) Dysfibrinogenemia

        (3) Deficiency of inhibitors to fibrinolysis (i.e., plasminogen activator inhibitor or α_2 plasmin inhibitor)

    b. Recommended work-up

        (1) Increased clot solubility in urea demonstrates factor XIII deficiency.

        (2) Increased thrombin time is evidence of a possible dysfibrinogenemia.

        (3) Rate of clot lysis tests and direct measurements of α_2 plasmin inhibitor levels can be performed to evaluate deficiency of inhibitors to fibrinolysis.

D. Other tests

    1. Dilute Russell's viper venom time (dRVVT). Russell's viper venom activates factor X without the usual help of factor V but still requires phospholipid. The dRVVT may therefore be prolonged when **antiphospholipid antibodies** are present.

    2. Thrombin time measures the time for the blood to clot after thrombin is directly added and therefore assesses thrombin's conversion of fibrinogen to fibrin. The thrombin time will be prolonged when thrombin is inhibited (as in **heparin therapy**), when there is low fibrinogen (as in **afibrinogenemia** or **DIC**), or when there is abnormal fibrinogen (as in **dysfibrinogenemia**).

3. **Reptilase time** is just like thrombin time, except it is not sensitive to the effect of heparin. If the thrombin time is prolonged, but the reptilase time is normal, then a **heparin effect** is diagnosed. If the reptilase time is also prolonged, then afibrinogenemia, DIC, or dysfibrinogenemia should be considered.

IV TREATMENT

A. **Platelet problems**
1. **Quantitative problems.** The treatment of thrombocytopenia is discussed in Chapter 60.
2. **Qualitative problems** are usually only treated when the patient is acutely bleeding or surgery is planned. Specific therapies may include dialysis for uremia, myelosuppression for myeloproliferative disorders, or steroids for immune disorders. Other commonly used treatments include:
   a. **Desmopressin** (0.3 μg/kg per day) works presumably by increasing the release of stored vWF from endothelial cells and is useful as prophylaxis before surgery in patients with type I vWD. For unclear reasons, it is also useful in other disorders of platelet dysfunction (e.g., uremia, storage pool disease).
      (1) Stores of vWF are depleted in 2–3 days, so desmopressin is usually only effective as short-term treatment.
      (2) Desmopressin is ineffective in type III vWD. In type IIb vWD, large multimers of vWF are already stuck to platelets, and exposure to desmopressin can trigger paradoxical thromboses and thrombocytopenia (from splenic removal). Therefore, the use of desmopressin should be avoided in patients with these subtypes.
   b. **Cryoprecipitate** (10–15 units every 12 hours) is effective in raising vWF levels 30%–50% (approximately 3% per unit), and is therefore useful in patients with vWD.
   c. **Platelet transfusions** can be used for refractory bleeding.
B. **Coagulation problems**
1. **Increased PT/normal PTT** and **increased PT/increased PTT**
   a. **With significant acute bleeding**
      (1) **Fresh frozen plasma** is given to normalize the PT/PTT regardless of the underlying etiology.
      (2) **Cryoprecipitate** can be used for patients with DIC to restore the fibrinogen level to > 150 mg/dl.

(3) Vitamin K (10 mg subcutaneously daily for 3 days) should be routinely administered in case vitamin K deficiency plays a primary or contributing role in the patient's coagulopathy.

HOT

KEY

Fresh frozen plasma contains all factors but only small amounts of fibrinogen. Cryoprecipitate contains concentrated factor VIII, vWF, and fibrinogen.

---

b. Without significant acute bleeding. Treatment takes into account the underlying cause.

    (1) DIC. In patients with DIC but no acute bleeding, the elevated PT is not treated. Instead, treatment is aimed at the cause of the DIC (e.g., antibiotics for sepsis).

    (2) Warfarin therapy

        (a) If the PT is higher than desired, the **warfarin dose** is usually **decreased** or **withheld,** and the PT is rechecked daily.

HOT

KEY

Remember, there is approximately a 2- to 3-day lag between the changes in dose and the changes in the PT. If you have withheld the warfarin, do not wait until the PT is in the appropriate range to resume therapy, because the PT will continue to drop. Therapy is best reinitiated when the PT is slightly higher than desired.

        (b) Low doses of **vitamin K** (e.g., 1 mg by mouth) can be administered to gradually lower the PT in patients with significant PT elevations.

    (3) Vitamin K deficiency or **liver failure.** Frequently, it is unclear whether the patient's elevated PT is from vitamin K deficiency, liver disease, or both (especially in alcoholics, who are prone to both disorders). **Vitamin K therapy** is often both diagnostic and therapeutic.

    (4) Factor deficiency is rare and not treated unless bleeding is present or surgery is planned.

2. Normal PT/increased PTT

    a. Factor deficiency is only treated if the patient is acutely bleeding or about to undergo surgery. Hemophilia A and B are treated with **factor VIII** and **IX concentrates,** respectively; other factor deficiencies are replaced with **fresh frozen plasma.**

    b. Factor inhibitors

(1) Acute treatment. Factor inhibitors associated with active bleeding can be extremely difficult to treat.

    (a) Aggressive factor replacement (to "overwhelm" the inhibitor) and/or **plasmapheresis** (to remove the inhibitor) are used.

    (b) Activated factor IX or recombinant factor VIIa can be used in the presence of factor VIII inhibitors (i.e., to bypass the step in which factor VIII is needed).

(2) Chronic treatment. Steroids and/or immunosuppressant agents (usually cyclophosphamide) may be administered as chronic therapy.

c. Antiphospholipid antibodies have a tendency to cause thromboses, not bleeding. Therefore, treatment is anticoagulation therapy if significant clotting occurs (see Chapter 67).

References

Kumar S, Pruthi RK, Nichols WL. Acquired von Willebrand disease. Mayo Clin Proc 2002;77:181–187.

Mannucci PM, Tuddenham EGD. Medical progress: the hemophilias—from royal genes to gene therapy.N Engl J Med 2001;344:1773–1779.

67. Hypercoagulable States

I INTRODUCTION

A. Definition. Hypercoagulable states are **clinical disorders of the blood that increase the patient's risk for developing thromboembolic disease.** A cause of thrombosis can be identified in more than 80% of patients with a clot, and often there are multiple causes present.

B. Pathogenesis. Homeostasis in blood clotting is maintained by interrelationships between coagulant and anticoagulant proteins in the vascular endothelium and blood. The pathogenesis of thrombus formation is summarized by **Virchow's triad:**
   1. Defects in blood flow (stasis)
   2. Defects in vascular endothelium
   3. Defects in blood coagulation (leading to hypercoagulability)

II CLINICAL MANIFESTATIONS OF HYPERCOAGULABLE STATES. A hypercoagulable state should be suspected in a patient who develops:

A. Multiple or recurrent clots

B. Clots in unusual locations (e.g., the upper extremities, mesenteric vessels, arteries)

C. Thromboembolic disease at an early age

III CAUSES OF HYPERCOAGULABLE STATES are important to consider when a patient has a blood clot.

A. Inherited clotting disorders
   1. Factor V Leiden mutation is the most common inherited cause of hypercoagulability. This mutation causes resistance of Factor V to the cleaving action of activated protein C.
   2. Prothrombin 20210a mutation is the second most common cause of hereditary thrombophilia.
   3. Protein C and/or S deficiency are uncommon but dramatic causes of thrombophilia that usually present as recurrent thrombotic disease in younger patients.
   4. Antithrombin (ATIII) deficiency is a rare autosomal dominant disorder that can present as severe thrombotic disease in younger patients.
   5. Rare disorders include dysfibrinogenemia, plasminogen deficiency, heparin cofactor II deficiency, elevated clotting factor levels, and others.

B. Acquired clotting disorders

1. **Malignancy,** known or occult, is a common cause of thrombosis. Common offenders include cancers of the lung, pancreas, colon, kidney, and prostate.

2. **Medications**

   a. **Heparin-induced thrombocytopenia and thrombosis (HITT),** an acquired disorder associated with the formation of arterial or venous thrombi in the presence of thrombocytopenia, occurs in a small percentage of patients receiving intravenous or subcutaneous heparin therapy. Heparin should be stopped promptly if thrombocytopenia develops.

   b. **Oral contraceptives** increase the risk of thrombosis independently and in conjunction with other risk factors. The amount of increased risk varies with the formulation of the contraceptive.

   c. Other (e.g., hormone replacement therapy, tamoxifen)

3. **Pregnancy** is associated with increased rates of thrombosis that may be secondary to a progressive increase in activated protein C resistance as pregnancy progresses.

4. **Nephrotic syndrome** causes a hypercoagulable state by unclear mechanisms. It is thought that the loss of urinary proteins shifts the balance of coagulation.

5. **Trauma/surgery** causes increased risk of thrombosis for multiple reasons including decreased venous blood flow, increased levels of tissue factor, immobilization, and others. Orthopedic surgeries are particularly high-risk procedures.

6. **Hyperhomocysteinemia** is both an inherited and acquired defect in which there are high serum levels of homocysteine. Homocysteine is toxic to endothelial cells, and increased levels are associated with thromboembolic disease and atherosclerotic disease.

7. **Myeloproliferative disorders** such as polycythemia vera and essential thrombocythemia are associated with thrombophilia.

8. **Antiphospholipid antibody syndrome** is marked by the presence of antiphospholipid antibodies, hypercoagulability, and recurrent spontaneous abortions.

9. **Immobilization**

10. **Other causes** such as rheumatologic disease, paroxysmal nocturnal hemoglobinuria, hyperviscosity, and others are also associated with hypercoagulability.

C. The causes of the most important hypercoagulable states (both primary and secondary) can be recalled using the mnemonic, "DAMN THROMBUS."

IV APPROACH TO THE PATIENT

A. In a patient with a new deep venous thrombosis, the patient history, physical examination, complete blood count (CBC), uri-

Causes of Hypercoagulable States ("DAMN THROMBUS")

Deficiencies or alterations in coagulation factors (e.g., protein C, protein S, antithrombin III, factor V, prothrombin, fibrinogen, plasminogen)
Antiphospholipid antibody syndrome
Malignancy (e.g., Trousseau's syndrome)
Nephrotic syndrome

Trauma
Hyperhomocysteinemia or **H**eparin-induced thrombocytopenia and thrombosis (HITT) or **H**emoglobinuria [i.e., paroxysmal nocturnal hemoglobinuria (PNH)]
Rheumatologic causes (i.e., vasculitis)
Oral contraceptives (and other medications)
Myeloproliferative disorders
Baby-carriers (i.e., pregnancy)
Unknown
Surgery or postoperative states (particularly neurosurgical and orthopedic)

nalysis, prothrombin time (PT) and partial thromboplastin time (PTT), and chest radiograph are sufficient to rule out most secondary causes of hypercoagulability.

B. The following **laboratory studies** may help exclude specific causes of hypercoagulability:
1. Factor V Leiden mutation test
2. Prothrombin 20210a mutation test
3. Screening tests for the presence of antiphospholipid antibodies, which include PTT and dilute Russell's viper venom test (dRVVT). Specific antibody assays are also available and include anticardiolipin antibodies, lupus anticoagulant, and β_2 microglobulin.
4. Homocysteine level (test after overnight fast)
5. Functional and quantitative assays for proteins C and S, antithrombin III, and fibrinogen

HOT KEY

When checking protein C and S levels, draw serum before warfarin therapy is initiated. Warfarin reduces protein C levels before those of all other vitamin K-dependent factors, because protein C has the shortest half-life. Therefore, warfarin can lead to a falsely low result on a protein C assay.

V TREATMENT

A. Anticoagulation therapy

1. **Initial therapy** of a patient presenting with deep venous thrombosis or pulmonary embolism consists of both **heparin** and **warfarin**. Because protein C has the shortest half-life of all the vitamin K-dependent factors, warfarin therapy alone can lead to a deficiency of protein C relative to the other procoagulant factors (i.e., factors II, VII, IX, and X). Patients with an underlying protein C deficiency who are given warfarin may be susceptible to a transient hypercoagulable state, leading to "coumadin skin necrosis." Coumadin necrosis can be avoided by administering heparin along with warfarin. In addition, the concomitant use of heparin ensures that the patient's blood rapidly becomes anticoagulated, which may prevent further extension of the clot.

   a. **Unfractionated heparin** is given by continuous intravenous infusion, and dosing is adjusted to a goal PTT that is 1.5 to 2.5 times the normal range.

   b. **Low-molecular-weight heparin** is an alternative to unfractionated heparin. This subcutaneous depot form of heparin is dosed every 12–24 hours and can even be used in select patients for outpatient management of thromboembolic disease. Dosing is weight-based and should be adjusted in patients with renal insufficiency. Blood testing is rarely needed but can be checked if desired by measuring anti-factor Xa levels.

2. **Long-term therapy.** Heparin is continued until the PT reaches the therapeutic range [i.e., an international normalized ration (INR) between 2 and 3], which usually takes about 5 days. Warfarin is usually continued for 3–6 months. Patients with recurrent thromboses or thrombosis resulting from a hypercoagulable state may require lifelong anticoagulation therapy.

B. Inferior vena cava (IVC) filter. An IVC filter may be placed in patients at high risk for bleeding with anticoagulation therapy or in patients with recurrent pulmonary emboli despite therapy.

C. Thrombolytic therapy should only be considered in patients with pulmonary embolism who have circulatory or hemodynamic compromise.

References

Dolovich LR, Ginsberg JS, Douketis JD, et al. A meta-analysis comparing low-molecular-weight heparins with unfractionated heparin in the treatment of venous thromboembolism: examining some unanswered questions regarding location of treatment, product type, and dosing frequency. Arch Intern Med 2000;160:181–188.

Federman DG, Kirsner RS. An update on hypercoagulable disorders. Arch Intern Med 2001;161:1051–1056.

Makris M, Rosendaal FR, Preston FE. Familial thrombophilia: genetic risk factors and
    management. J Intern Med Suppl 1997;740:9–15.
Simioni P, Prandoni P, Lensing AW, et al. The risk of recurrent venous thromboem-
    bolism in patients with an Arg506—>Gln mutation in the gene for factor V (fac-
    tor V Leiden). N Engl J Med 1997;336:399–403.

68. Lymphadenopathy

I INTRODUCTION

A. Definition. Lymphadenopathy occurs when the **lymph nodes are of an abnormal consistency** or **increased size.** Lymphadenopathy can be **regional** (i.e., only one group or a few contiguous groups of nodes are involved) or **generalized** (i.e., involving more than two separate sites).

B. Lymphadenopathy **usually signals the presence of disease** and therefore warrants medical evaluation.

II APPROACH TO THE PATIENT

A. First, **make sure the lymph nodes are truly abnormal.** Certain lymph nodes (e.g., the submandibular and inguinal nodes) are commonly palpable.

B. Once lymphadenopathy is deemed abnormal, **generate a differential diagnosis** based on the location of the lymphadenopathy, the human immunodeficiency virus (HIV) status of the patient, the clinical scenario, and the physical attributes of the node. This information helps to guide the need for laboratory tests and other studies [e.g., complete blood count (CBC) and peripheral smear evaluation, Monospot test, hepatitis serologies, serum lactate dehydrogenase (LDH), erythrocyte sedimentation rate (ESR), Venereal Disease Research Laboratories (VDRL) test, and chest radiographs].

1. **Location of the lymphadenopathy.** The location of the lymphadenopathy allows you to form an initial differential diagnosis.

   a. If the lymphadenopathy is **generalized,** the most likely etiologies can be remembered with the mnemonic, "SHE HAS CUTE LAN" on the following page.

   b. If the lymphadenopathy is **localized,** refer to Table 68-1.

2. **HIV status** must always be considered whenever a patient has regional or generalized lymphadenopathy. In HIV-infected patients, generalized lymphadenopathy typically occurs early in the course of HIV disease. Lymphadenopathy can be caused either by the HIV itself or other systemic diseases that are common in HIV-infected patients.

3. **Clinical scenario.** Considering the patient's age and associated findings can help narrow the differential diagnosis.

   a. Patient age. Lymphadenopathy in patients younger than 30 years of age is most often benign (and caused by an in-

Causes of Generalized Lymphadenopathy ("SHE HAS CUTE LAN")

Syphilis
Hepatitis
Epstein-Barr virus infection

Histoplasmosis
AIDS/HIV infection
Serum sickness

Cytomegalovirus (CMV) infection
Unusual drugs (e.g., hydantoin derivatives, anti-thyroid medications, anti-leprosy medications, isoniazid)
Toxoplasmosis
Erythrophagocytic lymphohistiocytosis

Leishmaniasis
Arthritis (rheumatoid)
Neoplasm: leukemia and lymphoma

TABLE 68-1: Major Causes of Localized Lymphadenopathy	
Affected Lymph Nodes	**Causes of Lymphadenopathy**
Cervical	Head and neck malignancy or infection, mononucleosis, tuberculosis, lymphoma
Supraclavicular	Lung, breast, or gastrointestinal malignancy, lymphoma
Axillary	Hand or arm infections, trauma for bites, cat-scratch disease, lymphoma, brucellosis, breast cancer
Epitrochlear	Unilateral: hand infections, lymphoma, tularemia
Inguinal	Leg or foot infections, pelvic malignancy, lymphoma, sexually transmitted disease
Hilar/mediastinal	Sarcoidosis, tuberculosis, lymphoma, fungal infections, lung cancer
Abdominal	Lymphoma, tuberculosis, *Mycobacterium-avium* complex infection, metastatic malignancy

fection). In patients older than 30 years, the possibility of malignancy becomes much more worrisome.

b. Signs and symptoms. Symptoms of fever, chills, night sweats, and weight loss should always be sought and, if present, usually imply a serious systemic infection or malignancy. Symptoms or signs of a local infection (e.g., pharyngitis, conjunctivitis, otitis, skin infection, or trauma) usually imply an infectious etiology.

c. Historical data. Pertinent historical data should be ascertained including a history of smoking, tick bites, travel, high-risk behavior, tuberculosis exposure, and animal contact.

4. Characteristics of lymphadenopathy on palpation. The physical attributes of lymphadenopathy can help a little but may be misleading; therefore, these findings alone should not dissuade further evaluation. In general, abnormal nodes are greater than 1 cm in diameter and the following tend to be true:

a. Infections tend to cause **tender** lymphadenopathy because of rapid growth of the node and subsequent capsular stretching. The nodes tend to be **asymmetric** with erythematous skin overlying the node.

b. Lymphoma classically leads to **large, firm, rubbery, nontender** lymphadenopathy.

c. Metastatic cancer usually results in **very firm** (sometimes "rock hard"), **nontender** nodes that are **immobile** (i.e., fixed to the underlying tissue).

HOT **KEY** Infamous lymph nodes include **Virchow's node** (a left supraclavicular lymph node) and **Sister Mary Joseph's node** (a periumbilical lymph node), both of which can be seen with gastrointestinal malignancies.

C. Evaluation

1. If **lymphoma** or **metastatic malignancy** is strongly considered, proceed to **fine-needle aspiration,** which is quite sensitive for metastatic malignancies (and infections) but not for lymphomas. If lymphoma is a strong possibility, **excisional biopsy** is usually required.

2. If **bacterial infection** is the most likely diagnosis, a **period of observation** (2–3 weeks, with or without antibiotics) is reasonable. If there is no evidence of resolution, fine-needle aspiration, excisional biopsy, or both is usually required.

3. If the **etiology** of the lymphadenopathy is **unclear, close follow-up** is essential because a small but significant percentage of these patients develop lymphoma within 1 year.

TREATMENT varies considerably and depends on the underlying cause.

References
Ferrer R. Lymphadenopathy: differential diagnosis and evaluation. Am Fam Phys 1998;58:1313–1320.
Habermann TM, Steensma DP. Lymphadenopathy. Mayo Clin Proc 2000;75:723–732.

69. Lymphoma

I INTRODUCTION

A. **Definition.** Lymphoma is a **malignant disorder of the lympho-reticular system.**

B. **Classification.** There are two groups of lymphomas (Table 69-1). The distinction is based on the presence or absence of multinucleated giant cells called **Reed-Sternberg cells** in an appropriate cellular environment.
1. **Hodgkin's disease.** Reed-Sternberg cells are usually present.
2. **Non-Hodgkin's lymphoma (NHL).** Reed-Sternberg cells are absent.

II HODGKIN'S DISEASE

A. **Epidemiology**
1. **Incidence.** There are fewer than **10,000 cases** reported per year.
2. **Patient profile**
   a. **Age.** Hodgkin's disease has a **bimodal age distribution.** The incidence peaks in patients **aged 20–25 years** and again in patients **older than 55 years.** In young patients, Hodgkin's disease is associated with high socioeconomic status and small family size.
   b. **Gender.** Except for the nodular sclerosis subtype, Hodgkin's disease is more common in **men** than women.
   c. **Race.** Hodgkin's disease is more common in caucasians than African-Americans.

B. **Pathogenesis of Hodgkin's disease.** Disease progression is **orderly.** Initially, the malignancy spreads to anatomically adjacent lymph tissues. Hematogenous spread to the liver, bone marrow, and other viscera occurs only in advanced disease.

C. **Clinical manifestations of Hodgkin's disease**
1. **Painless, superficial adenopathy** (usually involving the neck or supraclavicular areas)

HOT KEY

Some patients with Hodgkin's disease report pain in lymphoid tissue following the ingestion of alcohol.

TABLE 69-1: Comparison of Hodgkin's Disease and Non-Hodgkin's Lymphoma (NHL)

Disease	Etiology	Malignant Cell Line	Site of Origin	Spread	Mediastinal Involvement	Bone Marrow Involvement	Systemic ("B") Symptoms	Best Prognostic Indicator
Hodgkin's disease	Unknown (viral etiology suspected)	Unclear	Nodal	Contiguous	Common	Uncommon	Very common	Stage
NHL	Unknown (Burkitt's lymphoma associated with Epstein-Barr virus)	90% B cell 10% T cell	Extranodal in up to 40% of patients	Non-contiguous	Rare	Low grade: very common High grade: unusual	Seen in less than 50% of patients	Grade

2. **Constitutional ("B") symptoms** (i.e., **fever, night sweats, weight loss**)
3. **Severe pruritus** (often confined to the lower extremities)
4. **Spinal cord compression** or **superior vena cava syndrome (rare)**
5. **Immunologic dysfunction,** which may develop simultaneously with the onset of the lymphoma and predispose the patient to infection
6. **Characteristic laboratory findings** include:
   a. Anemia
   b. Leukocytosis (initially), thrombocytosis
   c. Eosinophilia
   d. Elevated erythrocyte sedimentation rate (ESR)
   e. Elevated alkaline phosphatase level
D. Approach to the patient
1. **Diagnosis.** The finding of Reed-Sternberg cells on lymph tissue biopsy is characteristic of Hodgkin's disease.
   a. **Differential diagnosis.** Reed-Sternberg cells are also seen with phenytoin-induced lymphoid hyperplasia, some NHLs or solid tumors, and mononucleosis.
   b. **Subtypes.** There are **four main histologic subtypes** of Hodgkin's disease, which are distinguished by the relative number of lymphocytes and Reed-Sternberg cells and the amount of fibrous tissue (Table 69-2).
2. **Staging.** Survival is affected more by the clinical and pathological stage than by the histopathologic subtype.
   a. **Staging evaluation**
      (1) **Chest radiograph.** A chest radiograph should be performed to evaluate mediastinal involvement.
      (2) **Computed tomography (CT).** Abdominal and pelvic CT scans are routinely done to assess nodes in these areas.

TABLE 69-2: Histopathologic Subtypes of Hodgkin's Disease	
Histologic Subtype	**Comments**
Lymphocyte-predominant	Best prognosis; usually presents in an earlier stage
Mixed cellularity	Intermediate prognosis; patients are older
Lymphocyte-depleted	Worst prognosis; patients are older
Nodular sclerosis	Female predominance; patients are younger; usually involves lower cervical, supraclavicular and mediastinal nodes

          (3) Other studies. Some patients also undergo **lymphangiography, bilateral bone marrow biopsies,** and **staging laparotomy with splenectomy.**

     b. Staging classification. The staging system for Hodgkin's diseases is based on the **Ann Arbor classification system.** Like most oncologic staging systems, prognosis is best for stage I patients and worst for stage IV patients. Table 69-3 presents a simplified staging scheme based on the extent of lymph node involvement. Within these stages are substages that affect treatment and prognosis.

          (1) If patients have no "B" symptoms, the letter **"A"** is added to the stage.

          (2) If **weight loss (in excess of 10% of body weight), unexplained fever,** or **night sweats** is present, the letter **"B"** is added. In general, those with symptoms have a poorer prognosis.

E. Treatment. In general, Hodgkin's disease should be thought of as a curable cancer.

   1. Treatment depends on the stage. General approaches follow; an oncology reference can provide detailed information regarding regimens.

     a. Low-stage disease (e.g., **stage I** and **IIa**) is usually treated with **radiation.**

     b. High-stage disease (e.g., **stage IIIb** and **IV**) is usually treated with **combination chemotherapy and radiation to bulky nodes.**

     c. Intermediate-stage disease. The optimal treatment for stage **IIb** and **IIIa** disease is **controversial.**

     d. Patients with aggressive disease that relapse despite multiple therapies may be candidates for high-dose therapy with **autologous bone marrow or peripheral stem cell support.**

   2. Long-term complications of treatment

     a. Chemotherapy increases the risk for acute leukemia; this risk peaks 5 years after initiation of therapy and decreases after 10 years. The development of acute leukemia as a re-

---

TABLE 69-3: Staging System for Patients with Hodgkin's Disease

Stage	Definition
I	Limited to one area
II	Two or more areas but limited to one side of the diaphragm
III	Two or more areas on both sides of the diaphragm
IV	Involvement of extralymphatic tissue (i.e., disseminated disease)

sult of chemotherapy for Hodgkin's disease is much more common in older patients.

b. Radiation therapy leads to an increased incidence of solid tumors (e.g., breast, stomach, or thyroid tumors); this risk, unlike that of leukemia, continues to increase with time.

III **NHL** is the name given to a **heterogeneous group** of malignancies involving both B and T cells.

A. Epidemiology

1. Incidence. The incidence is four times greater than that of Hodgkin's disease. In addition, the HIV epidemic has, in part, led to an increase in the incidence of NHL over the past several years.

2. Patient profile

a. Age. The median age at the time of diagnosis is **50 years.**

b. Gender. NHL is more common in **men** than women.

c. Race. It is more common in caucasians than African-Americans.

d. Other factors

(1) NHL is more common in patients with **altered immunity** (e.g., HIV-positive patients, those receiving immunosuppressive therapy, and those with congenital immunodeficiencies or autoimmune disease).

(2) Some subtypes are associated with **chromosomal abnormalities.**

B. Pathogenesis of NHL. The spread of disease is not contiguous.

C. Clinical manifestations of NHL. Presentations depend on the site and subtype of tumor.

1. Common complaints include:

a. Asymptomatic superficial lymphadenopathy

b. "B" symptoms (much less common than in Hodgkin's disease)

c. Abdominal complaints

d. Bone pain or **pathologic fracture**

e. Symptoms related to pancytopenia

f. Acute emergencies (e.g., superior vena cava syndrome, spinal cord compression, airway compression)

2. Characteristic laboratory findings include:

a. Complete blood count (CBC) ranging from normal to a decrease in all cell lines (i.e., pancytopenia)

b. Elevated uric acid and lactate dehydrogenase (LDH) levels

c. Elevated alkaline phosphatase levels

D. Approach to the patient

1. Diagnosis. Biopsy of tissue allows a definitive diagnosis to be made. Depending on the classification system, the many **sub-**

FIGURE 69-1. General therapeutic measures for patients with non-Hodgkin's lymphoma (NHL).

types of NHL can be grouped into **three categories** based on the histologic grade of the tumor: **low-grade, intermediate-grade,** and **high-grade.**

2. **Staging**

   a. **Staging evaluation.** Bone marrow biopsy, chest radiographs, and abdominal and pelvic CT scans are often performed, and some patients require lumbar puncture or a bone scan. Staging laparotomy and lymphangiography are not usually indicated.

   b. **Staging classification.** The Ann Arbor staging system for Hodgkin's disease (see Table 69-3) is also used to stage NHLs; however, in NHL, the histologic type is the single best predictor of prognosis. Therefore, the Ann Arbor staging system is less useful for these patients.

E. **Treatment** depends primarily on histology, the extent of disease, and patient characteristics. Treatment options are diagrammed in Figure 69–1. In addition to standard chemotherapy, **immunotherapy** (i.e., anti CD20 antibody rituximab) has an increasingly important role in NHL therapy.

HOT KEY

There exists a curious irony to NHL: tumors that confer a favorable prognosis are the least likely to be cured because low-grade tumors are less responsive to chemotherapy. Patients with high-grade lymphomas generally have a poor prognosis, but the chance of cure is increased.

References

Colombat P, Salles G, Brousse N, et al. Rituximab (anti-CD20 monoclonal antibody) as single first-line therapy for patients with follicular lymphoma with a low tumor burden: clinical and molecular evaluation. Blood 2001;97:101–106.

Fung HC, Nademanee AP. Approach to Hodgkin's lymphoma in the new millennium. Hematol Oncol 2001;20:1–15.

70. Myeloproliferative Versus Myelodysplastic Syndromes

I **INTRODUCTION.** Myeloproliferative and myelodysplastic disorders are often confused. However, paying attention to the names will remind you that these are very different diseases.

A. Myeloproliferative disorders are a group of diseases in which early cells in the bone marrow replicate uncontrollably; generally, an **increase** in white blood cells (WBCs), red blood cells (RBCs), platelets, or a combination of these is noted (myelofibrosis is often an exception).

B. Myelodysplastic disorders involve ineffective hematopoiesis, causing hypercellular, normocellular, or hypocellular bone marrow. Generally, a **decrease** in WBCs, RBCs, platelets, or a combination of these is noted.

II **MYELOPROLIFERATIVE DISORDERS**

A. Introduction

1. **Types of disorders.** There are four myeloproliferative disorders. They all involve clonal proliferation of the hematopoietic stem cell, leading to both qualitative and quantitative changes in all cell lines. The type of disorder is therefore based on the predominant cell line that is affected.

   a. Chronic myelogenous leukemia (CML) is characterized by prominent proliferation of the WBC line.

   b. Polycythemia vera is characterized by prominent proliferation of the RBC line.

   c. Essential thrombocytosis is characterized by prominent proliferation of platelets.

   d. Myelofibrosis is characterized by prominent proliferation of fibroblasts.

2. **General approach to the patient.** A myeloproliferative disorder is usually suspected when typical abnormalities are found on the complete blood count (CBC).

   a. Primary abnormality

   (1) If the WBC is significantly elevated, CML is a possibility and the differential diagnosis is that of leukocytosis (see Chapter 64).

    (2) **If the RBC count is significantly elevated,** polycythemia (see Chapter 63) is diagnosed and polycythemia vera should be considered.

    (3) **If the platelets are markedly elevated,** consider the differential diagnoses for thrombocytosis (see Chapter 61), including essential thrombocytosis.

b. Multiple abnormalities. More than one abnormality (e.g., an increased hematocrit and platelet count) is helpful in that it implies a myeloproliferative disorder; however, more than one myeloproliferative disorder may need to be considered. The following features can help diagnose a specific myeloproliferative disorder:

    (1) **Massive splenomegaly** (see Chapter 31) implies either CML or myelofibrosis.

    (2) A **decreased leukocyte alkaline phosphatase (LAP) score** is noted in CML.

    (3) **Nucleated RBCs, early WBCs,** and **abnormal RBC** morphology (i.e., **teardrop cells**) are characteristic of a **leukoerythroblastic smear** and are seen in myelofibrosis.

    (4) An **increased hematocrit** is only seen in polycythemia vera.

    (5) **Increased platelets** out of proportion to the WBC elevation and an **increased LAP score** allow differentiation of essential thrombocytosis from CML.

HOT KEY

A bone marrow biopsy is usually not necessary to diagnose a myeloproliferative disorder, with the possible exception of myelofibrosis.

B. CML

  1. Approach to the patient

    a. Patient history

      (1) Common complaints include **fevers, sweats, fatigue,** and **abdominal fullness** (from splenomegaly).

      (2) Significant leukocytosis (e.g., a WBC count > 300,000 cells/μl) may cause **leukostasis** in approximately 1% of patients with CML. Symptoms of leukostasis include **blurred vision, respiratory distress,** and **priapism.**

    b. Physical examination. Significant splenomegaly is a common finding.

    c. Laboratory studies

      (1) **WBC count.** The WBC count is significantly elevated (e.g., 150,000 cells/il). The white blood cell differential primarily consists of neutrophils, but **basophilia** can often be present.

(2) Peripheral blood smear. Typically, myeloid forms in varying degrees of maturation are seen.

(3) Vitamin B$_{12}$ and uric acid levels may be increased as a result of increased transcobalamin secretion and high cell turnover, respectively.

d. **Bone marrow biopsy.** If performed, a hypercellular marrow with left-shifted WBCs is usually seen. When the disease progresses to the accelerated (blast) phase, the bone marrow has more than 30% blasts.

e. **Cytogenetic studies.** Almost all patients with CML have a translocation between chromosomes 9 and 22 (i.e., the **Philadelphia chromosome** or the **bcr/abl fusion gene**) that may be detected by karyotype testing or by molecular testing.

2. **Treatment**

a. **Leukapheresis** is used if the patient has symptoms of leukostasis, which is a medical emergency.

b. **Pharmacologic therapy**

(1) Hydroxyurea is usually used to lower the WBC count to 5,000–10,000 cells/µl.

(2) Interferon-α (IFN-α) may offer palliation by suppressing the Philadelphia chromosome.

(3) Imatinib is a selective inhibitor of the bcr/abl tyrosine kinase. It has been shown to induce cytogenetic and hematologic remission in many CML patients. Although long-term results are unknown, this agent holds much promise for the treatment of CML.

c. **Bone marrow transplantation** offers the only possibility for cure. Patients should generally be younger than 55 years and have a human leukocyte antigen (HLA)-matched sibling.

3. **Prognosis.** The average survival from diagnosis is 3–4 years. The disease eventually progresses to an accelerated (blast) phase that results in progressive anemia and thrombocytopenia; at this point, the survival time usually decreases to a few months.

C. **Polycythemia vera**

1. **Approach to the patient**

a. **Patient history**

(1) Symptoms of **hyperviscosity** are common (e.g., **headaches, dizziness, blurred vision**).

(2) Both **thrombosis** and **bleeding** may result from abnormalities in platelet function.

(3) Increased basophils may result in increased histamine release and account for the high incidence of both **pruritus** and **peptic ulcers.**

HOT KEY Think of polycythemia vera when a patient is admitted with a bleeding peptic ulcer but continues to have a normal or elevated hematocrit.

    b. Physical examination. Splenomegaly is commonly found on examination but is not as marked as in CML and myelofibrosis.

    c. Laboratory studies

        (1) Hematocrit. A hematocrit consistently greater than 60% in men and 55% in women is usually due to polycythemia vera.

        (2) Mean corpuscular volume (MCV). In approximately 25% of patients, there is an associated iron deficiency that causes a low MCV. Gastrointestinal bleeding from engorged vessels or peptic ulcer disease and increased demand from the elevated RBC mass are potential etiologies of the iron deficiency.

        (3) Vitamin B_{12} and **uric acid levels** are frequently elevated, as in CML.

        (4) Erythropoietin level. The erythropoietin level is usually low (< 20 mU/ml).

    d. Marrow progenitor cell culture. This may be the most sensitive test for polycythemia vera. Spontaneous cell growth in the absence of exogenous erythropoietin is diagnostic.

    e. Bone marrow biopsy. Although not necessary for diagnosis, a bone marrow biopsy will show panhyperplasia and, notably, increased megakaryocytes. Iron stores may be decreased.

2. Treatment

    a. Phlebotomy may be performed weekly until the hematocrit has been lowered to less than 45%; thereafter, maintenance phlebotomy may be performed as needed.

    b. Pharmacologic therapy

        (1) Hydroxyurea is sometimes given to patients with marked thrombocytosis (e.g., a platelet count $>$ 700,00 cells/μl) with the goal of decreasing the risk of thrombosis. Hydroxyurea is also frequently administered to patients with intractable pruritus or a high phlebotomy requirement.

        (2) Aspirin in low doses (e.g., 325 mg per day) is sometimes given to patients who experience recurrent thromboses despite phlebotomy or hydroxyurea therapy.

        (3) Alkylating agents and **radiophosphorus** can be leukemogenic and are increasingly avoided.

3. **Prognosis.** The average survival with treatment is 10–15 years. Polycythemia vera can convert to CML, myelofibrosis, and, rarely, acute myelogenous leukemia (AML).

D. **Essential thrombocytosis**
   1. **Approach to the patient**
      a. **Patient history**
         (1) Abnormalities in platelet function can lead to both thromboses and bleeding. **Erythromelalgia** (i.e., intense, burning pain in dependent extremities often accompanied by skin warmth and mottling) results from microvascular occlusion. Although it can occur in all myeloproliferative disorders, erythromelalgia is especially common in patients with essential thrombocytosis.
         (2) Many patients (particularly young women) are **asymptomatic.**
      b. **Physical examination.** Splenomegaly occurs in two thirds of patients but is not as significant as in CML and myelofibrosis.
      c. **Laboratory studies**
         (1) **Platelet count.** The platelet count is invariably greater than 400,000 cells/μl and often exceeds 1,000,000 cells/μl.
         (2) **Peripheral blood smear.** The platelet morphology is frequently abnormal, with many large, hypogranular forms.
         (3) **Bleeding times** and **aggregation** studies may show abnormalities in platelet function.
      d. **Bone marrow biopsy.** If performed, bone marrow biopsy reveals an increased number of large, hyperploid megakaryocytes. This finding contrasts that of reactive thrombocytosis, in which the megakaryocytes are small and of lower ploidy.
   2. **Treatment**
      a. **Hydroxyurea** is often used for patients with symptomatic thromboses or platelet counts > 700,000 cells/μl.
      b. **Anagrelide** is also an effective oral agent to lower the platelet count.
      c. **IFN-α** can sometimes be used to control thrombocytosis if other agents are ineffective.
      d. **Aspirin.** Small daily doses (e.g., 325 mg per day) may be indicated for patients with recurrent thromboses or vasomotor symptoms despite adequate control of the platelet count with hydroxyurea.
      e. **Alkylating agents** and **radiophosphorus** are increasingly avoided.

3. Prognosis. Essential thrombocytosis is an indolent disease. The average survival is usually at least 10–15 years.
E. Myelofibrosis (or agnogenic myeloid metaplasia)
  1. Approach to the patient
    a. Patient history. Symptoms reflect anemia (**fatigue, dyspnea**), thrombocytopenia (**easy bruisability**), and marked splenomegaly (**abdominal fullness**).
    b. Physical examination. Splenomegaly is usually marked and hepatomegaly may also be present.
    c. Laboratory studies
      (1) Hematocrit. Anemia is almost always present.
      (2) Peripheral blood smear. The combination of **teardrop cells**, a **leukoerythroblastic smear** (nucleated RBCs and left-shifted WBCs), and **large, abnormal platelets** is virtually diagnostic of myelofibrosis.
    d. Bone marrow biopsy is diagnostic and reveals increased reticulin fibers in the early stages of disease and more severe fibrosis later in the course of the disease.
  2. Treatment
    a. Supportive measures include blood and platelet transfusions as needed. Erythropoietin, androgens, and novel therapy such as thalidomide or etanercept may be given in an attempt to decrease transfusion requirements or constitutional symptoms.
    b. Hydroxyurea can be useful in reducing spleen size or controlling thrombocytosis or leukocytosis.
    c. Splenectomy or **splenic irradiation** may be indicated for patients with refractory anemia or thrombocytopenia or in patients with recurrent pain from splenic enlargement.
    d. IFN-α may benefit some patients.
    e. Bone marrow transplant currently offers the only chance for cure.
  3. Prognosis. The illness usually results in bleeding from thrombocytopenia and progressive liver failure from extramedullary hematopoiesis; the average survival is 5 years.

III   MYELODYSPLASTIC SYNDROME (MDS) is a clonal disorder characterized by ineffective hematopoiesis. The bone marrow is often hypercellular, and cytopenias are noted on the peripheral smear. MDS is most often idiopathic but can be secondary to chemotherapy, toxins, or radiation.

A. Classification. The current classification scheme is far from perfect. It includes **chronic myelomonocytic leukemia (CMML),** which is more like a myeloproliferative disorder in its proliferation of the monocyte line. It is also impossible to predict which patients will progress to AML and which will follow a more benign course using the current classification scheme.

1. **Refractory anemia (RA);** less than 5% blasts in the bone marrow
2. **Refractory anemia** with **ringed sideroblasts (RARS);** less than 5% blasts and greater than 15% ringed sideroblasts.
3. **Refractory anemia** with **excess blasts (RAEB);** 5%–19% blasts
4. **RAEB in transformation (RAEB-t);** 20%–29% blasts
5. **CMML;** peripheral monocytosis (> 1,000 cells/uL), less than 20% blasts

B. **Approach to the patient**
1. **Patient history.** Patients are **frequently asymptomatic** at diagnosis. If symptoms and signs are present, they result from one of the cytopenias and therefore include **fatigue, infection,** and **bleeding.**
2. **Physical examination.** Splenomegaly may be present but often is not.
3. **Laboratory studies.** Abnormalities in two or three of the following cell lines are usually present.
   a. **RBC line.** Anemia, an increased MCV, macro-ovalocytes, and a decreased reticulocyte count
   b. **WBC line.** Neutropenia, hypogranular neutrophils, and the **Pelger-Huet anomaly** (bilobed nuclei)
   c. **Platelets.** Thrombocytopenia and hypogranular platelets.
4. **Bone marrow biopsy** is necessary to diagnose myelodysplastic syndromes. When there are **more than 30% blasts, acute leukemia** is diagnosed.

C. **Treatment**
1. **Supportive therapy.** Blood and platelet transfusions are given as needed, but may eventually be complicated by alloantibody formation, which decreases RBC and platelet survival.
2. **Pharmacologic therapy.** Virtually all therapy for MDS is either supportive or investigational. A few of the more commonly used agents are discussed here:
   a. **Growth factors**
      (1) **Erythropoietin** may decrease the transfusion requirement in some patients.
      (2) **Granulocyte colony-stimulating factor (G-CSF)** or **granulocyte-macrophage colony-stimulating factor (GM-CSF)** usually increase neutrophil counts and decrease the incidence of associated minor infections, but no significant survival benefit has been demonstrated.
   b. **Pyridoxine** is non-toxic and improves anemia in a small number of patients.

c. **Intensive chemotherapy** (with regimens similar to those for leukemia) has had mixed results.

3. **Bone marrow transplantation** offers the only possibility of cure for the small group of eligible patients. Patients must be younger than 55 years and have an HLA-matched sibling donor.

D. **Prognosis** is based on a variety of features including age, degree of cytopenias, cytogenetics, and an overall tendency to evolve into AML. Patients with mild cytopenias and favorable cytogenetics can survive for many years. Patients with less favorable findings (often classified as RAEB, RAEB-t, or CMML) have an increased risk of transforming to AML (20–50%) and survival time is much shorter (i.e., approximately 1 year).

References

Druker BJ, Talpaz M, Resta DJ, et al. Efficacy and safety of a specific inhibitor of the BCR-ABL tyrosine kinase in chronic myeloid leukemia. N Engl J Med 2001; 344:1031–1037.

Heaney ML, Golde DW. Myelodysplasia. N Engl J Med 1999;340: 1649–1660.

Faderl S, Talpaz M, Estrov Z, et al. The biology of chronic myeloid leukemia. N Engl J Med 1999;341:164–172.

Tefferi A. Myelofibrosis with myeloid metaplasia. N Engl J Med 2000;342:1255–1265.

71. Acute Leukemia

I INTRODUCTION

A. Leukemia results from the clonal proliferation of white blood cells (WBCs). Leukemias are classified according to the **cell line** involved (**lymphocytic** or **myelogenous**) and the **maturity of the malignant cell.** Because chronic myelogenous leukemia (CML) involves clonal proliferation of stem cells, it is better thought of as a myeloproliferative disorder and is discussed in Chapter 70.

B. Patients with acute leukemia are commonly hospitalized for chemotherapy or for complications associated with the leukemia itself or its treatment.

II ACUTE LEUKEMIA results from a hematopoietic progenitor cell losing its ability to differentiate while replicating uncontrollably.

A. Classification
1. **Acute lymphoblastic leukemia (ALL).** The progenitor cell is a **lymphocyte precursor.** ALL can be classified according to:
   a. Morphology
   (1) L1 = small lymphoblastic
   (2) L2 = large lymphoblastic
   (3) L3 = undifferentiated
   b. Immune subtype
   (1) Pre-B cell
   (2) B cell
   (3) T cell
2. **Acute myelogenous leukemia (AML),** also known as **acute nonlymphocytic leukemia,** is diagnosed when the progenitor cell is a **myelocyte precursor.** AML can be classified according to which cell in the myelogenous lineage underwent clonal expansion (Table 71-1).

B. Epidemiology
1. **ALL** represents 80% of childhood cases of acute leukemia (peak age: 3–7 years) and approximately 10%–20% of adult cases. The L1 morphology, which usually occurs in children, and the pre-B cell immune subtype carry a more favorable prognosis.
2. **AML** represents the majority of adult cases (approximately 60%–70%); the average age at onset is 50 years.
3. **Biphenotypic leukemia.** In another 10%–20% of adult cases, leukemia has features of both ALL and AML.

TABLE 71-1: Classification of Acute Myelogenous Leukemia (AML)	
Type	Name of Leukemia*
M1	Myeloblastic
M2	Myeloblastic with differentiation
M3	Promyelocytic
M4	Myelomonocytic
M5	Monocytic
M6	Erythroleukemia
M7	Thromboleukemia

*General progression is from early to mature cell types.

C. **Risk factors** for acute leukemia include prior radiation or chemotherapy, chemical exposures (e.g., benzene), myelodysplasia, myeloproliferative disorders, aplastic anemia, and congenital chromosomal disorders (e.g., Down's syndrome, Turner's syndrome, Klinefelter's syndrome). In most cases, no obvious predisposing condition is found.

D. **Clinical manifestations of acute leukemia.** Patients usually seek medical attention within days or weeks of the start of their illness. The pathologic processes outlined below (particularly pancytopenia) give rise to the most common findings on presentation.

1. **Pancytopenia** may result in **petechiae, fatigue** and **pallor,** or **clinically apparent infections** (e.g., cellulitis, pneumonia).

2. **Blast cell proliferation and invasion**
   a. **ALL. Bone pain, arthralgias, lymphadenopathy,** and **hepatosplenomegaly** are common with ALL.
   b. **AML.** AML type M5 is associated with **gingival, skin,** and **central nervous system (CNS)** involvement.

3. **Leukostasis** [i.e., vaso-occlusion by white blood cells (WBCs)] may occur with a leukocyte count greater than 100,000 cells/μl. CNS disorders (**headaches, strokes**) and pulmonary findings **(dyspnea, hypoxia)** are common manifestations of leukostasis.

4. **Disseminated intravascular coagulation (DIC)** may occur with AML types M3 and M5. It usually results in **excessive bleeding** rather than clotting.

HOT

▶ M3 causes DIC.

KEY

E. Approach to the patient
   1. Laboratory studies
      a. Complete blood count (CBC). Pancytopenia is usually present but may also be found in a variety of other disorders (see Chapter 59).
      b. Peripheral blood smear
         (1) Blasts are usually, but not universally, found on the peripheral blood smear.
         (2) Auer rods, eosinophilic rods that may be seen in the cytoplasm of blasts, are **pathognomonic for AML.**
      c. Coagulation tests. If DIC is present, a prolonged prothrombin time (PT), decreased fibrinogen level, and elevated levels of fibrin degradation products may be seen.
      d. Electrolyte panel. Metabolic abnormalities may result from spontaneous **tumor lysis syndrome** or, more commonly, with therapy-induced tumor lysis. High cell turnover can result in hyperuricemia, hyperkalemia, hyperphosphatemia, hypocalcemia, and/or acidosis.
      e. Cerebrospinal fluid (CSF) analysis may show abnormalities in patients with carcinomatous meningitis, which is most often associated with ALL and AML type M5.
   2. Radiography. A **chest radiograph** may show an anterior mediastinal mass in patients with ALL (especially the T cell variety).
   3. Bone marrow biopsy. The diagnosis of acute leukemia relies on the presence of **more than 30% blasts** in the bone marrow. Morphology, histochemical stains [i.e., peroxidase, periodic acid-Schiff (PAS)], surface markers [i.e., terminal deoxynucleotidal transferase (TdT)], and cytogenetics can all help determine whether the leukemia is ALL or AML as well as the prognosis.
      a. ALL. Remember that you "ALL PAST ('passed')" the test by using this mnemonic:

Differentiating ALL from AML ("ALL PAST")

ALL is associated with a positive **PAS** stain and a positive **TdT** enzymology (TdT is positive in 95% of ALL cases).

---

      b. AML is associated with a positive peroxidase stain. (Peroxidase stains the myeloid granules.)

F. Treatment
   1. Types of therapy
      a. Induction chemotherapy is high-dose, usually kills more than 99.9% of leukemic cells, and is meant to induce a **complete remission (CR).** A patient is in CR if there are fewer than 5% blasts in the bone marrow, no blasts in the peripheral blood, no evidence of extramedullary invasion, and normalization of the blood counts.
      b. Consolidation (early intensification) therapy is usually needed to prevent relapse.
      c. Maintenance therapy, which entails lower doses, may be indicated and is often continued for several years.
   2. General approaches to therapy
      a. ALL
         (1) Chemotherapy
            (a) Induction chemotherapy (often with daunorubicin, vincristine, and prednisone) can induce a CR in most patients with ALL.
            (b) CNS prophylaxis with cranial irradiation and intrathecal methotrexate is usually administered after remission because leukemic meningitis is the site of relapse in up to two thirds of patients who do not receive prophylactic therapy.
            (c) Maintenance therapy (or consolidation therapy for high-risk patients) is often given for 2–3 years.
         (2) Bone marrow transplantation. With standard chemotherapy, approximately two thirds of children and one half of adults will be cured. Because these rates are comparable to those observed with allogenic transplantation during the first remission, bone marrow transplantation is usually reserved for patients with poor prognostic features or for **relapsed patients who achieve a second remission.**
      b. AML
         (1) Chemotherapy
            (a) Induction chemotherapy (usually with daunorubicin and cytarabine) produces a CR in approximately two thirds of patients, but less than one half are cured.
            (b) CNS prophylaxis. Patients with symptoms suggestive of leukemic meningitis and asymptomatic patients with M4 or M5 AML usually undergo a CSF evaluation to rule out leukemic meningitis during remission.
            (c) Consolidation therapy is usually given, often with the same induction agents or cytarabine alone. In

contrast to the management of ALL, **maintenance therapy is not indicated.**

    (d) All-trans retinoic acid (ATRA) is used in addition to standard chemotherapy for M3 AML. These leukemic cells bear a characteristic translocation [t(15:17)] involving the retinoic acid receptor alpha gene. ATRA induces differentiation in M3 AML and improves both survival and remission rates.

  (2) Bone marrow transplantation may be preferable **following the first remission** in patients with AML because cure rates may be increased.

III COMPLICATIONS ASSOCIATED WITH ACUTE LEUKEMIA

A. Leukostasis with symptoms is more common in patients with AML than those with ALL and may necessitate emergent plasmapheresis.

B. Tumor lysis syndrome may occur de novo (most commonly with M3 or M5 AML) or with the initiation of therapy. Preventive and therapeutic measures usually include **vigorous hydration, allopurinol therapy, calcium replacement,** and **sodium bicarbonate administration** (to treat acidosis and hyperkalemia and facilitate the excretion of uric acid).

C. Anemia and **thrombocytopenia** should be managed as described in Chapter 59 V and Chapter 60, respectively. Menstruation should be suppressed to prevent excessive bleeding.

D. DIC frequently accompanies treatment for M3 AML. **Low-dose heparin therapy** may be used as prophylaxis.

E. Fever and **neutropenia.** The risks associated with neutropenia are highest when the absolute neutrophil count is less than 500 cells/μl. Neutropenic precautions should be taken (see Chapter 59 V A 3). Patients should be thoroughly evaluated for the source of their fever (see Chapter 48), and **broad-spectrum antibiotics** should be instituted as soon as blood cultures are drawn.

F. Complications associated with bone marrow transplant

  1. Graft versus host disease (GVHD) may accompany allogenic bone marrow transplant.

    a. Acute GVHD may manifest with a rash, diarrhea, and liver abnormalities. Immunoprophylaxis with **methotrexate** and **cyclosporine** may be beneficial.

    b. Chronic GVHD usually manifests with skin changes similar to scleroderma and is often treated with **prolonged immunosuppression.**

  2. *Pneumocystis carinii* **pneumonia (PCP)** is usually treated with **trimethoprim/sulfamethoxazole (TMP/SMX).** One double-strength tablet (160 mg/800 mg) daily or three times per week is effective prophylaxis.

3. **Cytomegalovirus (CMV) pneumonia** must be recognized and is often treated with **ganciclovir.**

4. **Herpes virus infections,** including herpes simplex virus and varicella-zoster virus reactivations, may be prevented and treated with **acyclovir.**

5. **Fungal infections,** including aspergillosis and candidiasis, confer an especially poor prognosis. Infections may be prevented with fluconazole and may be treated with fluconazole, voriconazole, or amphotericin B.

References

Lowenberg B, Downing JR, Burnett A. Medical progress: acute myeloid leukemia. N Engl J Med 1999;341:1051–1062.

Marr KA, Seidel K, Slavin MA, et al. Prolonged fluconazole prophylaxis is associated with persistent protection against candidiasis-related death in allogeneic marrow transplant recipients: long-term follow-up of a randomized, placebo-controlled trial. Blood 2000;96:2055–2061.

Tallman MS, Andersen JW, Schiffer CA, et al. All-trans-retinoic acid in acute promyelocytic leukemia. N Engl J Med 1997;337:1021–1028.

72. Plasma Cell Dyscrasias

I INTRODUCTION

A. Definition. Plasma cell dyscrasias (= monoclonal gammopathies = paraproteinemias) are malignancies of the B lymphocyte system. Common plasma cell dysplasias include **multiple myeloma** and **Waldenström's macroglobulinemia.**

B. Clinical manifestations of plasma cell dyscrasias

1. The clinical manifestations of all plasma cell dyscrasias result from:
   a. Proliferation of the neoplastic cells and invasion of various organs
   b. Secretion of cell products (either immunoglobulins or subunits)
   c. The host's response to the tumor

2. Patients with plasma cell dyscrasias often have **M (monoclonal) components** in their serum.
   a. The M component represents the immunoglobulin (or light or heavy chain) that is being secreted and can be quantitated by performing **serum protein electrophoresis.** Qualitative assessment is made using **immunoelectrophoresis.**
   b. M components are **not specific to plasma cell dyscrasias.** They are also seen in leukemia, lymphoma, sarcoidosis, rheumatoid arthritis, monoclonal gammopathy of uncertain significance (MGUS), and other diseases.

II MULTIPLE MYELOMA

A. Epidemiology. Myeloma accounts for 1% of all malignant disease and more than 10% of hematologic malignancies in the United States.

1. It is a disease of **older people;** the median age at diagnosis is 61 years.

2. The incidence in **African-Americans** is twice that in Whites.

B. Clinical manifestations of multiple myeloma. The most common presenting symptoms are **related to anemia, bone pain,** and **infection.** The important clinical manifestations of multiple myeloma can be remembered using the mnemonic, "PLASMA."

Important Clinical Manifestations of Multiple Myeloma
("PLASMA")

Proteinuria/renal insufficiency
Lytic bone lesions and hypercalcemia
Anemia and Abnormal bleeding
Sepsis and infections
Marrow involvement
Amyloidosis

1. **Proteinuria/renal insufficiency** is multifactorial in etiology, with causes including light-chain proteinuria, hypercalcemia, hyperuricemia, amyloidosis, and pyelonephritis.
2. **Lytic bone lesions** and **hypercalcemia.** Bone pain occurs in 70% of patients, usually involving the back and ribs. Because the lesions are lytic, plain radiographs are better than bone scans.
3. **Anemia** and **abnormal bleeding.** The majority of patients will have anemia (usually normocytic) due to various causes. Paraproteinemias may cause platelet dysfunction, leading to abnormal bleeding.
4. **Sepsis** and **infections.** Because of the excess production of abnormal immunoglobulins, myeloma patients usually have decreased levels of normal immunoglobulins leading to increased susceptibility of infections. Seventy-five percent of patients will have a serious infection at some time.
5. **Marrow involvement.** The bone marrow is infiltrated by plasma cells, which initially causes anemia and may lead to bone marrow failure. The extent of marrow plasmacytosis ranges from 5%-100%.
6. **Amyloidosis** develops in a minority of patients and occurs when light chains deposit in normal tissue. This may lead to carpal tunnel syndrome, congestive heart failure (CHF), and renal or liver disease.

C. **Laboratory findings**
1. **Proteinuria** may be evident on urinalysis, but the dipstick is often negative because it tests for albumin, not globulin.
2. **Anemia** is usually normocytic and normochromic, and **rouleau formation** may be noted on the peripheral smear.
3. **Narrow anion gap.** Because globulin is cationic, the increased unmeasured cations decrease the anion gap.
4. **Low serum bicarbonate.** A type 2 renal tubular acidosis may result from proximal tubular damage as a result of filtered light chains.

5. **Elevated creatinine** signifying renal damage may be present.
6. **Pseudohyponatremia** may result from increased paraprotein, which can cause laboratory errors.
7. **Hypercalcemia** may occur from increased osteoclast activity.
8. **Elevated erythrocyte sedimentation rate (ESR).** The ESR is frequently elevated, but this is a nonspecific finding.
D. **Approach to the patient**
   1. **Protein electrophoresis** on serum and urine is usually ordered based on suspicious symptoms, signs, or laboratory test results.
      a. **Procedure.** Albumin and α, β, and γ globulin are separated by differing mobilities in an electric field. In myeloma, increased paraprotein causes an abnormal spike (usually in the β or γ region).
      b. **Results.** When used together, serum and urine protein electrophoresis will miss approximately 1% of myeloma patients (those that are minimal or nonsecretors). However, of patients who have a variant of myeloma (solitary bone plasmacytoma or extramedullary plasmacytoma), fewer than 30% will have a positive protein electrophoresis.
         (1) Serum protein electrophoresis will confirm the diagnosis of myeloma in 80%–90% of patients. Approximately two thirds of patients with positive serum protein electrophoresis results will also test positive on urine protein electrophoresis.
         (2) Urine protein electrophoresis. In the remaining patients, only the light chain is secreted. The light chain can be detected using urine protein electrophoresis.

HOT KEY

The diagnosis of myeloma is usually established by the following triad:
- **Marrow plasmacytosis > 10%**
- **Lytic bone lesions**
- **M component** in **serum** (usually > 3 g/dl) or **urine**
  IgG (50% of patients)
  IgA (25% of patients)
  Light chains only (20% of patients)
  IgD (1% of patients)

---

2. **Immunoelectrophoresis** is then performed to determine if the abnormal spike is polyclonal or monoclonal.
   a. A **polyclonal spike** is seen in reactive conditions (e.g., infection, malignancy, collagen vascular disease).

     b. A **monoclonal (M component)** spike often signifies my-
eloma but may also be found in many other conditions
(e.g., chronic lymphocytic leukemia, lymphoma, sarcoidosis). Therefore, this test should not be used to screen
asymptomatic patients because the clinical setting is critical to interpreting the test correctly.

HOT

KEY

An IgG spike > 3.5 g/dl or an IgA spike > 2 g/dl almost always represents myeloma (and will therefore be monoclonal
when tested by immunoelectrophoresis).

---

   3. Differential diagnosis. The main disorder to distinguish from
myeloma is **MGUS.** Characteristics of MGUS usually include:
     a. M component usually < 2 g/dl
     b. Absence of Bence Jones proteinuria
     c. Marrow plasmacytosis < 5%
     d. Absence of anemia, renal disease, hypercalcemia, and
bone lesions

HOT

KEY

In approximately 10%–25% of patients, MGUS progresses to
multiple myeloma (over many years or decades).

E. Treatment. Unless the patient undergoes bone marrow transplant, the goal is primarily **palliation.**
   1. Chemotherapy usually consists of an alkylating agent (i.e.,
melphalan) and prednisone, or vincristine, doxorubicin, and
dexamethasone.
   2. Thalidomide is an active and effective agent.
   3. Radiation is also used for bone lesions.
   4. Bisphosphonates are administered monthly to improve
skeletal complications.
   5. Pneumococcal vaccination should be given to help prevent
infectious complications.
F. Prognosis is influenced by multiple factors. The serum **β2 microglobulin** level is an important prognostic indicator and
should be checked at diagnosis. **Tumor burden** is also a predictor of survival.
   1. Patients with a **low tumor burden** (i.e., IgG spike < 5 g/dl, no
more than one lytic lesion, and absence of severe anemia, re-

nal failure, or hypercalcemia) have a median survival of approximately 5 years.

2. Those with a **high tumor burden** (IgG spike > 7 g/dl, serum calcium > 12 mg/dl, more than three lytic lesions, or a hematocrit < 25%) have a median survival of approximately 1 year.

III WALDENSTRÖM'S MACROGLOBULINEMIA. In Waldenström's macroglobulinemia, the abnormal cells are a hybrid between lymphocytes and plasma cells.

A. **Clinical manifestations of Waldenström's macroglobulinemia.** The hybrid cells secrete IgM, which accounts for most of the clinical manifestations. The clinical manifestations **are similar to those of myeloma;** however, there are **important differences.**

1. **Hyperviscosity** is much more common in Waldenström's macroglobulinemia than in multiple myeloma. Symptoms may include altered mental status, visual disturbances, and mucosal bleeding.

2. **Hepatomegaly, adenopathy,** and **splenomegaly** are commonly seen in Waldenström's macroglobulinemia but not in myeloma.

3. Hypercalcemia, bony lesions, and renal insufficiency are much less common in Waldenström's macroglobulinemia.

4. A simple way to remember the features that may distinguish Waldenström's macroglobulinemia from multiple myeloma is to use the mnemonic, "Uncle Waldo loves HAMS."

Characteristics of Waldenström's Macroglobulinemia
("Uncle Waldo loves HAMS")

Hyperviscosity
Adenopathy
Ig**M**
Splenomegaly

B. **Treatment** usually involves alkylating agents (i.e., chlorambucil) or nucleoside analogs (i.e., fludarabine). Plasmapheresis may also be needed frequently to treat symptoms of hyperviscosity.

References
Bataille R, Harousseau JL. Multiple myeloma. N Engl J Med 1997;336(23):1657–1664.
Dimopoulos MA, Panayiotidis P, Moulopoulos LA, et al. Waldenström's macroglobulinemia: clinical features, complications, and management. J Clin Oncol 2000;18: 214–226.
Berenson JR, Lichtenstein A, Porter L, et al. Long-term pamidronate treatment of advanced multiple myeloma patients reduces skeletal events. Myeloma Aredia Study Group. J Clin Oncol 1998;16:593–602.

73. Metastatic Neoplasms

I INTRODUCTION

A. Detection of malignancies. Malignancies are usually detected in one of three main ways:
1. **Screening** (e.g., as with breast, cervical, prostate, and colorectal cancer)
2. As a result of **local symptoms** or **findings** (e.g., pain, a change in bowel habits, hematuria, a lump)
3. As a result of **systemic symptoms** or **findings** (e.g., metastatic disease, paraneoplastic syndromes)

B. Common sites of metastasis. This chapter will help you remember the malignancies that commonly metastasize to the **bone, brain, liver,** and **lung.** If no primary source of metastasis is found, the term **carcinoma of unknown primary (CUP)** is used and treatment is centered around the most likely cause.

C. Common malignancies capable of metastasis. Although there are many malignancies capable of metastasizing to different areas, there is a core group that can usually go anywhere—**thyroid cancer, lung cancer, breast cancer, gastrointestinal malignancies, renal cell carcinoma, sarcoma, prostate cancer,** and **melanoma.**

II METASTASIS TO BONE

A. Common malignancies capable of metastasizing to bone are depicted in Figure 73–1.
1. **Melanoma** is not included in the diagram. Nevertheless, because melanoma can go anywhere, it should always be considered when a patient has a metastatic malignancy to **any organ.**
2. **Thyroid cancer**
3. **Lung cancer**
4. **Breast cancer**
5. **Gastrointestinal tract malignancies** (usually only the mucinous subtype goes to bone)
6. **Renal cell carcinoma**
7. **Sarcoma**[1]
8. **Prostate cancer**

---

[1]**Multiple myeloma** is not included on the diagram on the next page because it is a cancer that arises within the skeletal system rather than metastasizing to the skeletal system. Nevertheless, if you want to include myeloma on the "benzene ring" diagram, just place the sarcoma next to myeloma (myeloma commonly affects the iliac crest).

FIGURE 73-1. Despite the long lists of malignancies capable of metastasis contained in conventional textbooks, the most common cancers that involve the bone, brain, liver, and lungs can practically all be contained in an easy-to-remember, "benzene ring" diagram. The benzene ring represents the human body; the cancers are placed at their approximate anatomical position (*sarcoma can arise anywhere). Even though this diagram is set up to help you remember those cancers that metastasize to bone, the same diagram (with some slight modifications) can be used to recall the cancers that go to the brain, liver, and lung.

B. Sites of metastasis. The bones most commonly involved are the **vertebrae, femur, pelvis, ribs,** and **sternum** (in that order).

C. Signs of bone cancer. Cancers that involve the skeletal system can be asymptomatic or produce pain, deformity, pathologic fractures, and hypercalcemia.

D. Treatment. Along with malignancy-specific therapy, bone metastases can be treated palliatively with local radiation, surgical stabilization, and possibly bisphosphonates.

III METASTASIS TO THE BRAIN

A. Common malignancies capable of metastasizing to the brain. This list is the same as the one for cancers that metastasize to bone, with one exception: prostate cancer tends not to go to the brain (or lung).
  1. **Thyroid cancer**
  2. **Lung cancer** (most common)
  3. **Breast cancer**
  4. **Gastrointestinal tract malignancies**
  5. **Renal cell carcinoma**
  6. **Sarcoma**

B. Sites of metastasis. Most metastases are **supratentorial** and are often **multiple.**

C. Signs of brain cancer include evidence of **increased intracranial pressure** or **brain disturbances** (focal or diffuse).

D. Treatment. Cranial irradiation is currently the mainstay of therapy for brain metastases, although in some cases systemic chemotherapy can be useful. Steroids (usually **dexamethasone**) can be effective in acutely controlling symptoms of cerebral edema. Surgical resection or stereotactic radiosurgery can sometimes be used depending on the number and distribution of metastasis.

 METASTASIS TO THE LIVER. Metastatic involvement of the liver is very common and can involve virtually any cancer (except primary brain cancer). In the United States, the incidence of metastatic cancer to the liver is much more common than primary hepatocellular carcinoma. Only cirrhosis causes more cases of fatal liver disease.

A. **Common malignancies capable of metastasizing to the liver.** Again, this list is very similar to that for cancers that metastasize to the bone. The major difference is that pancreatic cancer commonly goes to the liver (which is not surprising, given the proximity of the two organs), whereas renal cell carcinoma, prostate cancer, and sarcomas involve the liver to a lesser extent (but still can).
   1. **Thyroid cancer**
   2. **Lung cancer**
   3. **Breast cancer**
   4. **Gastrointestinal tract malignancies**
   5. **Pancreatic malignancy**
   6. **Renal cell carcinoma**
   7. **Sarcoma**
   8. **Prostate cancer**
B. **Signs of liver cancer.** Often the first (and sometimes only) serum abnormality seen is an elevated alkaline phosphatase.
C. **Treatment.** Systemic or hepatic intraarterial chemotherapy are commonly used modalities. Surgical resection, percutaneous injection, cryosurgery, and hyperthermic coagulation also have roles in therapy depending on the size and distribution of lesions. External hepatic radiation therapy is limited by its effect on normal liver.

H O T

 In patients with isolated elevations of alkaline phosphatase, always consider metastatic involvement of the liver as a cause.

K E Y

V **METASTASIS TO THE LUNG**

A. **Common malignancies capable of metastasizing to the lung.** Although almost any malignancy can involve the lung, the most common include:

    1. Thyroid cancer
    2. Breast cancer
    3. Gastrointestinal tract malignancies
    4. Renal cell carcinoma
    5. Testicular cancer (instead of prostate cancer)
  B. Sites of metastasis. Classically, lung metastases tend to be multiple and involve the peripheral areas of the lung parenchyma; lesions are most common in the lower lobes. Endobronchial metastases are very unusual.
  C. Signs of lung cancer. Metastases are often detected by imaging studies.
  D. Treatment. Chemotherapy, radiation, and surgery are all viable options for therapy.

References

Diel IJ, Solomayer EF, Costa SD, et al. Reduction in new metastases in breast cancer with adjuvant clodronate treatment. N Engl J Med 1998;339:357–363.

Kemeny N, Huang Y, Cohen AM, et al. Hepatic arterial infusion of chemotherapy after resection of hepatic metastases from colorectal cancer. N Engl J Med 1999;341:2039–2048.

Major PP, Lipton A, Berenson J, Hortobagyi G. Oral bisphosphonates: a review of clinical use in patients with bone metastases. Cancer 2000;88:6–14.

Vermeulen SS. Whole brain radiotherapy in the treatment of metastatic brain tumors. Semin Surg Oncol 1998;14:64–69.

PART VIII

RHEUMATOLOGY

74. Monoarticular Arthritis

I **INTRODUCTION.** By addressing the following **three questions** in a patient with joint complaints, you will focus the differential diagnosis while dictating the pace and nature of the evaluation.

A. Does the patient have **true arthritis?** Joint pain (i.e., arthralgia) must be accompanied by signs of inflammation to be a considered true arthritis.

B. Is the arthritis **monoarticular or polyarticular?** It is crucial to perform a complete musculoskeletal examination because a patient, distracted by knee pain for example, may overlook swelling and tenderness of other joints or soft tissues. The **number of joints involved** will change your differential diagnosis.

C. Are there any hints of **systemic involvement**? Historical points such as fevers, unintended weight loss, fatigue, or physical signs such as new skin lesions suggest multi-system disease.

II **CAUSES OF MONOARTICULAR ARTHRITIS.** Once you have established true arthritis of one joint, **you must rule out an infectious etiology** because if left untreated this could lead to permanent joint damage and, in some cases, sepsis. With this caveat in mind, the mnemonic "If I Make The Diagnosis, No More Harm" will help you recall the common causes of monoarticular arthritis, with infection being first on the list.

Causes of Monoarticular Arthritis ("If **I** Make **The** Diagnosis, No More Harm")

Infectious disease
Inflammatory disease
Metabolic disorders
Trauma
Neoplasm
Miscellaneous (foreign body synovitis, avascular necrosis)
Hemarthrosis

A. **Infection**
  1. Common joint pathogens include **Staphylococcal** and **Streptococcal infection,** particularly in the setting of **skin breakdown. Gonorrheal infections** should be considered when arthritis is accompanied by pustules and/or tendonitis.
B. **Inflammatory disorders** (e.g., **psoriatic arthritis, rheumatoid arthritis, Reiter's syndrome,** and other **collagen vascular diseases**). Although these diseases are usually polyarticular and often accompanied by hints of systemic involvement, they may begin as a monoarticular swelling and thus have to be considered when the other causes are ruled out.
C. **Metabolic disorders** [e.g., **gout, pseudogout** (calcium pyrophosphate deposition disease, CPPD)].
  1. **Acute gout can be indistinguishable from a septic joint.** Both give prominent systemic symptoms, and both may have very high white blood cell count in joint fluid. Light microscopic examination of synovial fluid reveals urate crystals seen as yellow crystals when parallel to the condenser (i.e., negative birefringence) and of course, gout is treated by allopurinol (but not acutely). Gout can also be superinfected with a bacterial pathogen. Pseudogout usually has a less acute presentation and tends to be accompanied by chondrocalcinosis that may be visible radiographically. These rhomboid-shaped pseudogout crystals give positive birefringence pattern.
D. **Trauma** to a joint (e.g., torn ligament, bone fracture) can lead to hemarthrosis or internal joint derangement. The patient should always be asked specifically about a history of trauma to the affected joint.
E. **DJD,** a very common disorder, when present in the elderly often causes polyarthritis (see Chapter 75). Monoarticular DJD usually is posttraumatic (e.g., old football injury).
F. **Neoplasm** is a rare cause of monoarticular swelling but should be considered. Examples include **osteoid osteoma** and **pigmented villonodular synovitis.**

G. Miscellaneous. This category includes **foreign body synovitis** and **avascular necrosis** (e.g., due to trauma, steroid use, or alcohol).

H. Hemarthrosis. Bleeding into a joint, when not related to trauma, is usually seen in patients with clotting abnormalities or those receiving anticoagulants.

III APPROACH TO THE PATIENT

A. Patient history
   1. Determine if there are any hints of **systemic disease.**
   2. Determine if arthritis has primarily an **inflammatory or mechanical component.**
      a. Inflammatory. Pain and stiffness worse at day's beginning or with disuse, then "loosens up"; associated with swelling and redness that are often appreciated by others.
      b. Mechanical. Pain worse with use or at the end of the day; recent trauma or overuse; minimal swelling.
B. Physical examination
   1. Determine if the patient has true arthritis (i.e., look for periarticular processes that may mimic arthritis [e.g., cellulitis, bursitis, tendinitis]).
   2. Determine the number of joints involved.
      a. Monoarticular. Infection and crystalline arthropathy most common.
      b. Oligoarticular (i.e., two to three joints involved). Consider gonococcal infection, crystal deposition, or rheumatoid arthritis.
      c. Polyarticular (i.e., more than three joints involved). See Chapter 75.
   3. Look for signs of systemic disease (e.g., cardiac murmur, skin lesions, nail changes).
C. Other diagnostic modalities
   1. **Plain radiographs** in the acute setting have a very low yield when there is no history of trauma or prominent bone pain on examination. Remember, infections require about 10 days before changes to the bone will be detectable by plain radiographs.
   2. **Arthrocentesis** with **joint fluid analysis** is the **mainstay of diagnosis** and should be performed in all patients with a palpable effusion.
      a. Send fluid for white blood cell (WBC) count with differential, Gram stain and culture, and crystal examination.
      b. Based on the results of the joint fluid analysis, the disorder can be categorized as noninflammatory, inflammatory, or septic (Table 74-1).

TABLE 74-1: Joint Fluid Analysis*

	Normal	Noninflammatory	Inflammatory	Septic
WBCs/mm³	< 200	200–10,000	10,000–25,000	> 25,000
%PMN	< 25%	< 25%	50%–90%	50%–100%
Possible Causes	. . .	DJD, trauma, aseptic necrosis	Collagen-vascular diseases, crystal-induced disease, TB, mycotic infections	Pyogenic bacterial infections

DJD = degenerative joint disease; *PMNs* = polymorphonuclear neutrophils; *TB* = tuberculosis; *WBC* = white blood cells.
*Results in different diseases may be variable.

HOT KEY

Always consider infection, regardless of the joint fluid analysis results, because a low cell count may represent early or partially treated infection.

References

Sack K. Monoarthritis: differential diagnosis. Am J Med 1997;102(1A):30S-34S.
Till SH, Snaith ML. Assessment, investigation, and management of acute monoarthritis. J Accid Emerg Med 1999;16(5):355–361.

75. Polyarticular Arthritis

I **INTRODUCTION.** Once you have established that a **polyarticular process (true arthritis of more than three joints)** is present, you must then address the following questions:

A. What is the **distribution of affected joints**?
   1. **Symmetric processes** involve paired joints bilaterally (e.g., bilateral wrists, bilateral shoulders, bilateral small proximal joints of hands).
   2. **Asymmetric processes** will involve non-paired joints (e.g., left knee with right wrist).
B. Is there any evidence of **systemic involvement (e.g., fever, chills, weight loss)**?

II **CAUSES OF POLYARTICULAR ARTHRITIS.** There are three main categories: symmetric, asymmetric, and miscellaneous (Table 75-1).

A. **Symmetric seropositive arthritis.** In addition to the characteristic joint distribution, a patient often will have accompanying **autoantibodies and frequently will also have systemic signs and symptoms.**
   1. **Rheumatoid arthritis**
      a. **Epidemiology.** The disease affects women twice as often as men, and the usual age at onset is 20–40 years.
      b. **Clinical manifestations.** The onset is **insidious,** but 20% will have brisk progression. **Major symptoms** include malaise, fever, and morning stiffness relieved with hot bath and exercise. **Joints classically involved** include proximal interphalangeal joints (PIPs), metacarpal phalangeal joints (MCPs), wrists, shoulders, knees, ankles, and metatarsal phalangeal joints (MTPs). **Extra-articular manifestations,** most common in patients with high titer rheumatoid factor (RF), may include subcutaneous nodules, pulmonary interstitial infiltrates, lymphadenopathy, and cutaneous ulcers. The classic bone **radiographic findings** include periarticular osteoporosis and marginal joint erosions.

HOT KEY

Eighty-five percent of patients with rheumatoid arthritis are RF-positive.

TABLE 75-1. Common Causes of Polyarticular Arthritis

Symmetric seropositive polyarthritis
  Rheumatoid arthritis
  Systemic lupus erythematosus (SLE)
  Systemic sclerosis
  Polymyositis
  Overlap syndrome
Asymmetric seronegative spondyloarthropathy
  Ankylosing spondylitis
  Psoriatic arthritis
  Reiter's syndrome
  Arthritis related to enteric disorders
Miscellaneous
  1 Gonorrheal—disseminated gonococcal infection
  2 Spirochetal—Lyme disease, secondary syphilis
  3 Viral—HIV, hepatitis B, parvovirus
  4 Other—infiltrative diseases, Still's disease, rheumatic fever,
    vasculitis

---

2. **Systemic lupus erythematosus (SLE)** is a multisystem autoimmune disorder.
   a. **Epidemiology.** Eighty-five percent of all patients are women 20–40 years of age.
   b. **Clinical manifestations.** Because SLE can **affect most organ systems,** diagnosis can be based on the presence of 4 of 11 characteristics. To receive a passing grade in our medical school, we needed to know the 11 criteria for SLE; therefore, we were all in "P-MOAD"—7 Ps and M O A D. The first two Ps are positive lab tests; the next five Ps are arranged from head to toe (see mnemonic next page).
3. **Systemic sclerosis (scleroderma)** is characterized by the presence of a positive ANA, early Raynaud's phenomenon (90% of patients), and fibrosis of the skin and internal organs which falls into two forms: diffuse and limited (CREST syndrome)
   a. **Clinical manifestations.** The diffuse form (affecting 20% of patients) has widespread skin thickening with frequent interstitial lung disease and an increased risk of suffering a renal crisis.
   b. The **limited** form (CREST syndrome) is characterized by **c**alcinosis, **R**aynaud's phenomenon, **e**sophageal motility dysfunction, **s**clerodactyly, and **t**elangiectasia. Those with CREST syndrome have a decreased risk of renal involve-

Criteria for the Diagnosis of SLE ("P-MOAD")

Positive antinuclear antibody (ANA): seen in 99% of patients
Positive other immunologic test [antibody (Ab) to double-stranded DNA, Ab to Smith, LE cell preparation, or false-positive syphilis serology]
Psychosis, seizures, or other neurologic abnormalities
Photosensitivity rash
Polyserositis (pleuritis, pericarditis, or peritonitis)
Proteinuria or renal involvement
Pancytopenia or single-cell line "penia" (anemia, thrombocytopenia, leukopenia)
Malar rash
Oral ulcers (painful)
Arthritis
Discoid rash (heaped-up borders, almost cheloid in appearance)

ment, a higher risk of pulmonary hypertension, and correlation with serum anti-centromere antibodies.

4. **Myositis-related arthritis,** when present, most commonly occurs in the hands and wrists.

   a. **Polymyositis.** Arthritis associated with true weakness of proximal muscles (e.g., deltoids and quadriceps).

   b. **Dermatomyositis** has accompanying violaceous skin lesions with arthritis and weakness.

B. **Asymmetric seronegative arthritis.** The classic seronegative spondyloarthropathies are characterized by **asymmetric involvement of the spine and peripheral joints, early onset of disease** (usually before age 40), an **absence of RF or ANA** (hence the term "seronegative"), and a strong association with **HLA-B27.** Consider pelvic films to assess the sacroiliac joint involvement that characterizes this group of disorders.

   1. **Ankylosing spondylitis.** This chronic inflammatory disease leads to pain and stiffening of the spine, affects men more than women, and usually occurs in the second or third decades of life.

   2. **Psoriatic arthritis.** Look for subtle skin changes at belly button, gluteal crease, and hairline.

   3. **Reactive arthritis.** Usually follows episode of infectious diarrhea or venereal infection with chlamydia. **Reiter's syndrome** is classically characterized by the clinical triad of **conjunctivitis, urethritis,** and **arthritis**—the patient cannot "see, pee, or bend at the knees."

4. **Arthritis related to enteric disorders** [e.g., inflammatory bowel disease (IBD), Whipple's disease, enteric infection]
C. **Miscellaneous causes.** There are many other causes of polyarthritis. Most can easily be remembered in the following manner: one gonorrheal, two spirochetal, three viral, and four others.
   1. **Gonorrheal. Disseminated gonococcal infection** (as a result of *Neisseria gonorrhoeae* infection) may result in migratory polyarthralgias of the ankles, knees, and fingers; tenosynovitis; fever; and/or a pustular rash often on the dorsum of the hands.
   2. **Spirochetal**
      a. **Lyme disease** (caused by *Borrelia burgdorferi* infection) is characterized by flu-like symptoms, erythema migrans, and unilateral knee arthritis. Late stages include neurologic problems (e.g., seventh nerve palsy, meningitis), cardiac conduction abnormalities, and/or chronic large joint arthritis.
      b. **Secondary syphilis** can involve almost any part of the body, including the joints.
   3. **Viral.** The three common viral etiologies include human immunodeficiency virus (**HIV), hepatitis B virus,** and **parvovirus.**
   4. **Other**
      a. **Infiltrative diseases** include **sarcoidosis, amyloidosis,** and polyarticular **tophaceous gout;** biopsy is usually necessary to make the diagnosis.
      b. **Still's disease** is a form of juvenile rheumatoid arthritis that affects adults. It is characterized by spiking fevers, arthritis, and an evanescent, salmon-colored rash.
      c. **Rheumatic fever** is discussed in Chapter 53.
      d. **Vasculitis** is discussed in Chapter 76.

HOT KEY

Degenerative joint disease (DJD), the most common cause of polyarticular arthritis, is a slowly progressive non-inflammatory process that destroys articular cartilage (it is a mechanical arthritis). Its natural history, distribution of involved joints (i.e., primarily distal interphalangeal joints (DIPs), shoulders, knees, and hips), and characteristic radiologic findings (i.e., joint space narrowing, bone spurs and sclerosis) make this a relatively straightforward diagnosis.

References

Boumpas DT, et al. Systemic lupus erythematosus: emerging concepts. Part 1, 2. Ann Intern Med 1995;122:940–950.

Felson DT, Lawrence RC, Dieppe PA, et al. Osteoarthritis: new insights. Part 1: the disease and its risk factors. Ann Intern Med 2000;133(8):635–646.

Felson DT, Lawrence RC, Hochberg MC, et al. Osteoarthritis: new insights. Part 2: treatment approaches. Ann Intern Med 2000;133(9):726–737.

Khan MA. Update on spondyloarthropathies. Ann Intern Med 2002;136:897–907.

Lee DM, Weinblatt ME. Rheumatoid arthritis. Lancet 2001;358(9285):903–911.

Pisetsky DS, St Clair EW. Progress in the treatment of rheumatoid arthritis. JAMA 2001;286(22):2787–2790.

76. Vasculitis

I **INTRODUCTION.** The vasculitides are characterized by inflammation of the blood vessels disrupting blood flow with resultant ischemic damage. Because of the broad distribution and varied nature of blood vessels, the clinical manifestations of vasculitis similarly are quite varied and often subtle.

II **CLINICAL MANIFESTATIONS OF VASCULITIS.** The vasculitides can present with any combination of the following (although disease presentation is primarily influenced by specific vessel involvement):

A. **Constitutional symptoms** (e.g., fever, fatigue, anorexia, weight loss)
B. **Arthralgias**
C. **Symptoms of organ ischemia** referable to affected viscera (e.g., pulmonary hemorrhage, glomerulonephritis)
D. **Peripheral neuropathy** from small vessel involvement
E. **Skin findings** (e.g., palpable purpura, livedo reticularis, necrotic lesions, infarcts of the tips of digits)

HOT

KEY

Palpable purpura is pathognomonic of a cutaneous, small vessel vasculitis of any etiology. Inflammation of the vessel allows extravasation of blood and fluid, resulting in palpable edema. Because the blood is no longer intravascular, the lesion is purpuric (nonblanchable) rather than erythematous (blanchable).

III **CAUSES OF VASCULITIS.** To help organize your approach, consider the vasculitides affecting large, medium, and small blood vessels. Because there are a large number of entities that can cause small vessel vasculitis, a mnemonic to make it easier to remember the different causes will be provided.

A. **Large vessel vasculitides.** These diseases affect vessels that have elastic lamina.
1. **Giant cell (temporal) arteritis**
   a. **Epidemiology.** Giant cell arteritis is rare in patients younger than 50 years. Women are affected more often than men.

    b. Clinical manifestations. Headache and/or scalp tenderness is the most common clinical finding, whereas jaw claudication is the most specific symptom. Sudden blindness is the most dreaded complication, so early diagnosis and treatment with corticosteroids are crucial. There is a close association with polymyalgia rheumatica, which is characterized by proximal muscle pain and stiffness.

    c. Diagnosis. Suspect in an elderly patient who complains of a headache and has an erythrocyte sedimentation rate (ESR) greater than 50 mm/hour. A temporal artery biopsy of at least 2 cm in length, to account for skip lesions, is needed for definitive diagnosis.

2. Takayasu's aortitis

    a. Epidemiology. Takayasu's aortitis is rare. Young Asian women are most commonly affected.

    b. Clinical manifestations. Patients have findings resulting from involvement of the aortic arch and its primary branches; thus, transient ischemic attacks and absent radial pulses yielding the moniker "pulseless disease" are most common.

    c. Diagnosis. Clinical suspicion must be supported by diagnostic angiography.

B. Medium vessel vasculitis

1. Polyarteritis nodosa (PAN)

    a. Epidemiology. The average age at onset is approximately 45 years. Men are affected more often than women. In 30% of patients, PAN is associated with hepatitis B antigenemia.

    b. Clinical manifestations. Virtually any organ system can be involved, making description of a "classic" case of PAN difficult. Due to the significant inflammation, fever and weight loss are common. Diffuse vessel involvement can cause new-onset hypertension, whereas involvement of specific medium arteries supplying the kidneys yields renal failure with a bland urinary sediment; mesenteric vessel involvement yields abdominal pain; disruption of blood to muscles causes myalgia and weakness; and neuropathies occur secondary to nerve ischemia.

    c. Diagnosis. Definitive diagnosis is made by biopsy of involved organs or by visceral angiography, which may reveal aneurysms, areas of stenosis, or obliteration of vessels.

C. Small vessel vasculitides. The mnemonic "VAASCULITIS" can help you remember the diverse and large number of causes of this group.

Causes of Small Vessel Vasculitis ("VAASCULITIS")

Various drugs
ANCA associated
Autoimmune disorders
Serum sickness
Cryoglobulinemia
Ulcerative colitis
Low complement (hypocomplementemic urticarial vasculitis)
Infections
Tumors
IgA nephropathy (Henoch-Schönlein purpura)
Smoking-related (thromboangiitis obliterans)

1. **Various drugs.** Penicillins, sulfa drugs, and propylthiouracil are just a few of the many drugs that can cause hypersensitivity vasculitis.
2. **ANCA associated**
   a. **Wegener's granulomatosis**
      (1) **Clinical manifestations.** Pulmonary involvement with cough, dyspnea, hemoptysis, or asymptomatic infiltrates occurs in approximately 95% of patients. The upper and lower respiratory tract are involved, resulting in ulcerations of the nasal mucosa, saddle nose deformity (secondary to perforation of the nasal septum), chronic sinusitis, serous otitis, or pulmonary infiltrates or cavities. The kidney is involved in approximately 85% of patients, leading to hematuria, proteinuria, and/or glomerulonephritis with rapidly progressive renal failure if treatment is delayed.
      (2) **Diagnosis.** Biopsy, preferably lung or kidney, reveals necrotizing granulomas in small arteries and veins. Serum antibodies yield a C-ANCA pattern with ELISA positive for proteinase-3.
   b. **Churg-Strauss syndrome** (allergic angiitis and granulomatosis)
      (1) **Epidemiology.** Associated with reactive airway disease.
      (2) **Clinical manifestations.** Pulmonary involvement (with asthma and, occasionally, fleeting pulmonary infiltrates) is most common. Mononeuritis multiplex is also well described. Peripheral eosinophilia can be significant.

    (3) Diagnosis. Biopsy (usually of lung tissue) shows small vessel vasculitis, extravascular granulomas, and eosinophil infiltration. P-ANCA pattern associated with positive ELISA for myeloperoxidase molecules.

  c. Microscopic polyangiitis (MPAN)

    (1) Clinical manifestations. Most important distinctions from classic PAN: rapidly progressive glomerulonephritis and small vessel involvement of the lung yielding alveolitis and hemorrhage.

    (2) Diagnosis. Biopsy shows necrotizing inflammation of capillaries, venules, and arterioles with no granulomas. P-ANCA pattern characteristic.

  d. Pauci-immune necrotizing glomerulonephritis

    (1) Identical to MPAN except no lung involvement.

3. Autoimmune disorders. Systemic lupus erythematosus (SLE) and rheumatoid arthritis may cause a vasculitis.

4. Serum sickness occurs 7–10 days after a primary exposure to an antigen (e.g., penicillin), or 2–4 days after a secondary exposure.

5. Cryoglobulinemia is characterized by immunoglobulins that precipitate in cold temperatures. Condition correlated with hepatitis C infection, acute or chronic.

  a. Type I cryoglobulins are monoclonal and usually associated with multiple myeloma, Waldenström's macroglobulinemia, or other lymphoproliferative disorders.

  b. Type II cryoglobulins, which have one monoclonal component and one polyclonal component, and **type III cryoglobulins,** which have two polyclonal components, are both considered mixed cryoglobulins. They are often associated with infections (e.g., hepatitis), connective tissue diseases, or lymphoproliferative disorders; patients are rheumatoid-factor-positive. **Essential mixed cryoglobulinemia** is diagnosed when no precipitating condition can be elicited.

6. Ulcerative colitis is occasionally associated with a secondary vasculitis.

7. Low complement. Hypocomplementemic urticarial vasculitis occurs predominantly in young women. Recurrent bouts of urticarial lesions, most commonly found on the trunk and extremities, are the most notable feature. All serum complement levels are low.

8. Infections should always be considered as a cause of small vessel vasculitis because they may be life-threatening.

  a. Bacterial. *Neisseria* species, *Staphylococcus aureus, Streptococcus* species, and *Pseudomonas aeruginosa* infections are most commonly associated with vasculitis. Syphilis and Lyme disease should also be considered.

   b. Viral. The most commonly implicated viruses are hepatitis B and C virus, Epstein-Barr virus, and cytomegalovirus (CMV).
   c. Rickettsial. Rocky Mountain spotted fever may be associated with vasculitis. The characteristic rash usually appears on the extremities 2–6 days after the onset of fever.
9. Tumors. Lymphoma and **multiple myeloma** are the malignancies most often associated with vasculitis.
10. IgA nephropathy (Henoch-Schönlein purpura) usually occurs in children or young adults. Classically, palpable purpura appears over the lower extremities, followed by abdominal pain, arthritis, and renal involvement. IgA deposits can be found in the skin and kidney.

HOT KEY Leukocytoclastic changes are indicative of vasculitis but do not indicate the specific cause. However, IgA deposits may be found on skin biopsy in patients with Henoch-Schönlein purpura, making this the only vasculitis that can be diagnosed by simple skin biopsy.

---

11. Smoking-related. Thromboangiitis obliterans (Buerger's disease) Described first in men but also seen in women, who are younger than 40 years and heavy smokers. It is likely that a significant vasospastic component causes vessel wall damage and inflammation leading to impaired arterial blood supply, Raynaud's phenomenon, thrombophlebitis, or deep venous thrombosis. Smoking cessation is the mainstay of therapy.

HOT KEY There are several additional types of vasculitis of which you may be aware. These involve either small vessels (e.g., Goodpasture's syndrome, Behçet's disease) or medium vessels (e.g., Kawasaki's disease, primary granulomatous central nervous system vasculitis).

IV APPROACH TO THE PATIENT

A. Patient history. A travel history and medication history may provide insight into the cause of the vasculitis (e.g., infection, drug therapy).
B. Laboratory studies. With the exception of the SLE, RA and ANCA associated vasculitides, no specific tests will focus the diagnosis. Notably, an elevated ESR only suggests that inflammation of any cause is present in the patient. Use the laboratory

to characterize the distribution and magnitude of end-organ involvement.

1. **Complete blood count (CBC).** Look for leukocytosis, anemia, or thrombocytosis.
2. **Renal panel.** Look for elevated creatinine levels.
3. **Urinalysis.** Look for hematuria or proteinuria.
4. **ESR** (usually elevated)
5. **ANA** and **rheumatoid factor (RF) levels**
6. **ANCA and if available specific ELISA for myeloperoxidase and proteinase-3.**
7. **Cryoglobulins**
8. **Complement levels**
9. **Blood cultures** (especially to rule out endocarditis)
10. **Cultures for gonococcal infection** (e.g., oral, anal, cervical, urethral)
11. **Serologies for hepatitis B** and **C virus, Epstein-Barr virus, CMV,** *Treponema pallidum,* or *Borrelia burgdorferi*

C. Diagnosis is very difficult to make conclusively without tissue biopsy. Use the history and physical examination to guide you to tissues most likely to be affected (e.g., skin, lung, peripheral nervous system).

V **TREATMENT.** A rheumatology consult is often useful when treating a patient with vasculitis. These diseases are uncommon; therefore, it is crucial to recognize that many infections, neoplasms, metabolic disorders, and drug reactions can serve as mimickers.

HOT

KEY
Because therapy involves immunosuppression, always ask yourself, "Am I about to start treating an infection with steroids?"

A. **Large, medium, and ANCA associated small vessel vasculitides** are often treated initially with **glucocorticoids** (e.g., prednisone, 1 mg/kg per day). In general, temporal arteritis responds to steroids alone, and its timely administration can be vision saving.
B. **Small vessel vasculitides**
   1. The **underlying condition** must be treated. Empiric antibiotics may be given if an infection (e.g., meningococcemia, endocarditis, Rocky Mountain spotted fever) is suspected. Stop use of any possible offending drugs (e.g., propylthiouracil).
   2. In certain cases, **steroids** with or without the addition of a cy-

totoxic agent may be used, following consultation with a rheumatologist.

References
Bonsib SM. Polyarteritis nodosa. Semin Diagn Pathol 2001;18(1):14–23.
Jennette JC, Falk R. Small-vessel vasculitis. N Engl J Med 1997;337:1651–1657.
Levine SM, Hellmann DB. Giant cell arteritis. Curr Opin Rheumatol 2002;14:3–10.

PART IX

ENDOCRINOLOGY

77. Hypercalcemia

I   INTRODUCTION

A. Definition. Hypercalcemia is an elevated level of ionized calcium in the blood. Hypercalcemia is a common problem in both inpatients and outpatients. In the former, hypercalcemia is usually secondary to malignancy; in the latter, hyperparathyroidism is more common.

B. Because **albumin binds calcium,** it is important to make sure that hypercalcemia is real and not just a reflection of hyperalbuminemia.

> **HOT**
> ▶
> **KEY**
>
> For every 1-mg increase in albumin (the normal albumin level is 4 mg/dl), you must decrease the calcium level by 0.8 mg/dl. The converse is true for hypoalbuminemia. For example, if the serum calcium is 11 mg/dl and the albumin is 5 mg/dl, the corrected calcium is 10.2 mg/dl (and the patient is not hypercalcemic).

II   CLINICAL MANIFESTATIONS OF HYPERCALCEMIA

A. Symptoms are usually nonspecific and tend to occur when the serum calcium level exceeds 12 mg/dl. The severity of symptoms is also dependent on the acuity of the calcium elevation. **"Abdominal moan, psychiatric groan, kidney stone,** and **urination zone** (i.e., the bathroom)," is a way to recall common symptoms.

1. Gastrointestinal symptoms include constipation, nausea, vomiting, and anorexia. Patients may develop acute pancreatitis.

2. Central nervous system (CNS) symptoms may range from depression and fatigue to confusion, lethargy, and weakness. Progression to coma and death may occur with severe hypercalcemia.

3. **Renal** symptoms include nephrolithiasis, renal failure, and polyuria leading to dehydration. Hypercalcemia interferes with antidiuretic hormone (ADH) action, leading to frequent urination.

B. **Signs** of hypercalcemia include hypertension, hypotonia, decreased deep tendon reflexes, and a shortened QT interval on the electrocardiogram (ECG).

III **CAUSES OF HYPERCALCEMIA.** There are many causes of hypercalcemia. The mnemonic "MISHAP + F" will help you remember the most important ones.

Causes of Hypercalcemia ("MISHAP + F")

Malignancy
Intoxication (vitamin D)
Sarcoidosis (and other granulomatous diseases)
Hospitalization and **H**ydrochlorothiazide
Adrenal disease and milk-**A**lkali syndrome
Primary hyperparathyroidism and **P**aget's disease
+
Familial hypocalciuric hypercalcemia (FHH)

A. **Malignancy.** Hypercalcemia occurs secondary to **local osteolysis** (seen with extensive bone involvement by the tumor) or **humoral influences** [induced by parathyroid hormone (PTH)-related peptide]. **Lymphomas** may produce excess 1,25-dihydroxyvitamin D.

B. **Intoxication with vitamin D.** Some patients take large amounts of vitamin D for unclear reasons; serum 25-hydroxyvitamin D or 1,25-dihydroxyvitamin D levels (depending on what form of vitamin D was ingested) will confirm this diagnosis.

C. **Sarcoid** and **other granulomatous diseases** (e.g., **tuberculosis, berylliosis**). Hypercalcemia results from increased formation of 1,25-dihydroxyvitamin D in granulomatous tissues.

D. **Hospitalization.** Hypercalcemia occurs in the setting of **prolonged immobilization.** Most commonly seen in patients with active bone turnover, such as younger patients with maturing bone.

E. **Hydrochlorothiazide.** Patients receiving this diuretic may have elevated serum calcium levels.

F. **Adrenal disease. Addison's disease** and **pheochromocytoma** are uncommon causes of hypercalcemia.

G. **Alkali ingestion.** Hypercalcemia occurs secondary to excess calcium carbonate ingestion (usually seen in patients with peptic ulcers).

H. Primary hyperparathyroidism. Primary hyperparathyroidism is caused by solitary adenomas (85% of patients), four-gland hyperplasia (10% of patients), or carcinoma (less than 5% of patients). Patients are usually asymptomatic at the time of diagnosis. Serum phosphate levels are often low.

I. Paget's disease, a metabolic bone disease of unknown etiology, is characterized by excessive bone destruction and unorganized repair that leads to skeletal deformities (e.g., kyphosis, bowing of the tibias, enlargement of the skull).

J. Familial hypocalciuric hypercalcemia (FHH) is a benign, autosomal dominant genetic disease characterized by hypercalcemia, hypocalciuria (<50 mg/24 hours), and occasionally hypermagnesemia. The serum PTH level is often slightly increased, which can lead to a mistaken diagnosis of hyperparathyroidism.

IV TREATMENT is warranted if symptoms are present or if serum calcium exceeds 12 mg/dl.

A. Initial therapy entails fluids, fluids, and more fluids, **followed** by diuretics primarily to prevent fluid overload. Other therapies include **bisphosphonates, calcitonin, plicamycin,** and **corticosteroids.**

B. Definitive treatment will, of course, depend on the underlying cause.

References

Bushinsky DA, Monk RD. Calcium. Lancet 1998;352(9124):306–311.

Grill V, Martin TJ. Hypercalcemia of malignancy. Rev Endocr Metab Disord 2000;1(4):253–263.

Kinder BK, Stewart AF. Hypercalcemia. Curr Probl Surg 2001;39(4):349–448.

78. Hypocalcemia

I INTRODUCTION

A. **Definition.** Hypocalcemia is a decreased ionized calcium level. Hypocalcemia is a common occurrence in very ill, hospitalized patients.

B. Because **albumin binds calcium,** it is important to make sure that hypocalcemia is real and not just a reflection of hypoalbuminemia.

> **HOT KEY**
>
> For every 1-mg decrease in albumin (the normal albumin level is 4 mg/dl), you must increase the calcium by 0.8 mg/dl. For example, if the serum calcium is 7.5 mg/dl and the albumin is 2 mg/dl, then the corrected serum calcium is 9.1 mg/dl (and the patient is not hypocalcemic).

C. In patients with respiratory alkalosis, the total serum calcium is normal but the ionized calcium is low; therefore, the patient may have signs and symptoms of hypocalcemia.

II CLINICAL MANIFESTATIONS OF HYPOCALCEMIA. Because hypocalcemia leads to enhanced excitation of the nervous system and muscle cells, the symptoms and signs primarily involve the **neuromuscular** and **cardiovascular** systems.

A. **Symptoms** include muscular cramps (which can progress to tetany), inspiratory wheezing (stridor due to laryngospasm), and paresthesias of the lips and extremities.

B. **Signs** include **hypotension, Chvostek's sign** (tapping the facial nerve leads to contraction of the facial muscles), and **Trousseau's sign** (occlusion of the brachial artery with a blood pressure cuff leads to carpal spasm). The **electrocardiogram** (ECG) may show a prolonged QT interval or atrioventricular (AV) block.

III CAUSES OF HYPOCALCEMIA. There are many causes of hypocalcemia; the mnemonic "HIPOCAL" will help you remember the most important ones.

Causes of Hypocalcemia ("HIPOCAL")

Hypoparathyroidism
Infection
Pancreatitis
Overload states
Chronic renal failure
Absorption abnormalities
Loop diuretics

A. Hypoparathyroidism. The major causes of hypoparathyroidism are **thyroidectomy** and **autoimmune destruction** of the parathyroid gland. Unusual causes include DiGeorge's syndrome and damage to the parathyroid as a result of infection, heavy metals, or irradiation. Functional hypoparathyroidism [i.e., decreased secretion of parathyroid hormone (PTH)] may occur secondary to magnesium deficiency.

B. Infection. Up to 20% of patients with **gram-negative sepsis** are hypocalcemic due to acquired defects in the parathyroid-vitamin D axis. This hypocalcemia may cause hypotension that is responsive to calcium replacement.

C. Pancreatitis. Serum calcium less than 8 mg/dl is one of Ranson's criteria; the calcium level may correlate with the severity of acute pancreatitis.

D. Overload states. Occasionally, hypocalcemia may be seen in cases of rapid intravascular **volume expansion.**

E. Chronic renal failure. Vitamin D is metabolized in the normal kidney to 1,25-dihydroxyvitamin D, which promotes intestinal calcium absorption. With renal failure, intestinal calcium absorption decreases and the patient becomes hypocalcemic.

F. Absorption abnormalities. Patients with malabsorption (due to any cause) of calcium, magnesium, or vitamin D will often have hypocalcemia.

G. Loop diuretics. Unlike thiazide diuretics (which can cause hypercalcemia), furosemide and other loop diuretics lead to enhanced renal excretion of calcium.

IV TREATMENT

A. If the patient has tetany, arrhythmias, or seizures, immediate therapy with **intravenous calcium gluconate** is indicated.

B. If the patient has asymptomatic hypocalcemia, **oral calcium** and **vitamin D** are usually sufficient.

C. If the patient has hypomagnesemia, replacement of magnesium is required to correct hypocalcemia.

References
Bushinsky DA, Monk RD. Calcium. Lancet 1998;352(9124):306–311.
RuDusky BM. ECG abnormalities associated with hypocalcemia. Chest 2001;119(2):
    668–669.

79. Diabetic Ketoacidosis (DKA)

I INTRODUCTION

A. **Definition.** Diabetic ketoacidosis (DKA) is a life-threatening complication of diabetes mellitus caused by a relative or absolute deficiency of insulin along with an excess of "stress hormones" (i.e., glucagon, epinephrine, and cortisol). This imbalance results in impaired cellular uptake of glucose, gluconeogenesis, lipolysis, and ketogenesis. Patients present with hyperglycemia, hyperosmolarity, significant dehydration from a glucose-induced osmotic diuresis, and acidosis from ketone production. DKA can be seen in both type 1 and type 2 diabetes, and initial management is the same for both disorders.

B. **Causes.** Infection, surgery, myocardial infarction (MI), or noncompliance with insulin therapy may all lead to DKA in patients with diabetes.

II CLINICAL MANIFESTATIONS OF DKA

A. **Signs and symptoms.** DKA may present with any of the following signs and symptoms.

1. **Hypotension** and **tachycardia** often reflect volume depletion, but sepsis should always be considered, especially if fever is present.

2. **Tachypnea** is common and often reflects the hyperventilation needed to compensate for the metabolic acidosis.

3. **Mild hypothermia** is usually present. Even a mild temperature elevation is a strong indicator of an underlying infection.

4. **Neurologic abnormalities,** including **seizures** and **altered mental status,** may be present. (Stroke may also precipitate DKA.)

5. **Abdominal pain** associated with **nausea** or **vomiting** may occur as a result of the ketoacidosis itself or as a result of intraabdominal pathology (e.g., cholecystitis).

6. **Polyuria** and **polydipsia** often precede other symptoms by 1–2 days and reflect the osmotic diuresis generated by glycosuria. The **differential diagnosis for polyuria** can be remembered as the **"6 Ds"**:

Differential Diagnoses for Polyuria ("6 Ds")

Diabetes mellitus
Diabetes insipidus
Diuretics
Diuretic phase of acute tubular necrosis (ATN)
Drinking too much
Darn! Too much calcium

B. Laboratory findings
   1. **Blood glucose levels greater than 300 mg/dl** are usually found in conjunction with **4+ glycosuria.**
   2. **Ketonemia** and **ketonuria** are present.
   3. **Anion gap acidosis** with a pH less than 7.3 is typical.
   4. **Hyponatremia** usually results from the hyperglycemia, which exerts an osmotic pull of water into the intravascular space, thereby decreasing sodium concentration. Vomiting with fluid losses accompanied by free water replacement may also contribute to hyponatremia. Significant hyperlipidemia may accompany DKA, resulting in pseudohyponatremia (see Chapter 43).
   5. **Profound potassium, magnesium,** and **phosphate depletion** are typically present. The acidosis of DKA results in a compensatory movement of hydrogen ions intracellularly pushing potassium ions into the extracellular (i.e., intravascular) space; this may normalize or even elevate the serum potassium despite significant total body depletion.
   6. An **elevated blood urea nitrogen (BUN)** and **creatinine level** usually result from **prerenal azotemia.**
   7. An **elevated white blood cell (WBC) count** with a **left shift** can occur even without infection.
   8. An **increased amylase level** is common but reflects both salivary and pancreatic sources; therefore, it is not a good marker for pancreatitis.

III **APPROACH TO THE PATIENT**

A. Diagnose DKA. The diagnosis of DKA is made by the association of **acidosis, hyperglycemia,** and **serum ketonemia.**
B. Identify treatable underlying causes.
   1. The possibility of an underlying infection should be investigated, even if the patient does not have a fever. A chest radiograph, urinalysis, and urine and blood cultures are usually obtained; other evaluation depends on the clinical presentation.

> **HOT**
> ▶
> **KEY**
>
> Because immediate serum ketone determinations are not always available, understanding the implications of urine ketone and serum electrolyte determinations is extremely useful:
> - **Urine ketones.** Ketones are concentrated in the urine, so the **absence of ketonuria usually rules out DKA.** Urine ketones are, however, nonspecific; therefore, a diagnosis of DKA requires other clinical criteria (i.e., acidosis, hyperglycemia).
> - **Serum electrolytes.** The **absence of an anion gap acidosis usually rules out DKA.**

2. Whether to image the abdomen in patients with DKA and abdominal pain is an extremely difficult decision that must be based on associated findings (e.g., fever, significant leukocytosis, liver test abnormalities) and clinical judgment.
3. Patients with diabetes are at increased risk for myocardial infarction (with or without chest pain). This may be the cause, or the result, of DKA, and should always be considered early in the evaluation of a patient with DKA.

IV TREATMENT

A. **Fluid replacement.** Aggressive intravenous fluid replacement is the first line of action to help correct both volume depletion (5–6 L on average) and hyperglycemia.
   1. **How much?** The most common mistake is not giving enough fluids. At least 1 L should be given in the first hour, often followed by 0.5–1 L/hr intravenously thereafter. Patients with cardiac dysfunction should have frequent lung examinations and oxygen saturation measurements to assess the possibility of pulmonary edema.
   2. **What kind?** A useful way of deciding between normal saline and half normal saline is to determine the **corrected sodium concentration,** which corrects for the dilution caused by hyperglycemia. For every extra 100 mg/dl of glucose over normal (e.g., 100 mg/dl), the serum sodium concentration needs to be increased by approximately 1.5 mg/dl:

   $$\text{Corrected Sodium} = \frac{(\text{Serum Glucose} - 100)}{100} \times 1.5 + \text{Serum Sodium}$$

   a. **Normal saline** is often used if the corrected sodium is less than or equal to 142 mg/dl or if hypotension is present.
   b. **Half normal** saline may be a better choice for patients with a corrected serum sodium that is greater than 142

mg/dl. In these patients, normal saline (with a sodium concentration of 150 mg/dl) would keep the sodium high and contribute to persistent hyperosmolarity, which is correlated with poor outcome.

B. Insulin. Because patients with DKA are significantly volume depleted, insulin is best given following or during aggressive fluid replacement. Giving insulin first may precipitate significant hypotension by moving glucose and water from the intravascular space to the intracellular space.

   1. Insulin bolus. Regular insulin in a dose of 0.1–0.3 units/kg should be administered intravenously. A dose of 10 units avoids overdosage and is usually adequate.

   2. Insulin drip

   a. Initiation. A starting dose of 0.1 units/kg/hr is effective and can be titrated to keep the glucose level at 200–300 mg/dl.

   b. Continuation. The insulin drip needs to be continued until the anion gap is back to normal, even if the glucose level has fallen to near normal levels. Once the glucose level is below 250 mg/dl, change the fluids to 5% dextrose in normal saline solution or 5% dextrose in half normal saline solution and continue the insulin drip (adjusting the drip rate to keep the glucose level at 200–300 mg/dl).

HOT

KEY
Changing to subcutaneous insulin prematurely will result in a rebound of ketoacidosis.

---

   c. Termination. The half-life of intravenous insulin is only 8 minutes, so subcutaneous insulin should be administered well before the insulin drip is stopped.

   3. Subcutaneous insulin. Both long acting (e.g., NPH) and short acting (e.g., regular, Humalog, NovoLog) insulin should be used during the transition from intravenous to subcutaneous insulin therapy. The patient's glucose level is checked every 4–6 hours initially and every 6–8 hours thereafter. Short acting subcutaneous insulin may be administered on a sliding scale; the approximate doses are given in Table 79-1.

C. Electrolyte replacement

   1. Potassium repletion is essential to prevent hypokalemia and potentially life-threatening arrhythmias. The potassium level universally falls during the treatment of DKA as a result of fluid replacement and correction of acidosis.

   a. A potassium level **below 4.5 mEq/L** is usually **the trigger for initiating replacement therapy.** A potassium level **be-**

TABLE 79-1. Subcutaneous Insulin Doses in the Treatment of Diabetic Ketoacidosis (DKA)

Glucose Level (mg/dl)*	Dose (Regular Insulin)
<150	0 units
>150 but <250	3 units
>250 but <350	5 units
>350 but <450	7 units
>450	9 units; call house officer

*If the glucose level is greater than 60 mg/dl but less than 100 mg/dl, the patient may be given 1 cup of orange juice. If the glucose level is less than 60 mg/dl and the patient cannot take fluids orally, administer 0.5 ampule of 50% dextrose (D50) and call the house officer.

low 4 mEq/L should alert you to aggressively replete potassium, because the level is likely to continue falling with therapy.

b. A potassium level of **4–5 mEq/L** is the **goal.**

   (1) Often, 20–40 mEq of potassium are given in each liter of intravenous fluid, depending on the rate of intravenous fluid administration. Extra potassium can be given to keep the potassium level in the desired range.

HOT KEY Generally, each 10 mEq of potassium given will raise the potassium level approximately 0.1 mEq/L (assuming normal renal function and no major change in volume or acid-base status).

   (2) Patients with renal insufficiency, hypotension, or significant volume depletion require careful potassium repletion to avoid causing hyperkalemia. Hypotensive or significantly volume depleted patients should probably not have a standing potassium dose given in their intravenous fluids, because they may inadvertently receive an excessive amount of potassium with large volume replacement.

HOT KEY Always confirm that the patient has adequate urine output before administering potassium.

2. **Magnesium replacement** is frequently necessary and will also help correct hypokalemia associated with hypomagnesemia. If the magnesium level is **less than 1.6 mEq/L,** intravenous magnesium sulfate may be given and repeated as needed. Magnesium repletion also needs to be titrated carefully in the presence of renal failure.

3. **Phosphate replacement** is often not required, but a level **less than 1 mg/dl** may be an indication for replacement with potassium phosphate (usually 9–15 mmol given at a maximal rate of 3 mmol/hr, repeated as needed). If the patient is able to take fluids orally, milk is very high in phosphate and an effective treatment of hypophosphatemia.

D. **pH Regulation.** Patients with a symptomatic acidosis (e.g., cardiac pump dysfunction) or a severe asymptomatic acidosis (pH less than 7.0) are sometimes administered sodium bicarbonate to keep the pH greater than 7.0. In general, however, sodium bicarbonate is contraindicated because it increases hypokalemia, shifts the oxygen dissociation curve to the left (increasing tissue hypoxia), increases intracellular acidosis, and is not associated with any survival advantage.

E. **Frequent monitoring** is the key to treating patients with DKA.

   1. An arterial line is often useful because frequent arterial blood gas and electrolyte measurements are needed.

      a. **pH.** The pH may be checked multiple times in the first hour (especially if it is significantly low) and hourly thereafter until a steady upward trend is noted. At this point, less frequent evaluation should be instituted (e.g., every 2–4 hours).

      b. **Electrolytes** (including glucose) are usually checked each hour initially and may be followed by checks every 2–4 hours after improvement is noted.

   2. Following the electrolytes and the anion gap is more useful than following the serum ketones, because serum ketone measurements may not include β-hydroxybutyrate.

      a. In patients with DKA and concomitant tissue hypoxia or circulatory collapse (e.g., sepsis), β-hydroxybutyrate is produced preferentially, so serum ketones may appear falsely low when the patient is very sick.

      b. With therapy, β-hydroxybutyrate (which is not measured) may be converted to acetoacetate (which is measured). Thus, serum ketone measurements may appear to increase despite clinical and biochemical improvement.

References
American Diabetes Association. Hyperglycemic crises in patients with diabetes mellitus. Diabetes Care 2001;24(11):1988–1996.

Kitabchi AE, Umpierrez GE, Murphy MB, et al. Management of hyperglycemic crises in patients with diabetes. Diabetes Care 2001;24(1):131–153.

Magee MF, Bhatt BA. Management of decompensated diabetes. Diabetic ketoacidosis and hyperglycemic hyperosmolar syndrome. Crit Care Clin 2001;17(1):75–106.

Trence DL, Hirsch IB. Hyperglycemic crises in diabetes mellitus type 2. Endocrinol Metab Clin North Am 2001;30(4):817–831.

80. Thyroid Disease

I **APPROACH TO THE PATIENT.** Because thyroid hormone affects virtually all body functions, abnormal thyroid function has **protean manifestations.** The simplest approach is to:

A. Decide whether the patient is hypothyroid or thyrotoxic based on both **clinical manifestations** and the results of **thyroid function tests.**
B. List the possible causes of the abnormal thyroid function and begin the process of elimination, using the clinical scenario and laboratory data. Determining the etiology of thyrotoxicosis may also require a radioactive iodine uptake study.

II **HYPOTHYROIDISM**

A. **Causes**
   1. **Primary hypothyroidism** results from a thyroid abnormality. Common causes include:
      a. **Hashimoto's disease** (the most common cause and a chronic process)
      b. **Thyroiditis** (subacute, postpartum)
      c. **Drugs** (thionamides, amiodarone [can cause hypothyroidism or thyrotoxicosis], iodide, lithium)
      d. **Surgical excision** or **radiation** of the thyroid gland
   2. **Secondary hypothyroidism** results from pituitary disorders.
   3. **Tertiary hypothyroidism** has a hypothalamic basis.
B. **Clinical manifestations of hypothyroidism**
   1. **Symptoms**
      a. Weakness, fatigue, and lethargy
      b. Arthralgias or myalgias
      c. Cold intolerance

HOT

 Remember: hypothyroidism produces cold intolerance.

KEY

---

      d. Skin dryness or edema
      e. Slow speech or hoarseness
      f. Menstrual irregularities, galactorrhea, or both
      g. Weight gain (usually no more than 10 pounds)

     h. Constipation
     i. Decreased sense of taste, smell, and hearing
     j. Peripheral neuropathy and carpal tunnel syndrome
  2. Signs
     a. Thin, brittle nails or thin, coarse hair
     b. Delayed return phase of deep tendon reflexes
     c. Puffiness of the face and eyelids or thickened tongue
     d. Pitting edema
     e. Effusions (anywhere)
     f. Hypothermia, bradycardia, or hypotension in severe cases. (However, diastolic blood pressure may be mildly elevated with moderate hypothyroidism)
     g. True obesity is rare
     h. Goiter is variably present

HOT

KEY

Goiter refers only to thyroid enlargement, not to the etiology. It may be present in either hypothyroidism or thyrotoxicosis.

---

  3. Laboratory studies
     a. Elevated levels of thyroid-stimulating hormone (TSH) and decreased levels of free thyroxine (T_4) are diagnostic of primary hypothyroidism; both parameters are low with secondary or tertiary hypothyroidism.
     b. Serum levels of cholesterol, creatine kinase, prolactin, and liver enzymes may be increased.
     c. Anemia, usually normocytic or macrocytic
     d. Hypoglycemia and hyponatremia
     e. Positive antithyroid antibody (i.e., anti-TPO [formerly called antimicrosomal] and antithyroglobulin) titers in patients with Hashimoto's disease
     f. Sinus bradycardia, low-voltage QRS complexes, and nonspecific T-wave abnormalities
C. Treatment
  1. Primary hypothyroidism. Replacement therapy with L-**thyroxine** is the treatment of choice in almost all cases of primary hypothyroidism.
     a. If the free T_4 is normal and the patient has only mild symptoms, start therapy at just below the expected final replacement dose (1.5 μg/kg/day of L-thyroxine).
     b. If the free T_4 is low or the patient is significantly symptomatic, start with a low dose of thyroxine and increase it slowly (every 2–4 weeks) until the maintenance dose level is achieved.

    c. TSH levels should be monitored every 5–6 weeks until the patient is biochemically euthyroid. Thereafter, monitoring can take place on an as-needed basis.

  2. Secondary or **tertiary hypothyroidism.** L-Thyroxine should be administered only after adrenal insufficiency has been excluded or treated.

D. Myxedema coma is a **life-threatening manifestation of hypothyroidism;** usually patients are stuporous, hypothermic, bradycardic, hypotensive, hypoxemic, and hypercapnic.

  1. Approach to the patient. Since the hypothyroidism is almost always longstanding, make sure to search for a precipitating cause (e.g., infection, ischemia, stroke, acute abdomen, pulmonary embolus) and treat the precipitating cause aggressively.

  2. Treatment. Patients often require ventilatory support and should be admitted to the intensive care unit (ICU). Intravenous L-thyroxine may be administered after adrenal insufficiency has been excluded or treated.

III THYROTOXICOSIS

A. There are many causes of **"thyrotoxicosis"** (a term that simply implies **symptoms and signs attributed to increased levels of thyroid hormones**). The causes can be subdivided into those that are attributable to thyroid hyperfunction (hyperthyroidism) and those that are not. A **radioactive iodine uptake** will reveal the functional status of the gland, expressed as the percentage of radioactive iodine captured by the thyroid.

  1. Hyperfunctioning thyroid (hyperthyroidism). The scan will reveal **high radioactive iodine uptake.**

    a. TSH-secreting tumor. This pituitary tumor is rare and should be considered in thyrotoxic patients with normal (or moderately elevated) TSH levels.

    b. Autonomous toxic adenoma(s). Hyperthyroidism may be caused by a single adenoma or by a toxic multinodular goiter. There are no associated eye findings, antithyroid antibodies, or thyroid-stimulating immunoglobulins (TSIs), which helps to distinguish this disorder from Graves' disease.

    c. Graves' disease, an autoimmune disorder that causes diffuse thyroid enlargement, is the most common cause of hyperthyroidism. Women 20–40 years of age are most commonly affected. Graves' disease may be associated with an infiltrative ophthalmopathy, dermopathy, or systemic autoimmune disorders and is usually associated with elevated TSI (and other antithyroid antibody) levels.

Causes of Thyrotoxicosis—Hyperfunctioning Gland ("TAG")

TSH-secreting tumor
Autonomous toxic adenoma
Graves' disease

2. **Damaged or nonfunctioning thyroid.** The thyroid uptake will reveal **low radioactive iodine uptake** (think of a "fist" obscuring the view—see below).
   a. **Factitious thyrotoxicosis** results from the ingestion of large amounts of exogenous thyroid hormone.
   b. **Iodine-induced thyrotoxicosis (Jod-Basedow disease)** occurs when a patient with a multinodular goiter receives a large iodine load (e.g., following radiographic contrast studies or amiodarone therapy).
   c. **Struma ovarii.** A exceedingly small percentage of ovarian dermoid tumors and teratomas contain thyroid tissue, which may autonomously secrete thyroid hormone.
   d. **Thyroiditis** is an autoimmune disease resulting in thyroid destruction. In the early phase, thyrotoxicosis may result from leakage of thyroid hormone. Hypothyroidism typically follows and may be transient or permanent.

Causes of Thyrotoxicosis—Decreased or Absent Thyroid Function ("FIST")

Factitious thyrotoxicosis
Iodine-induced thyrotoxicosis
Struma ovarii
Thyroiditis

B. **Clinical manifestations of thyrotoxicosis**
   1. **Symptoms**
      a. Nervousness, emotional lability, and restlessness
      b. Heat intolerance and increased sweating
      c. Fatigue, weakness, and muscle cramps
      d. Palpitations and angina
      e. Weight loss (despite hyperphagia) and hyperdefecation

2. Signs
  a. Agitation and anxiety
  b. Warm, moist palms
  c. Stare and lid lag
  d. Fine tremor and hyperreflexia
  e. Irregularly irregular pulse (a sign of atrial fibrillation—think of the first President Bush), widened pulse pressure, and, occasionally, evidence of high-output heart failure
3. Laboratory studies
  a. Serum free T_4 and free T_3 are usually increased, and serum TSH is decreased (except when a TSH-secreting tumor is responsible for hyperthyroidism).
  b. Hypercalcemia, anemia, and increased alkaline phosphatase levels may be seen in hyperthyroidism.
C. Treatment. There are many potential ways to treat thyrotoxic patients—the best way depends on the cause and clinical setting.
  1. Symptomatic relief is provided by **β blockers** (e.g., propranolol). β blockers do not decrease thyroid hormone secretion but reduce adrenergic stimulation.
  2. Reduction of thyroid hormone secretion can be accomplished using **thiourea drugs** (e.g., methimazole, propylthiouracil), **iodinated agents, radioactive iodine,** or **thyroid surgery.**
  3. Thyroiditis. Patients with thyrotoxicosis secondary to thyroiditis are best treated symptomatically (typically with β blockers) until the condition resolves spontaneously. These patients will then usually require treatment for **hypo**thyroidism, either transiently (if thyroid function returns) or permanently.
D. Thyroid storm is a **life-threatening exacerbation of thyrotoxicosis.**
  1. Approach to the patient. Always look for a precipitating cause of clinical decompensation as well as the etiology of thyrotoxicosis (e.g., myocardial infarction, infection, surgery).
  2. Clinical manifestations include the usual features of thyrotoxicosis and the precipitating event, plus **fever** and **psychosis** (hallmarks of **thyroid storm**), nausea, vomiting, and seizures.
  3. Treatment goals include suppression of the effects of thyroid hormone and rapid reduction of circulating thyroid hormone levels.
    a. These goals are usually accomplished by intravenous administration of a β blocker, a thiourea, an iodide (following thiourea therapy), and corticosteroids.

b. Definitive treatment occurs once the patient is rendered euthyroid.

References

Dayan CM. Interpretation of thyroid function tests. Lancet 2001;357(9256):619–624.

Umpierrez GE. Euthyroid sick syndrome. South Med J 2002;95(5):506–513.

Weetman AP. Graves' disease. N Engl J Med 2000;343(17):1236–1248.

Woeber KA. Update on the management of hyperthyroidism and hypothyroidism. Arch Intern Med 2000;160(8):1067–1071.

81. Adrenal Insufficiency

I INTRODUCTION

A. **Definitions.** Adrenal insufficiency is defined as the inadequate production of glucocorticoids, mineralocorticoids, or both. However, glucocorticoid deficiency has the greater clinical manifestations and is therefore the focus of this chapter

1. **Glucocorticoid insufficiency** occurs when **glucocorticoid production** by the adrenal gland **is deficient.** This may be due to adrenal gland dysfunction (primary adrenal insufficiency) or inadequate secretion of adrenocorticotropic hormone (ACTH) (secondary adrenal insufficiency).

2. **Hypoaldosteronism** occurs when **mineralocorticoid production is impaired.** It can occur with adrenal insufficiency (as in Addison's disease) or as an isolated finding; when hypoaldosteronism occurs as an isolated finding, it is usually the result of defective renin secretion.

II CAUSES OF ADRENAL INSUFFICIENCY

A. **Primary adrenal insufficiency (Addison's disease)** results from destruction of the adrenal glands and is therefore accompanied by hypoaldosteronism. One way to remember the common causes of primary adrenal insufficiency is to use the mnemonic "ADDISON'S":

> Causes of Addison's Disease ("ADDISON'S")
>
> **A**myloidosis
> **D**estruction (autoimmune or hemorrhage following trauma)
> **D**rugs (anticoagulants leading to bilateral adrenal hemorrhage)
> **I**nfections [bacterial sepsis (especially meningococcus), tuberculosis, disseminated fungal infections, cytomegalovirus (CMV) in AIDS patients, syphilitic gummas]
> **S**arcoidosis
> **O**verload of iron (hemochromatosis)
> **N**eoplasm (bilateral metastatic disease, usually from the lung)
> **S**urgical (hemorrhage during open-heart surgery or following bilateral adrenalectomy)

B. Secondary adrenal insufficiency is caused by pituitary dysfunction. There are many causes of secondary adrenal insufficiency, but the most important are summarized in Table 81-1. All these causes affect the pituitary gland and lead to **hypopituitarism;** the most common disorders are ACTH suppression due to **withdrawal of chronic exogenous corticosteroids** and **ACTH deficiency due to pituitary tumors.**

C. Tertiary adrenocortical insufficiency occurs with **hypothalamic disorders, pituitary stalk destruction,** and certain **central nervous system (CNS) diseases.**

III CLINICAL MANIFESTATIONS OF ADRENAL INSUFFICIENCY

A. Primary adrenal insufficiency. The clinical manifestations vary depending on the time course of adrenal destruction.

   1. Chronic insufficiency. Most patients (75%) present with chronic insufficiency due to gradual destruction of the adrenal gland. More than 90% of the gland must be destroyed before symptoms occur; therefore, symptoms occur over many months and, in some cases, years. Table 81-2 can be used to determine "WWHHOOO" may have chronic insufficiency.

HOT

KEY

Hyperpigmentation may precede other manifestations. It tends to be generalized but is accentuated in sun-exposed areas, pressure points (e.g., knees and knuckles), and on the nail beds, nipples, and palmar creases. In dark-skinned patients, the only signs of hyperpigmentation may be on the tongue and in the perilimbal region of the eyes.

TABLE 81-1. Causes of Secondary Adrenal Insufficiency

Category	Specific Cause
Congenital	Familial hypopituitarism
Hematologic	Pituitary apoplexy (hemorrhage)
Pregnancy-related	Sheehan's syndrome
Drugs	Withdrawal of chronic exogenous corticosteroids
Metabolic/endocrine	Chronic renal failure, diabetes mellitus, hemochromatosis
Infectious	Tuberculosis, syphilis, fungal disease
Iatrogenic	Irradiation of the pituitary gland
Idiopathic	Empty sella syndrome, sarcoidosis
Neoplasm	Pituitary tumors
Surgical	Surgical destruction

TABLE 81-2. Clinical Manifestations of Chronic Adrenal Insufficiency ("WWHHOOO")

Clinical Manifestation	Incidence
Weakness	Common
Weight loss	Common
Hyperpigmentation	Common
Hypotension	Variable
Obstipation and other gastrointestinal symptoms (nausea, vomiting, diarrhea, pain)	Variable
Orthostasis	Variable
Other (hyponatremia, hyperkalemia, nonanion gap metabolic acidosis, hypoglycemia, eosinophilia)	Variable

    2. Acute insufficiency (adrenal crisis). Only 25% of patients with adrenal insufficiency will present acutely, but when it occurs, it can be **life-threatening.** Adrenal crisis is usually seen in a patient with adrenal insufficiency (known or not) who experiences a significant stress (e.g., infection, cardiac ischemia, surgery). It may also be seen in a previously healthy patient if acute adrenal destruction occurs (e.g., adrenal hemorrhage due to sepsis or anticoagulation therapy).

      a. Signs and symptoms

        (1) Profound anorexia, nausea, and **vomiting** may be seen.

        (2) Abdominal pain may be mistaken for a "surgical abdomen."

        (3) Hypotension may be severe and is typically unresponsive to saline hydration.

        (4) Fever may occur, even in the absence of an initiating infection.

        (5) Hypoglycemia. Remember, *gluco*corticoids stimulate *gluco*neogenesis.

        (6) Hyperpigmentation may occur but is not as common as in chronic insufficiency.

      b. Laboratory findings are similar to the findings in chronic insufficiency (see Table 81-2).

B. Secondary adrenal insufficiency. The development of signs and symptoms can be chronic or acute. The clinical manifestations are the same as in primary adrenal insufficiency, with the following exceptions:

    1. Patients may have **other evidence of pituitary dysfunction**

(e.g., hypothyroidism, hyperprolactinemia, diabetes insipidus, gonadotropin deficiency).

2. **Hyperkalemia** and a **non-anion gap metabolic acidosis** are usually **not present** (because aldosterone is sill secreted **appropriately**).

3. **Hyperpigmentation** usually **does not occur.**

IV APPROACH TO THE PATIENT

A. The most difficult aspect of diagnosing adrenal insufficiency is **considering the diagnosis.** The pattern of clinical manifestations and lab findings should alert you to the possibility of adrenal insufficiency. When a patient presents with hypotension, weakness, abdominal pain, unexplained fever, hypoglycemia, or nonspecific findings, consider Addison's disease.

B. Confirmation of the diagnosis is straightforward.

1. **Plasma cortisol assay.** If the plasma cortisol level is greater than 20 μg/dl, adrenal insufficiency is very unlikely.

2. **Rapid ACTH stimulation test.** If the plasma cortisol level is less than 20 μg/dl, perform a rapid ACTH stimulation test. A normal response rules out primary (but not secondary) adrenal insufficiency.

3. **Plasma ACTH level.** Measure the plasma ACTH if secondary adrenal insufficiency is still a consideration. A plasma ACTH level less than 20 pg/ml in the setting of cortisol deficiency usually confirms the diagnosis.

V TREATMENT

A. Acute insufficiency (adrenal crisis). If there is strong clinical suspicion for adrenal crisis, appropriate treatment should not be delayed until diagnostic testing is completed.

HOT KEY

Dexamethasone does not interfere with the plasma cortisol assay and can be used initially.

---

1. **Intravenous glucocorticoids.** High doses of glucocorticoids (e.g., hydrocortisone, 100 mg every 8 hours) are administered initially; mineralocorticoids may also be used but are not routinely given until the cortisol dose has been tapered to lower levels. (High doses of hydrocortisone have sufficient mineralocorticoid activity.)

2. **Supportive treatment** (e.g., intravenous fluids, oxygen) should also be instituted in a monitored setting.

3. Precipitating causes should be treated.

B. Chronic insufficiency

1. Primary adrenal insufficiency. Both glucocorticoids and mineralocorticoids are administered.

   a. Doses vary, but a rough estimate for a maintenance dose is 20–25 mg of cortisol daily and 0.1–0.2 mg of fludrocortisone daily.

   b. Patients should be counseled that treatment is **lifelong** and that doses should be increased during times of stress. Patients should also carry a wallet card or wear a bracelet bearing their diagnosis.

2. Secondary or **tertiary insufficiency.** Usually only glucocorticoids are needed.

References

Lamberts SW, de Herder WW, van der Lely AJ. Pituitary insufficiency. Lancet 1998; 352(9122):127–134.

Mayo J, Collazos J, Martinez E, Ibarra S. Adrenal function in the human immunodeficiency virus-infected patient. Arch Intern Med 2002;162(10):1095–1098.

Shenker Y, Skatrud JB. Adrenal insufficiency in critically ill patients. Am J Respir Crit Care Med 2001;163(7):1520–1523.

Ten S, New M, Maclaren N. Clinical review 130: Addison's disease 2001. J Clin Endocrinol Metab 2001;86(7):2909–2922.

82. Altered Mental Status

I **INTRODUCTION.** Altered mental status is a disorder of cognitive function that is broadly classified as a disturbance in either the level or content of consciousness.

A. A disturbance in the **level of consciousness** usually represents an abrupt change in awareness that spans the spectrum from alertness, through mild confusional states, frank delirium, and, finally, coma.

B. A disturbance in the **content of consciousness** usually presents as a slow deterioration or change in any or all of the following: memory, judgment, abstract thinking, recognition, language skills, or personality. A global change in the content of consciousness represents **dementia.**

II **CAUSES OF ALTERED MENTAL STATUS.** The mnemonic "MIST-P" is a useful way to help remember a long list of differential diagnoses and roughly divides the causes into three broad classes:

A. **M**etabolic, **I**nfectious, **I**nflammatory, and **I**nherited disorders (which is a very broad category);

B. **S**eizures and **S**tructural problems (stroke/vascular disorders, **T**umor, **T**rauma); and

C. **P**sychiatric disorders.

> **HOT KEY** Although a single cause of altered mental status is sought, a combination of factors is often responsible (e.g., a urinary tract infection in an elderly person who has Alzheimer's disease and is receiving multiple medications).

III **APPROACH TO THE PATIENT.** Given the overlap in the differential diagnoses for mild confusional states, delirium,

Causes of Altered Mental Status (MIST-P)

Metabolic
    Medicines: either medications that are directly psychoactive (e.g., benzodiazepines) or that have significant cognitive side effects
    Electrolyte derangements (e.g., disorders of sodium, glucose, or calcium) or **E**ndocrine disorders (increased or decreased levels of glucose, cortisol, thyroid hormone)
    Temperature derangements (i.e., hypothermia or hyperthermia)
    Alcohol and other drugs, either in toxicity or causing a withdrawal syndrome
    B$_{12}$ and other vitamin deficiencies, [e.g., niacin deficiency (pellagra) or thiamine deficiency (Wernicke-Korsakoff syndrome)]
    Oxygen deficiency to the brain may result from insufficient oxygen in the blood (i.e., hypoxemia), an inadequate number of red blood cells (RBCs) to carry the oxygen (i.e., anemia), or insufficient forward flow (i.e., decreased cardiac output)

    Liver or kidney disease causing encephalopathy
Infectious disorders either affecting the central nervous system (CNS) directly (e.g., encephalitis, brain abscess) or due to a systemic infection (e.g., urosepsis)
Inflammatory (e.g., collagen vascular diseases, sarcoidosis)
Inherited or degenerative diseases (e.g., Huntington's disease, Alzheimer's disease)
Seizures (actively seizing or due to a postictal state)
Strokes and other vascular disorders
    Ischemic infarcts (from emboli, thromboses, or vasculitis)
    Bleeds (epidural, subdural, subarachnoid, or intracerebral)
    Hypertensive encephalopathy
    Thrombotic thrombocytopenic purpura (TTP) or disseminated intravascular coagulation (DIC)
    Hyperviscosity syndrome (seen with plasma cell dyscrasias or significantly elevated RBC counts)
Tumors: malignant processes may lead to altered mental status either because of an intracranial lesion or because of a paraneoplastic process
Trauma (e.g., concussion)
Psychiatric disorders
Porphyria

coma, and dementia as well as the potential consequences of an incorrect or delayed diagnosis, all patients with altered mental status should be evaluated in a thorough and systematic manner.

A. Perform the ABCs.
   1. **Airway.** Consider intubation.
   2. **Breathing.** Consider intubation.
   3. **Circulation.** Check vital signs.
B. Assess the need for intravenous access and **fluids, oxygen,** and **electrocardiographic monitoring.**
C. Rule out easily reversible conditions.
   1. **Thiamine** (100 mg intravenously) is usually given.
   2. **50% dextrose (D50)** is usually given empirically when a fingerstick test for glucose is not readily available.
   3. **Naloxone hydrochloride** should be administered if an opiate overdose is suspected.

 H O T
KEY
Remember to always carefully consider all the medications a patient has been receiving as a potential cause of altered mental status.

D. Rule out common, immediately life-threatening conditions. Check the pupils, oculocephalic reflex, motor response, meningeal signs, and vital signs, looking for evidence of any of the following disorders:
   1. **Mass effect** (e.g., tumor, infarct, bleed, or abscess). If mass effect is suspected, make arrangements for emergent neuroimaging and an emergent neurosurgical consult. Mannitol, steroids, or intubation with hyperventilation may be indicated.
   2. **Meningitis.** Initial measures include blood cultures and early empiric antibacterial therapy followed by a lumbar puncture (see Chapter 88).
   3. **Status epilepticus.** Lorazepam, fosphenytoin, and, if necessary, phenobarbital are administered (see Chapter 86).
   4. **Hypertensive encephalopathy.** Nitroprusside is often administered.
   5. **Hyperthermia.** Cooling measures should be initiated.
E. Continue the work-up if the cause of altered mental status is still not apparent.
   1. **Patient history** and **physical examination.** Perform a thorough examination, with particular focus on the neurologic examination.

2. **Laboratory studies.** The following studies are often useful:
   a. **Complete blood count (CBC)**
   b. **Electrolyte panel** (including glucose and calcium)
   c. **Blood urea nitrogen (BUN)** and **creatinine levels**
   d. **Liver tests**
   e. **Prothrombin time (PT)** and **partial thromboplastin time (PTT)**
   f. **Arterial blood gases** (possibly including carboxyhemoglobin)
   g. **Toxicology screen**
   h. **Urinalysis**
3. **Other studies.** An electrocardiogram (ECG), chest radiograph, lumbar puncture (with an opening pressure), and head computed tomography (CT) or magnetic resonance imaging (MRI) scan may be appropriate.
4. **Neurology consult.** Consultation with a neurologist may be necessary if the diagnosis still cannot be made.
F. **Initiate treatment** according to the cause.

References

Inouye SK. Prevention of delirium in hospitalized older patients: risk factors and targeted intervention strategies. Ann Med 2000;32(4):257–263.

Meagher DJ. Delirium: optimising management. Br Med J 2001;322(7279):144–149.

Samuels SC, Evers MM, Delirium. Pragmatic guidance for managing a common, confounding, and sometimes lethal condition. Geriatrics 2002;57(6):33–38.

83. Peripheral Neuropathy

I INTRODUCTION

A. **Clinical syndromes.** Peripheral neuropathies can be divided into three clinical syndromes:

1. **Polyneuropathies** present with **symmetrical** abnormalities in sensation, motor strength, or both.

2. **Mononeuritis multiplex** is an **initially asymmetric** abnormality in more than one nerve trunk occurring either simultaneously or over days to years.

3. **Mononeuropathies** imply **focal** involvement of a single nerve (e.g., carpal tunnel syndrome) and usually result from local nerve compression or stretch.

B. Because **polyneuropathy** is the most common peripheral neuropathy and poses the greatest difficulty in differential diagnosis, it is the **focus of this chapter.**

II CLINICAL MANIFESTATIONS OF POLYNEUROPATHY

A. **Sensory abnormalities** in the feet are usually the first symptom of polyneuropathy.

1. **Hypesthesia** (decreased sensation), **anesthesia** (absent sensation), **paresthesia** ("pins and needles" sensation without any stimuli), **dysesthesia** (burning sensation with or without stimuli), and **hyperpathia** (exaggerated pain perception) may all be noted. Initially, subjective complaints may be unaccompanied by objective findings.

2. Later, a pansensory loss in the feet may occur and progress centrally. Finger involvement often occurs once the shins are affected; eventually, the classic **"stocking-glove"** pattern may be seen.

B. **Motor abnormalities** may also occur. The extensors are usually more involved than the flexors (i.e., weakness of dorsiflexion of the toes is a common finding). The ankle reflex is often diminished early in the course of the disease, and a diminished knee reflex and foot drop are seen with progression.

III CAUSES OF POLYNEUROPATHY.
Polyneuropathies may result from a variety of disorders. The mnemonic, "MOVE, STUPID," can be used.

Causes of Polyneuropathy ("MOVE, STUPID")

Metabolic disorders (diabetes mellitus)
Other (rare heredofamilial disorders)
Vasculitis or **V**itamin deficiency (vitamin B_{12}, thiamine, pyridoxine, folate)
Endocrine disorders (hypothyroidism)

Syphilis or **S**arcoid
Tumor-related (i.e., paraneoplastic syndrome)
Uremia or liver disease
Paraproteinemia/amyloidosis,[1] **P**orphyria, **P**rimary biliary cirrhosis, or **P**olycythemia vera
Infections[2] or **I**diopathic causes [e.g., Guillain-Barré syndrome, chronic inflammatory demyelinating polyneuropathy (CIDP)]
Drugs or toxins (including alcohol)

IV **APPROACH TO THE PATIENT.** Many of the disorders that can cause polyneuropathies are potentially life-threatening if not appropriately diagnosed and treated. Because the differential diagnosis is extensive and the etiology may or may not be obvious, the evaluation needs to be tailored to the situation. If the diagnosis is not initially apparent, a four-step process may be used to cover most of the possibilities.

A. Take a thorough patient history.
   1. Make sure to ask about **recent events** that may provide a clue to the diagnosis. Specifically, inquire about recent viral illnesses (which may suggest Guillain-Barré syndrome), the presence of similar symptoms in family members or coworkers (which may suggest a toxic exposure), and systemic symptoms (e.g., weight loss, which may raise suspicion for an occult malignancy).
   2. Obtain a **medication history.** Some drugs that may be responsible for polyneuropathy include amiodarone, dapsone,

---

[1]Amyloidosis may cause peripheral neuropathy without an accompanying paraproteinemia but is listed with paraproteinemia because these disorders are often thought of together.

[2]Peripheral neuropathy can be associated with infection (e.g., Lyme disease, leprosy, or AIDS). Patients with AIDS may develop polyradiculopathy with abnormalities on cerebrospinal fluid analysis that may be secondary to cytomegalovirus infection.

hydralazine, isoniazid, metronidazole, nitrofurantoin, phenytoin, vincristine, and high doses of pyridoxine.

3. Inquire about **toxin exposures.** The most common toxins include heavy metals (e.g., arsenic, lead, mercury, thallium), industrial agents, and pesticides (e.g., organophosphates); diphtheria toxin should also be considered but is quite rare.

H O T

K E Y

Remember, common things are common. If diabetes or uremia is present or the patient is a long-time alcoholic, you may not need to look any further.

B. **Assess the time course.** Only a few disorders commonly result in an **acute polyneuropathy** (i.e., one that occurs over a few days). Furthermore, unlike subacute or chronic polyneuropathies, acute disorders usually produce predictable patterns on **electrodiagnostic evaluation** (i.e., **electromyography, nerve conduction studies**).

1. **Acute axonal polyneuropathies** have relatively preserved nerve conduction and are usually caused by **porphyria** or **intoxications** (e.g., arsenic).

2. **Acute demyelinating polyneuropathies** display a significant decrease in nerve conduction and are essentially synonymous with **Guillain-Barré syndrome,** although **diphtheria** and **toxic berry** (buckthorn) **ingestion** may rarely produce the same clinical picture.

C. **Perform appropriate laboratory studies** if the diagnosis is still not evident. Review the list of possible causes and obtain the laboratory tests that will help shorten the list. Tests that may be requested include:

1. Complete blood count (CBC)
2. Erythrocyte sedimentation rate (ESR)
3. Renal panel with electrolytes
4. Fasting glucose level
5. Vitamin B_{12} level
6. Thyroid function tests
7. Liver tests
8. Venereal Disease Research Laboratory (VDRL) test for syphilis
9. Serum and urine protein electrophoresis and serum immunofixation

D. **Consider occult disorders.** The simple laboratory tests outlined in IV C may not rule out some of the more occult processes (e.g., tumor, vasculitis, sarcoidosis), but they may provide evidence for or against a possible diagnosis (e.g., a normal ESR makes vasculitis less likely). The following tests may be useful in certain clinical settings:

1. **Antinuclear antibody (ANA), rheumatoid factor (RF),** and **serum cryoglobulin** assessments may be used in the evaluation of suspected vasculitis (see Chapter 76).
2. **Radiography**
   a. **Chest radiographs** may show evidence of sarcoidosis or an occult tumor.
   b. A **computed tomography (CT) scan** may be performed if an intra-abdominal malignancy is suspected.
3. **Urinary heavy metal** and **porphobilinogen levels** can be used to evaluate the possibility of toxic metal exposures and acute intermittent porphyria, respectively.
4. **Lyme titers** are only useful in the appropriate clinical setting because they lack specificity.
5. **Cerebrospinal fluid evaluation**
   a. Findings include high protein levels and a normal cell count in patients with Guillain-Barré syndrome or CIDP.
   b. In AIDS patients with cytomegalovirus polyradiculopathy, findings include neutrophilic pleocytosis, high protein levels, and low glucose levels.
6. **Electrodiagnostic studies** may be performed (if they have not been already) to help categorize whether there is primarily axonal degeneration or demyelination. These studies may be especially helpful in diagnosing CIDP.
7. **Sural nerve biopsy.** The ankle is the easiest place to obtain a cutaneous nerve biopsy.
   a. Nerve biopsy is of low yield in symmetric polyneuropathies but should be considered in patients with suspected **mononeuritis multiplex** because a vasculitis may be more likely. The yield of biopsy is also increased in patients with suspected **vasculitis, amyloidosis, sarcoidosis,** or **leprosy** and in those with palpably thickened nerves.
   b. Because **heredofamilial disorders** often present at an early age and have a characteristic histopathology, a sural nerve biopsy should also be considered in **children.**

V   TREATMENT is generally aimed at the underlying disorder. Some general measures and specific therapies are discussed here.

A. **General measures.** Relief of neuropathic pain is usually not easily accomplished. **Tricyclic antidepressants** (e.g., desipramine, amitriptyline) or the **anticonvulsant gabapentin** are often tried. Other anticonvulsants or **topical capsaicin** may also be helpful in some cases.

B. Specific therapies

1. Guillain-Barré syndrome

a. Most patients require hospitalization for observation and **supportive care** (e.g., intubation for respiratory failure).

b. **Plasmapheresis** or **intravenous immunoglobulin (IVIG)** is beneficial (especially within the first 2 weeks of illness). Steroids are not usually effective.

c. Approximately 85% of patients will recover completely or have only mild residual defects. The mortality rate is approximately 3%-4%.

2. CIDP may be treated with **steroids, immunosuppressants,** and **IVIG** or **plasmapheresis** if ambulation is threatened.

3. Isoniazid overdose can be treated with **intravenous pyridoxine** (1 g for each gram of isoniazid ingested).

4. Acute intermittent porphyria

a. Acute treatment. Intravenous **glucose** and **hematin** may be needed for acute attacks.

b. Chronic treatment entails **avoiding precipitating factors** (e.g., sulfa drugs) and **adhering to a high-carbohydrate diet.**

References

Hughes RA. Peripheral neuropathy. Br Med J 2002;324(7335):466–469.

Parry GJ. Management of diabetic neuropathy. Am J Med 1999;107(2B):27S-33S.

Poncelet AN. An algorithm for the evaluation of peripheral neuropathy. Am Fam Phys 1998;57(4):755–764.

84. Vertigo

....

I INTRODUCTION

A. **Definitions**
   1. **Dizziness** is a term used to describe an unusual head sensation or gait unsteadiness. Faintness and vertigo are forms of dizziness.
   2. **Faintness** is usually described as a sense of light-headedness and is usually caused by an insufficient supply of oxygen, blood, or glucose to the brain. Faintness often occurs with hyperventilation, hypoglycemia, or just before a syncopal event.
   3. **Vertigo,** the topic of this chapter, is the illusion of movement (usually spinning). The patient may describe the environment as moving while he or she remains stationary, or vice versa.
B. **Clinical manifestations of vertigo**
   1. **Nausea** and **vomiting** usually accompany vertigo.
   2. **Gait unsteadiness** and **ataxia** are common.
   3. Vertigo **worsens with head movement.**
C. **Etiology.** Vertigo most commonly results from a defect in the vestibular system, but defects in the visual system or the somatosensory system can cause vertigo as well.

II TYPES OF VERTIGO. Prognostically, it is important to distinguish **central** vertigo from **peripheral** vertigo.

A. **Central vertigo** often has a **poorer prognosis** than peripheral vertigo.
   1. **Clinical manifestations of central vertigo**
      a. Central vertigo is usually accompanied by other **brain stem** or **cerebellar** (occasionally even **cerebral hemispheric**) **signs** (e.g., headache, limb ataxia, true weakness, paresthesias, dysarthria, diplopia). **Nystagmus** may be present and can take any form: horizontal, vertical, or multidirectional.
      b. Central vertigo is usually not accompanied by tinnitus or hearing loss.
   2. **Causes of central vertigo.** The most common causes of central vertigo can be remembered with the mnemonic, "MAIM." (Often, patients with central vertigo are "maimed" because of their poor prognosis.)

Causes of Central Vertigo ("MAIM")

Multiple sclerosis
Acoustic neuroma
Ischemia or central nervous system (CNS) lesions [especially basilar transient ischemic attack (TIA)]
Migraine (especially basilar)

B. Peripheral vertigo
   1. Clinical manifestations of peripheral vertigo tend to cause more patient distress than those of central vertigo; however, the episodes are briefer because the CNS tends to adapt.
   a. Tinnitus and **hearing loss** are common.
   b. Nystagmus, which is usually present, occurs unidirectionally and is horizontal. The fast component is toward the side of the unaffected ear. Unlike the nystagmus of central vertigo, the nystagmus of peripheral vertigo is inhibited by visual fixation. **Otherwise, the neurologic examination is completely normal.**
   2. Causes of peripheral vertigo. Peripheral vertigo is usually a result of processes that involve the **labyrinth** (inner ear) or **eighth cranial nerve.** Causes include:
   a. Acoustic neuroma (also causes central vertigo)
   b. Ménière's disease (vertigo, hearing loss, and tinnitus)
   c. Benign paroxysmal positional vertigo (BPPV), very brief (e.g., less than 1 minute) episodes of vertigo, usually brought on by head movement and often following ear trauma or infection
   d. Labyrinthitis leads to acute, severe vertigo, nausea, and vomiting in patients who have had a recent viral syndrome.
   e. Inner ear infections
   f. Head trauma (recent)
   g. Psychogenic causes (considered in patients with a normal neurologic examination and lacking nystagmus during an episode of vertigo)
   h. Aminoglycoside antibiotics and other drugs
   i. Endocrine disorders (e.g., hypothyroidism, diabetes)

III APPROACH TO THE PATIENT

A. Patient history. In many patients, the cause of vertigo can be determined from the history alone.

Common Causes of Peripheral Vertigo ("AMPLITUDE")

Acoustic neuroma
Ménière's disease
Positional (BPPV)
Labyrinthitis
Infection of the inner ear
Trauma (head)
Ψchogenic causes
Drugs
Endocrine disorders

B. Physical examination. The examination should focus on the ears, eyes, and nervous system.
   1. The presence or absence of an **ear infection, nystagmus,** and **neurologic deficits** should be ascertained.
   2. The **Nylen-Bárány maneuver** is important in the assessment of BPPV. The seated patient turns his or her head to one side while quickly lying down so that the head hangs over the edge of the table. If vertigo is reproduced (along with nystagmus), the patient is likely to have BPPV.
C. Special tests should be ordered in the following situations:
   1. If hearing loss or tinnitus is a major component, an audiogram is useful to evaluate for Ménière's disease or acoustic neuroma.
   2. If thyroid disease or diabetes mellitus is suspected, **blood work** is useful.
      a. Thyroid-stimulating hormone (TSH) levels may be useful if thyroid disease is suspected.
      b. Serum glucose values may prove useful if diabetes is suspected.
   3. If peripheral causes seem unlikely or if the patient has neurologic abnormalities, brain **magnetic resonance imaging (MRI)** and **magnetic resonance angiography (MRA)** are indicated.

IV TREATMENT

A. Central vertigo. Treatment depends on the cause. For patients suspected of having vertebrobasilar TIAs, see Chapter 87.
B. Peripheral vertigo. For acute peripheral vertigo of almost any cause, the patient should be prescribed bed rest and given antihistamines, anticholinergics, and/or benzodiazepines. The patient should be cautioned regarding falls.

   1. Medications may prevent CNS adaptation to peripheral vertigo and, therefore, should not be used for an extended period.

   2. A mild exercise program can expedite the adaptation process.

References

Furman JM, Cass SP. Benign paroxysmal positional vertigo. N Engl J Med 1999;
341(21):1590–1596.

Palaniappan R. Balance disorders in adults: an overview. Hosp Med (London) 2002;
63(5):278–281.

Tusa RJ. Vertigo. Neurol Clin 2001;19(1):23–55.

85. Singultus

I **INTRODUCTION.** A hiccough is an inspiratory sound caused by the abrupt closure of the glottis in the setting of rhythmic spasm of the diaphragm and respiratory muscles. Hiccoughs can occur at any age and can last for years (but usually only last for a few minutes). There is a strong male predominance.

II **CAUSES OF SINGULTUS.** Singultus may be caused by a wide variety of conditions that have one thing in common—they involve the reflex arc shown in Figure 85–1. Causes can be classified as **peripheral** (i.e., involving the vagus or phrenic nerves or structures adjacent to the diaphragm) or central.

Common Causes of Singultus ("SINGULTUS")

Surgery (following abdominal, thoracic, or neck surgery)
Infection of structures adjacent to the diaphragm (e.g., lower lobe pneumonia, subphrenic abscess, peritonitis)
Nervous system disorders (e.g., stroke, meningitis, brain tumor, multiple sclerosis)
Gastric distention (very common cause)
Uremia
Low serum calcium, sodium, or potassium
Tumor of the pancreas
Ψchiatric disorders
Steroids and other drugs (e.g., alcohol, benzodiazepines, barbiturates)

III **TREATMENT.** Treating the underlying disorder is the best course of action.

A. Several benign strategies to relieve hiccoughs have been anecdotally successful. These include (in no particular order):

   1. Having the patient swallow a tablespoon of granulated sugar.

   2. Massaging the soft palate or applying traction to the tongue.

   3. Placing a nasogastric tube or a nasopharyngeal catheter.

   4. The age-old scare tactic.

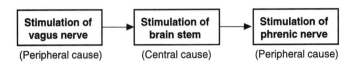

FIGURE 85–1. The many causes of singultus involve this reflex arc in some way.

B. Pharmacologic therapy (e.g., with chlorpromazine or metoclopramide) may be instituted if the benign strategies fail.

References

Friedman NL. Hiccups: a treatment review. Pharmacotherapy 1996;16(6):986–995.

Goldstein R. Practice tips. Simple method for curing hiccups. Can Fam Physician 1999;45:1459.

Rousseau P. Hiccups. South Med J 1995;88(2):175–181.

86. Seizure Disorders

I. INTRODUCTION

A. Definitions

1. A **seizure** is a paroxysmal abnormality of cerebral function caused by uncontrolled, excessive discharges from a group of neurons.

2. **Epilepsy** is the tendency to have recurrent (unprovoked) seizures.

3. **Status epilepticus** is continuous seizure activity. Practically, any seizure lasting more than 5 minutes or occurrence of more than two subsequent seizures without returning to baseline between seizures may be considered status epilepticus. (Most seizures last 30 seconds to 2 minutes.)

HOT KEY

A prolonged seizure is a medical emergency.

---

4. An **aura** is subjective sensation experienced before a seizure. In fact, these represent simple partial seizures (see III A).

5. **Automatisms** are repetitive movements such as lip-smacking, chewing, and scratching that often accompany complex partial seizures.

6. **Postictal** refers to "after the ictus (or event)." Patients are often tired and disoriented after a seizure and may have a transient focal paralysis secondary to seizure activity, called Todd's paralysis. Typically, all symptoms improve over the course of minutes to hours.

B. Epidemiology. Epilepsy is a relatively common neurological problem, affecting about 0.5% of the population.

II. DIFFERENTIAL DIAGNOSIS

A. Syncope. This condition is most often confused with seizures because it involves loss of consciousness and is accompanied by brief "seizure-like" movements that may occur with the loss of consciousness. Some factors that help distinguish syncope from seizures include the following:

454

1. **Precipitating factors. Seizures** usually have **no immediate precipitating factors** and **no premonitory symptoms except for an aura.** In contrast, syncope is often associated with emotional stress, Valsalva maneuvers, or cardiac conditions and it may be preceded by tiredness, nausea, diaphoresis, and "graying out" of vision. Syncope usually begins with an erect posture, whereas seizures are variable.

2. **Course. Seizures** usually lead to **immediate unconsciousness, lasting for several minutes,** with a **period of sleepiness or disorientation for minutes to hours after the event.** Syncope usually leads to unconsciousness, lasting for several seconds, with a rapid return (seconds to several minutes) to full consciousness and alertness (if the patient has been allowed to assume a recumbent position).

B. **Other conditions.** Migraine, transient ischemic attack, stroke, movement disorders, and psychiatric disorders are also diagnostic possibilities.

III **TYPES OF SEIZURES** The most important distinction to make when evaluating a patient who has had a seizure is deciding if the event is a partial or a generalized seizure. This distinction helps determine etiology, location of brain abnormality, prognosis, and subsequent treatment.

A. **Partial seizures.** Partial seizures are those that **begin in one "part" of the brain** and are the **most common type of seizure.** In adults, they most often **occur following brain injury** (e.g., tumor, trauma, stroke). Partial seizures are also known as "localization-related seizures."

1. **Simple partial seizures** result in a **focal neurologic deficit without alteration of awareness.** These seizures may include shaking of a limb, numbness on one side, rising epigastric sensation, odd smell or taste, auditory or visual phenomena, a sense of familiarity (déjà vu), or a sense of strangeness (jamais vu).

2. **Complex partial seizures** result in a **loss of awareness. Complex partial seizures with secondary generalization** refer to a seizure that begins focally and then spreads to involve the brain diffusely, leading to a generalized seizure.

HOT

KEY

Most generalized seizures occurring in adults are secondarily generalized.

B. Generalized seizures. Generalized seizures **begin with a diffusely abnormal discharge of neurons leading to widespread cortical involvement.** These seizures occur in the **inherited epilepsies** or **secondary to diffuse brain injury.**

    1. Tonic-clonic seizures are one of the **most widely recognized generalized seizures.**

        a. They usually begin with **alteration of consciousness.**

        b. Then **bilateral stiffening** (tonic phase) of limbs, often with a clenched jaw, occurs, followed by **rhythmic shaking of limbs** (clonic phase), followed by **complete loss of tone.**

        c. Afterward, patients may be difficult to arouse and it may take minutes to hours to return to baseline.

    2. Tonic seizures involve **tonic stiffening,** usually for about 10 seconds, often causing individuals to fall.

    3. Clonic seizures involve **rhythmic shaking,** with no tonic phase.

    4. Atonic seizures involve **sudden and sometimes complete loss of body tone.** They often lead to a fall.

    5. Absence seizures involve **"staring spells,"** which last for several seconds.

        a. Onset is abrupt and cause individuals to stop what they are doing. Absence seizures often occur **many times per day** and **more frequently in children** compared with adults.

        b. Although individuals are not responsive during an episode, they **often return to baseline level of consciousness immediately.**

        c. Associated symptoms may include **eye blinking, lip smacking,** or **swallowing.**

    6. Myoclonic seizures are myoclonic jerks, which are brief, lightning-fast jerks of a group of muscles. These movements are associated with a generalized electrical discharge. Myoclonic seizures may be associated with an inherited epilepsy syndrome, progressive epilepsy syndromes, or neurodegenerative disorders.

HOT KEY It is important to distinguish myoclonic seizures from the more common medical causes of myoclonic jerks, such as transitions in and out of sleep, severe hypoxic injury, and metabolic derangements.

IV APPROACH TO THE PATIENT

A. Assess and protect the airway. Both during and after a seizure, patients should be positioned on their side to avoid aspiration.

B. Always consider whether the patient may still be seizing. If the patient is seizing for more than 5 minutes, acute intervention to stop the seizure should be taken (see V B). A patient often does not return to baseline mental status immediately after a seizure, but the typical course is that of constant improvement.

C. Do not forcefully restrict limbs, but make sure that obstacles such as beds or chairs are cleared out of the way to avoid injury. All hospitalized patients with a recent history of seizures should have padded bed rails to help decrease injury.

D. Obtain a detailed history and perform a detailed physical examination, which most often help distinguish between seizure and other disorders with transient neurologic deficits. The evaluation of a patient with a known seizure disorder who has a seizure typical of that condition obviously differs from the evaluation of a patient with a first-time seizure.

E. Obtain several laboratory studies, because metabolic derangements (e.g., hyponatremia) may provoke seizures. A **glucose level** should be obtained immediately. It may often be appropriate to treat a patient with intravenous glucose (and thiamine) presumptively. **Other laboratory studies** should include complete blood count, electrolyte panel, blood urea nitrogen, creatinine, calcium, magnesium, phosphorous, liver panel, anticonvulsant medication levels (if appropriate), and toxicology screen (including ethanol level).

HOT

KEY
Almost all patients briefly stop breathing during a generalized seizure and therefore become acidemic.

F. Consider performing an infectious work-up in all patients with a seizure. In patients with a known seizure disorder, an intercurrent infection is a common cause of worsening of seizures.

G. Consider performing cerebrospinal fluid (CSF) studies. Although not every patient with a seizure needs a lumbar puncture, the likelihood of a causal central nervous system (CNS) infection should always be strongly considered.

HOT

KEY
CNS infections commonly present with seizures and may be especially difficult to recognize without CSF studies in immunosuppressed or elderly patients.

H. Obtain brain imaging if the episode is a new-onset seizure or represents a change in the type of seizure for a patient with epilepsy. A **magnetic resonance imaging (MRI) scan of the brain is the imaging modality of choice.** The acuity of the presentation and rapidity with which an MRI can be obtained often determine if computed tomography (CT) is obtained before the MRI. Immediate CT is indicated if the patient is at high risk for an acute intracranial process (e.g., hemorrhage, infection, stroke, hydrocephalus).

I. Consider obtaining an electroencephalogram (EEG). In some circumstances, an EEG may be useful acutely to determine if a patient is seizing without overt clinical signs (nonconvulsive status). For an outpatient, the EEG may help distinguish between types of epilepsy or direct attention to a given area.

 TREATMENT

A. Nonmedication-related management

1. **Seizure precautions** should be instituted for all inpatients.
2. Patients should be told to use common sense and to **avoid activities that would be dangerous if they were to have another seizure** (e.g., swimming alone, working on ladders, driving a motorized vehicle). In many states, a seizure must be reported to state public health agencies, who will in turn notify the department of motor vehicles. All patients with seizures should be told specifically not to drive until the seizure disorder is under adequate control, as determined by the treating physician and, in many states, the department of motor vehicles.

B. Medications

1. **Status epilepticus.** Patients should be in a monitored setting and may require intubation for airway protection.
   a. Give **intravenous thiamine** (100 mg) and **glucose** (50 ml of 50% dextrose).
   b. Give 0.1 mg/kg **lorazepam** (Ativan), the first-line acute anticonvulsant medication, at 2 mg/min via intravenous push. Note that lorazepam only temporarily (for about 15–20 minutes) halts status epilepticus, but this often allows enough time to begin determining the etiology.
   c. If the seizure does not stop immediately, give 20 mg/kg **fosphenytoin** at 150 mg/min. Watch for hypotension.
   d. In some cases, higher doses of the above medications, additional medications, or general anesthesia may be required to control seizures.
2. **Epilepsy.** Almost all anticonvulsant drugs treat partial seizures (and the generalized seizures that begin in a partial manner). A subset of anticonvulsant drugs specifically treat

generalized seizures (e.g., valproic acid). Side effect profile and ease of administration are most important in the treatment of partial seizures. Table 86-1 lists some medications commonly used to control seizures, along with their potential side effects.

a. Monitor for side effects

    (1) Almost all anticonvulsant drugs have **potential serious side effects,** including an allergic reaction, hematologic and liver toxicity, and hyponatremia. Rash, fever, or other reactions should be evaluated immediately. A complete blood count, liver enzymes, and an electrolyte panel are followed frequently when starting a new anticonvulsant drug.

TABLE 86–1. Pharmacologic Agents Commonly Used for Seizures

Agent	Seizure Type	Adverse Effects
Phenytoin (fosphenytoin, Dilantin)	Partial, tonic-clonic	Dizziness, diplopia, ataxia, incoordination, confusion, slurred speech, rash, gingival hyperplasia, hirsutism, blood dyscrasias, toxic hepatitis, facial coarsening
Carbamazepine (Tegretol)	Partial, tonic-clonic	Ataxia, dizziness, diplopia, vertigo, nausea, aplastic anemia, hyponatremia, blood dyscrasias, toxic hepatitis,
Valproic acid (Depakote, Depacon, Depakene)	All	Ataxia, sedation, tremor, toxic hepatitis, thrombocytopenia, hair loss, weight gain, nausea
Phenobarbital	Partial, tonic-clonic	Somnolence, cognitive and behavioral changes, rash, blood dyscrasias
Topiramate (Topamax)	Partial, tonic-clonic, others	Psychomotor slowing, sedation, fatigue, paresthesias, speech or language problems, weight loss, kidney stones
Lamotrigine (Lamictal)	Partial, tonic-clonic, others	Dizziness, diplopia, sedation, headache, ataxia, rash
Neurontin	Partial	Sedation, dizziness, ataxia
Ethosuximide	Absence	Nausea, anorexia, rash, blood dyscrasias, somnolence

      (2) Almost all anticonvulsant drugs have some **non-life-threatening CNS side effects** (e.g., sedation, nausea, nystagmus, ataxia), drug interactions, and potential teratogenicity.

   b. Build dose gradually. To minimize side effects, most anticonvulsant drugs are started at a low dose and are gradually increased to either maximum tolerated dose or control of seizures.

   c. Try other medications if needed. Approximately 65% of patients achieve full seizure control with the first medication tried. Other patients will need to change medications or take more than one medication.

C. Other therapies. In specialized cases in which medications fail to provide adequate control, the following may be considered: undergoing surgery to remove a seizure focus, implanting a device that delivers recurrent low-dose electrical stimuli to the vagus nerve (vagus nerve stimulator), or following a restrictive (i.e., ketogenic) diet.

References

Ahmed S, Chadwick D, Walker RJ. The management of alcohol-related seizures: an overview. Hosp Med (London) 2000;61(11):793–796.

Lowenstein DH, Alldredge BK. Status epilepticus. N Engl J Med 1998;338(14): 970–976.

Marks WJ Jr, Garcia PA. Management of seizures and epilepsy. Am Fam Phys 1998; 57(7):1589–1600.

87. Stroke

I INTRODUCTION

A. Definitions. A stroke is an acute focal neurologic deficit produced by a disturbance in cerebral circulation that results in ischemic infarction, hemorrhage, or both. If the deficit resolves within 24 hours, the incident is a **transient ischemic attack (TIA).**

B. Epidemiology. Stroke is the third leading cause of death and a leading cause of disability in the United States. Mortality rates from stroke have fallen by more than 50% in the past 30 years, probably due to better control of hypertension and other risk factors.

II CAUSES OF STROKE

A. Ischemic infarction

1. **Distribution.** Cerebral infarcts can be classified according to the type of vessel involved.

   a. Small vessel. Chronic stress to vessels produces lipohyalinosis, leading to stenosis and occlusion.

   b. Large vessel. Embolism from a vessel, valve, or cardiac chamber or thrombosis (often caused by a ruptured atherosclerotic plaque) leads to stenosis and inadequate perfusion. Affected arteries include the:

   (1) Middle cerebral artery
   (2) Anterior cerebral artery
   (3) Carotid artery
   (4) Posterior cerebral artery
   (5) Vertebrobasilar circulation

   c. Watershed infarctions may occur at the junction of the anterior and middle cerebral arteries or the junction of the posterior and middle cerebral arteries during systemic hypotension.

   d. Venous. Thrombosis occurring in the superior sagittal sinus or other large cerebral veins may also result in cerebral infarction.

2. **Source.** Small vessel, large vessel, watershed, and venous infarctions may be produced by local processes or disease in the systemic circulation. It is helpful to remember the sources of infarcts by beginning in the arterioles of the brain, working backward to the heart, and then through the venous system to the brain again (Table 87-1).

TABLE 87-1. Sources of Cerebral Infarcts

Source	Distribution	Risk Factors	Useful Data
Small arteries	Small vessel	Hypertension, diabetes mellitus	Glucose, Hg-A1C
Large and medium arteries	Large vessel	Diabetes mellitus, elevated cholesterol, vasculitis, Asian decent, syphilis, dissection	Glucose, Hg-A1C, cholesterol panel, ESR, toxicology screen, MHA-TP, MRA or angiography
Carotid stenosis	Large vessel	Diabetes mellitus, elevated cholesterol	Glucose, Hg-A1C, cholesterol panel; MRA, Doppler ultrasound, or angiography
Aortic arch	Large vessel	Elevated cholesterol, coronary artery disease	Transesophageal echocardiogram
Left ventricle	Large vessel	History of anterior myocardial infarction, ejection fraction <30%	ECG, cardiac monitoring, echocardiogram
Heart valves	Large vessel	Abnormal or prosthetic valves, endocarditis	Echocardiogram, ESR, blood cultures
Left atrium	Large vessel	Atrial fibrillation, left atrial enlargement	ECG, echocardiogram
Hypotension	Watershed	Coronary artery disease, arrhythmia, shock	ECG, cardiac monitoring, CBC
Hematologic	Venous; large or small vessel	Polycythemia, thrombocytosis, leukocytosis, hypercoagulable states, sickle cell anemia	CBC, PT, PTT, anticardiolipin antibody, Russell viper venom test, protein C and S, antithrombin III, IgM, viscosity studies
Systemic veins	Large vessel	Deep venous thrombosis with patent foramen ovale or atrial septal defect	Echocardiogram with contrast, lower extremity Doppler ultrasound
Cerebral veins or sinuses	Venous	Dehydration, hypercoagulable state, otitis, sinusitis	Magnetic resonance venogram, conventional venogram

CBC = complete blood count; ECG = electrocardiogram; ESR = erythrocyte sedimentation rate; Hg-A1C = glycosylated hemoglobin; MHA-TP = microhemagglutination-Treponema pallidum; MRA = magnetic resonance angiogram; PT = prothrombin time; PTT = partial thromboplastin time.

B. Hemorrhage

1. **Intraparenchymal hemorrhage** is usually caused by hypertension; an underlying vascular malformation or tumor may also result in intraparenchymal hemorrhage.

2. **Subarachnoid hemorrhage** is usually caused by ruptured cerebral aneurysms. A sudden onset of headache and neck stiffness is characteristic.

3. **Subdural hematoma** can occur with or without a history of preceding trauma.

4. **Epidural hematoma** is almost always sudden and post-traumatic.

5. **Hemorrhagic transformation.** Bleeding occurs into an ischemic infarct.

III APPROACH TO THE PATIENT

A. Consider differential diagnoses

1. **Migraine**
2. **Postictal state**[1]
3. **Hypoglycemia**
4. **Hypertensive encephalopathy**

B. Brain imaging

1. **Infarction.** In the first 6 hours after ischemic infarction, head computed tomography (CT) and magnetic resonance imaging (MRI) may be unrevealing; therefore, the patient history and physical examination findings are particularly important. Localization of the lesion helps to identify the infarction as large vessel, small vessel, watershed, or venous, thereby limiting the differential diagnosis and directing treatment. Table 87-2 summarizes the clinical manifestations and findings on imaging studies for each type of cerebral infarct.

2. **Hemorrhages** will usually be apparent immediately using CT or MRI, although lumbar puncture may be required to rule out subarachnoid hemorrhage, which may not be seen on imaging.

C. Search for an underlying cause

1. Almost all patients should undergo the studies summarized in Table 87-3. Local practice varies greatly regarding whether patients with TIA need to be admitted to the hospital for evaluation and/or observation. Recent evidence suggests that certain subgroups of patients with TIA may be at relatively higher short-term risk for stroke: age older than 60 years,

---

[1]Focal weakness following a seizure (i.e., Todd's paralysis) is occasionally seen.

87-2. Clinical Manifestations of Cerebral Infarcts*

Type	Clinical Manifestations	Imaging Study Findings
Small vessel	Lacunar syndrome (e.g., pure motor hemiparesis, ataxic hemiparesis, pure sensory deficit, clumsy hand dysarthria)	Small, often round, lesions in the white matter, deep gray matter, and brain stem
Large vessel		
Middle cerebral artery	Hemiparesis and hemisensory deficit (face = arm > leg)	Infarction in wedge of cortex and underlying white matter
Anterior cerebral artery	Same as for middle cerebral artery infarction except leg > arm, sparing face	
Carotid artery	Signs of middle cerebral artery infarct plus or minus signs of anterior cerebral artery infarct or amaurosis fugax	
Posterior cerebral artery	Visual field cut	
Vertebrobasilar circulation	Cranial nerve palsies, ataxia, coma	
Watershed	"Man in the barrel" with proximal arm and leg weakness and numbness	Infarction in cortex and underlying white matter in a line from the eyes to the occiput
Venous	Variable; headache often present; legs often affected	Infarction and hemorrhage near the superior sagittal sinus or in the temporal lobe

*Specific neurologic deficits in a given patient are often more complex and depend on the exact location of the infarct.

TABLE 87-3. Initial Work-Up for the Evaluation of Stroke Patients

Tests	Purpose
CBC, PT, PTT	Rule out hematologic problem
ESR, MHA-TP	Rule out vasculitis, syphilis
ECG	Rule out arrhythmia, myocardial infarction
Head CT or MRI scan	Rule out non-stroke, differentiate ischemic infarction from hemorrhage*

CBC = complete blood count; CT = computed tomography; ECG = electrocardiogram; ESR = erythrocyte sedimentation rate; MHA-TP = microhemagglutination-*Treponema pallidum*; MRI = magnetic resonance imaging; PT = prothrombin time; PTT = partial thromboplastin time.
*Head CT may not show evidence of ischemic infarction until 6 hours postinfarction, but is relatively sensitive for hemorrhage immediately. Contrast is rarely helpful. MRI is more sensitive for ischemic infarct, especially in the brain stem and cerebellum where bone obscures the CT view, but is more expensive and time consuming.

presence of diabetes mellitus, episode longer than 10 minutes, and presence of motor weakness or speech impairment.
2. The following studies are indicated in certain circumstances:
   a. Carotid Doppler ultrasound is indicated following a large vessel TIA or stroke when endarterectomy or stent is being considered.
   b. Cardiac echocardiography is indicated following a large vessel TIA or stroke.
   c. CT angiography is often considered in the setting of an acute stroke when knowledge of intracranial vasculature may affect treatment.
   d. Magnetic resonance angiography. A magnetic resonance angiogram (MRA) of the head is indicated for patients with possible intracranial large vessel disease or suspected arterial dissection. MRA of the neck can also confirm abnormal carotid Doppler ultrasound findings.
   e. Conventional angiography may be appropriate if carotid endarterectomy is being considered or when vasculitis, aortic dissection, or subarachnoid hemorrhage is suspected.
   f. Transcranial Doppler ultrasound is often indicated for patients with possible intracranial large vessel disease or vasospasm following subarachnoid hemorrhage.
   g. Lumbar puncture is indicated if subarachnoid hemorrhage is a possibility and not visualized on CT scan.
   h. Hypercoagulability studies (see Chapter 67) are appropriate in young patients (i.e., those younger than 45 years) with no other risk factors for stroke.

i. **Toxicology screen.** A toxicology screen is often performed in young patients with stroke to rule out cocaine use.

IV TREATMENT

A. Ischemic infarction. Treatment has been primarily supportive and focused on secondary prevention, but therapies directed at dissolving clots and protecting the patient from cerebral ischemia have been evolving rapidly.

1. **Generally accepted therapies**
   a. **Pharmacologic therapy**
      (1) **Heparin** followed by **warfarin** reduces the risk of a recurrent event by approximately 65% for patients with a known cardiac source of embolus (e.g., atrial fibrillation, mechanical heart valve, mural thrombus). The timing and level of treatment are debated.
      (2) **Aspirin** or another antiplatelet agent is usually indicated for stroke prophylaxis in patients who are not receiving anticoagulants.
      (3) **t-PA.** Intravenous administration of tissue plasminogen activator (t-PA) may be beneficial for patients with a cerebral infarct who can be **treated** within 3 hours of symptom onset (defined as the time the patient can be last **confirmed** to be **normal**). Although this treatment does not currently appear to decrease mortality rates, t-PA may lead to a 50% relative increase in patients who are neurologically normal at 3 months. Importantly, t-PA may be associated with a 6% risk of serious intracranial hemorrhage (50% of which were fatal). Therefore, the risks and benefits of this drug remain debated.
   b. **Supportive measures**
      (1) Hold or decrease antihypertensive agents and consider intravenous hydration to increase blood flow to the ischemic area around the infarct.
      (2) Watch for aspiration, deep venous thrombosis, and other complications.
   c. **Specific treatment** that addresses the cause of the stroke (e.g., carotid endarterectomy) should be carried out if indicated.
   d. **Physical, occupational,** and **speech therapy** are necessary.
2. **Evolving therapies**
   a. **Anticoagulation.** Antiplatelet versus warfarin therapy continues to be reevaluated in a variety of clinical settings (e.g., aortic arch disease and intracranial atherosclerosis).

    b. Intra-arterial thrombolysis. Thrombolytic agents may be beneficial if administered intra-arterially during cerebral angiogram within 6 hours of infarct onset.

    c. Neuroprotection. A variety of neuroprotectant therapies are being investigated as a way of minimizing ischemic damage.

B. Hemorrhage

  1. Hemorrhagic transformation. The treatment is the same as that for ischemic infarction, except heparin and aspirin are withheld.

  2. Intraparenchymal hemorrhage. Surgical evacuation may be possible, depending on the size and location of the hemorrhage.

  3. Subarachnoid hemorrhage

    a. Consultation with a neurosurgeon or interventional radiologist is indicated to explore the possibility of early aneurysm clipping or coiling.

    b. Nimodipine therapy and hydration are indicated.

  4. Subdural and **epidural hemorrhages.** Consultation with a neurosurgeon to investigate the possibility of evacuation is appropriate.

References

Albers GW, Amarenco P, Easton JD, Sacco RL, Teal P. Antithrombotic and thrombolytic therapy for ischemic stroke. Chest 2001;119(Suppl 1):300S-320S.

Antithrombotic Trialists' Collaboration. Collaborative meta-analysis of randomised trials of antiplatelet therapy for prevention of death, myocardial infarction, and stroke in high risk patients. [Erratum appears in BMJ 2002;324(7330):141.] BMJ 2002;324(7329):71–86.

Brott T, Bogousslavsky J. Treatment of acute ischemic stroke. N Engl J Med 2000; 343(10):710–722.

Gage BF, Fihn SD, White RH. Warfarin therapy for an octogenarian who has atrial fibrillation. Ann Intern Med 2001;134(6):465–474.

88. Meningitis

INTRODUCTION. Meningitis may result from infection, malignancy (i.e., carcinomatous meningitis), or systemic illness (e.g., lupus, sarcoidosis). Infectious etiologies (particularly acute bacterial meningitis) are common, life-threatening causes of meningitis and are the major focus of this chapter. Infectious meningitis can be classified as easy as "A, B, C."

Classification of Infectious Meningitis ("A, B, C")

Aseptic meningitis
Bacterial meningitis (acute)
Chronic meningitis

II CAUSES OF INFECTIOUS MENINGITIS

A. Aseptic meningitis
   1. **Viral infections,** including mumps, herpes simplex virus 1, coxsackievirus, Epstein-Barr virus, and cytomegalovirus (CMV), are common causes of aseptic meningitis.
   2. **Spirochetal infections.** Secondary syphilis, Lyme disease, and leptospirosis may also cause aseptic meningitis.
   3. **Parameningeal focus.** An infection near the arachnoid layer—but not invading it—may produce inflammation in the cerebrospinal fluid (CSF) (e.g., spinal epidural abscess or intracranial abscess) despite persistently negative CSF cultures.

B. Acute bacterial meningitis
   1. *Streptococcus pneumoniae* is the most common cause of meningitis in adults.
   2. *Neisseria meningitidis* infection may be epidemic or sporadic and is rare in adults older than 50 years.
   3. *Haemophilus influenzae* infection, previously common in children younger than 6 years, has been significantly reduced by the *H. influenzae* vaccine.

4. *Listeria monocytogenes* infection is most often seen in infants, the elderly, the debilitated, alcoholics, and patients who are immunosuppressed.

5. *Staphylococcus aureus, Staphylococcus epidermidis,* and **gram-negative bacilli.** Infections with these organisms may occur following neurosurgical procedures, head trauma, or shunt infections. Left-sided endocarditis should always be considered when the infecting organism is *S. aureus.*

C. **Chronic meningitis**

1. **Fungal infections,** including *Coccidioides immitis* and *Cryptococcus neoformans* infections, are especially common causes of chronic meningitis. More virulent fungi and acute presentations may be seen in immunocompromised patients.

2. **Mycobacterial infections.** *Mycobacterium tuberculosis* is the most common mycobacterial cause of chronic meningitis.

3. **Spirochetal infections.** *Treponema pallidum* and *Borrelia burgdorferi,* the causes of syphilis and Lyme disease, respectively, may cause aseptic or chronic meningitis.

III CLINICAL MANIFESTATIONS OF INFECTIOUS MENINGITIS

A. **Fever** and **headache** should always raise the suspicion of meningitis.

B. **Neck stiffness,** positive **Kernig's** and **Brudzinski's signs,** and **photosensitivity** are also common findings, but are less likely with certain infections (e.g., cryptococcal meningitis).

C. **Altered mental status** (rare in aseptic meningitis), **focal neurologic abnormalities, seizures,** and **evidence of increased intracranial pressure** (e.g., papilledema) may all be seen.

D. **Signs related to the causative organism** may be present. For example, a petechial or purpuric rash caused by meningococcus infection is present in approximately 50% of patients with meningococcal meningitis.

HOT KEY

Infants, the elderly, and immunosuppressed patients may not generate a high fever or signs of meningismus. The sensitivities of neck stiffness and the other findings are not high enough to rule out meningitis clinically; therefore, all patients with a fever and altered mental status, and many patients with a fever and a headache, require further evaluation.

IV APPROACH TO THE PATIENT

A. **Patient history.** The time course of the patient's illness may provide a clue as to the type of meningitis; however, a lumbar puncture is always necessary.

1. **Aseptic meningitis** often presents acutely after a "flu-like" prodrome. More than 90% of patients are younger than 30 years.

2. **Acute bacterial meningitis** presents acutely (usually within hours to days) and typically with symptoms that are more severe than in **patients with aseptic meningitis.**

3. **Chronic** meningitis usually is more indolent; symptoms may not appear for days to weeks.

B. **Blood cultures** and **empiric therapy.** If acute meningitis is suspected, draw two sets of blood cultures and start empiric therapy with antibiotics (and possibly steroids) immediately (see V); the yield on Gram stain and culture of the CSF will probably not change within 4 hours of starting therapy. Blood cultures are positive in approximately 50% of patients with bacterial meningitis and should always be obtained because they may be diagnostic in patients with a negative CSF culture.

C. **Lumbar puncture** and **CSF fluid analysis.** Acute bacterial meningitis often cannot be distinguished from more benign processes (e.g., aseptic meningitis, common viral syndromes) on the basis of clinical criteria alone; therefore, a lumbar puncture should be performed whenever meningitis is a consideration.

1. **Lumbar puncture**

a. **Contraindications.** A lumbar puncture can usually be done safely in the presence of normal mental status and a nonfocal neurologic exam with no evidence of increased intracerebral pressure (e.g., papilledema). If there is evidence of altered mental status, a focal neurologic examination, or increased intracerebral pressure, empiric therapy should be initiated and a computed tomography (CT) scan obtained before lumbar puncture.

b. **Procedure**

(1) **Premedicate the patient.** Premedicating with low doses of a benzodiazepine (e.g., lorazepam; 0.5–2 mg intravenously) and morphine sulfate (e.g., 2–4 mg) often lessens the pain and anxiety associated with lumbar puncture. These agents should be avoided in patients with altered mental status.

(2) **Measure the opening pressure.** Opening pressure elevations are nonspecific, but significant elevations are common with acute bacterial meningitis. Normal or minimal elevations predominate in aseptic meningitis.

(3) **Draw four samples.** You will usually have four tubes.

(a) A **cell count** is usually performed on the CSF sample in tubes 1 and 4. If the last tube has a significantly decreased number of red blood cells (RBCs) in comparison to the first tube, a traumatic tap may be more likely than a true disease process (e.g., subarachnoid hemorrhage, herpes encephalitis).

   (b) Protein and **glucose levels** are often obtained from the sample sent in tube 1 or tube 4.

   (c) Gram staining and **culture.** The CSF sample in tube 2 is usually used for Gram staining and culture. Only a small amount of CSF (e.g., 1 ml) is required.

   (d) Cryptococcal antigen (CRAG) titer, an **India ink preparation,** and **fungal culture** can also be performed on the tube 2 sample in human immunodeficiency virus (HIV)-positive or immunocompromised patients; however, a serum CRAG is more sensitive than a CSF CRAG.

   (e) Other studies may be needed. Tube 3 is often filled and refrigerated pending the results of the standard tests.

2. CSF analysis

   a. Cell count. The normal cell count is 0–5 lymphocytes/μl. If pleocytosis is found, the predominant cell type helps to prioritize the differential diagnoses.

   (1) Neutrophilic [polymorphonuclear neutrophil (PMN)] pleocytosis

   (a) The patient should be considered to have **acute bacterial meningitis** until proven otherwise.

   (b) Early viral infections can also be neutrophil predominant, but the worst should always be assumed first.

   (c) PMN counts greater than 50,000 cells/μl should alert you to a possible **brain abscess with rupture into a ventricle.**

   (2) Lymphocytic pleocytosis. An elevated lymphocyte count can occur with **all three categories of infectious meningitis** (i.e., the ABCs) as well as with **other processes.**

   (a) ABCs. Aseptic and chronic meningitis typically have a lymphocytic predominance. Certain types of bacterial infections (e.g., early or partially treated bacterial meningitis, brain abscesses, parameningeal infections) may also cause lymphocytic pleocytosis.

   (b) Other causes. These patients will probably need "2 ICE" cubes to help their headaches (see mnemonic next page).

   b. Protein level. The normal protein level in adults is 15–45 mg/dl. Approximately 90% of patients with acute bacter-

Other Causes of Lymphocytic Meningitis ("2 ICE")

Infections (malaria, toxoplasmosis, fresh water amebiasis,
    cysticercosis, Rocky Mountain spotted fever)
Intoxications (salicylates, barbiturates, heavy metals)
Cancer (carcinomatous meningitis)
Collagen vascular disease [systemic lupus erythematosus
    (SLE)]
Endocrine disorder (pheochromocytoma)
Endocarditis

ial meningitis have an elevated CSF protein level, whereas
patients with aseptic meningitis often have a normal or
minimally elevated protein level.

  c. Glucose level. The normal glucose level is 45–85 mg/dl.
The CSF glucose may vary with the serum glucose.

    (1) The ratio of CSF to serum glucose is less than 0.4 (as-
suming that the serum glucose level is less than 250
mg/dl) in most patients with acute bacterial meningitis, but is normal (greater than 0.4) in patients with
aseptic meningitis.

    (2) Carcinomatous, fungal, and tuberculous meningitis
are other common causes of depressed CSF glucose.

  d. Gram stain and **culture**

    (1) Gram stain. The Gram stain is positive in the major-
ity of cases of untreated acute bacterial meningitis.
(*L. monocytogenes,* however, is notorious for not being identified.)

    (2) Culture. The CSF culture is positive in most cases of
bacterial meningitis.

D. Ancillary tests

  1. Patients with neutrophilic pleocytosis (i.e., a high probability of bacterial meningitis)

    a. Latex agglutination tests for bacterial antigen can be done on
patients who may have a partially treated culture-negative
bacterial meningitis.

    b. Head CT scan or **magnetic resonance imaging (MRI).**
Acute bacterial meningitis may be caused by direct extension from sinusitis, otitis, or mastoiditis. An imaging
study is necessary if extension is suspected.

  2. Patients with lymphocytic pleocytosis. By considering the
possible causes of a lymphocytic pleocytosis (i.e., the ABCs
and the 2 ICE cubes) and the clinical setting, you can determine which diagnostic tests may be useful.

    a. ABCs

      (1) Aseptic meningitis. Mumps virus, herpes simplex

virus, varicella-zoster virus, and CMV can be recovered from the CSF, and a Monospot test can be done for Epstein-Barr virus, but in most cases, the viral agent is not recovered. A **Venereal Disease Research Laboratory (VDRL) test** should always be sent and **Lyme titers, and PCR for HSV** are also a consideration in cases of suspected aseptic meningitis.

    (2) Bacterial meningitis. Acute bacterial infection resulting from a parameningeal focus is a possibility and, depending on the presentation, a **CT scan** or **MRI** may be considered.

    (3) Chronic meningitis. *M. tuberculosis* infection or fungal infection are possible etiologies. Commonly ordered tests include a **purified protein derivative (PPD) test,** a **CSF acid-fast bacillus stain** and **culture, CSF** and **serum CRAG titers,** and *Coccidioides* **serology** (other fungal serologies and cultures may also be ordered).

        (a) Multiple CSF samples increase the yield on acid-fast bacillus staining and culture, but the culture may still be negative in up to 25% of patients with tuberculous meningitis. A PCR-based test for tuberculosis (TB) is under investigation.

        (b) A history of TB, active TB, or basilar meningitis on MRI may support the diagnosis of tuberculous meningitis.

  b. Other causes. CSF cytology is frequently sent when carcinomatous meningitis is a consideration. Multiple (often three) CSF samples are needed to increase the yield.

V **TREATMENT.** Medication doses are given for **adults** with **normal renal** function.

A. Empiric antibacterial therapy for acute bacterial meningitis is critical.

  1. No penicillin allergy

    a. Ceftriaxone (often 2 g intravenously every 12 hours) or cefotaxime (2 g intravenously every 4 hours) is the best choice because these drugs cover gram-negative organisms (including *H. influenzae*) as well as the emerging penicillin-resistant **S. pneumoniae.**

    b. Ampicillin (12–18 g/day in divided doses) or **penicillin G** (18–24 million units intravenously/day divided or with continuous therapy) should be **added** in patients with epidemiologic risk factors for *L. monocytogenes* (immunocompromised, older than 50 years).

    c. Acyclovir should be added for cases suspicious for HSV (while awaiting results of HSV PCR).

    d. Vancomycin should be added to cover *S. aureus* in cases involving head trauma, recent neurosurgery, or manipulation of a CSF shunt. Vancomycin may also be needed if the local prevalence of drug-resistant *S. pneumococcus* is high.

    e. Fungal coverage should be considered in any immuno-compromised patient.

2. Penicillin allergy

    a. In patients who are allergic to penicillin and have a history of anaphylaxis, **chloramphenicol** may be used. Chloramphenicol is also effective against Listeria.

    b. If the patient is allergic to penicillin but has no history of anaphylaxis, ceftriaxone or cefotaxime may be tried. **Trimethoprim/sulfamethoxazole (TMP/SMX)** can be added if Listeria infection is a possibility.

B. Steroids may be given in the following situations:

    1. To decrease the incidence of deafness in children with *H. influenzae* infection.

    2. In most cases of adult bacterial meningitis.

    3. In some cases of tuberculous meningitis of moderate severity.

 PREVENTION. Rifampin prophylaxis (600 mg orally twice daily for 2 days for adults) is appropriate for close contacts of a patient with meningococcal meningitis. Household and daycare center contacts and hospital workers with intense exposure should all be given prophylaxis.

References

Aronin SI, Quagliarello VJ. New perspectives on pneumococcal meningitis. Hosp Pract (Off Ed) 2001;36(2):43–46, 49–50, 51.

de Gans J, van de Beek D. Dexamethasone in adults with bacterial meningitis. N Engl J Med 2002;347:1549–56.

Hussein AS, Shafran SD. Acute bacterial meningitis in adults: a 12-year review. Medicine 2000;79(6):360–368.

Roos KL. Pearls and pitfalls in the diagnosis and management of central nervous system infectious diseases. Semin Neurol 1998;18(2):185–196.

89. Spinal Cord Compression

I **INTRODUCTION.** Spinal cord compression is a true medical emergency that requires prompt intervention. The clinical diagnosis of cord compression may be difficult because early symptoms are often attributed to more common processes. Furthermore, the characteristic symptoms often occur too late to prevent irreversible damage. Clinical suspicion is therefore paramount.

II **CAUSES OF SPINAL CORD COMPRESSION**

A. **Malignancy,** most often from **metastatic disease,** is by far the most common cause of spinal cord compression. Consistent with the number of each type of vertebrae, the thoracic vertebrae are most often involved, followed by approximately equal involvement of the cervical and lumbosacral vertebrae.
   1. If you remember the cancers that involve the bone—breast, lung, thyroid, kidney, prostate, and multiple myeloma—you will remember the most common causes of spinal cord compression (see also Chapter 73). **Breast, lung,** and **prostate cancer** account for most cases of cord compression.
   2. Lymphomas, primary spinal tumors (i.e., meningiomas, neurofibromas), and many other malignancies can also cause spinal cord compression.
B. **Infections.** Epidural abscesses and osteomyelitis (e.g., from bacteria or tuberculosis) occasionally lead to cord compression.
C. **Herniated discs** that are large and central in location occasionally result in cord compression.
D. **Epidural hemorrhage** may occur spontaneously or result from arteriovenous malformations, trauma, anticoagulation therapy, or underlying tumors, resulting in cord compression.
E. **Rheumatologic disorders.** Arthritis (especially rheumatoid arthritis) with cervical involvement can result in cord compression from relatively minor trauma (e.g., whiplash or intubation). Ankylosing spondylitis may result in lumbar cord compression.

III **CLINICAL MANIFESTATIONS OF SPINAL CORD COMPRESSION**

A. **Back pain** is the most common symptom and is present in at least 80% of patients. The quality of the pain is variable and nonspecific and does not usually allow spinal cord compression to be distinguished from more benign disorders. **Point tenderness** over the involved vertebrae is common in spinal cord compression and should raise a red flag.

B. Neurologic findings are infrequent initially but become more prominent with time.

1. **Decreased sensation** and/or **weakness in the lower extremities,** a **sensory level, saddle anesthesia,** and **hyperreflexia** may all be found.

2. **Bladder** and **bowel dysfunction** may occur late in the course of disease. Urinary retention with overflow incontinence and constipation are often seen.

IV APPROACH TO THE PATIENT. Diagnosis depends on imaging studies.

A. Modalities

1. **Magnetic resonance imaging (MRI)** is extremely sensitive and noninvasive and is therefore the first choice. The entire cord needs to be evaluated because multiple skip lesions are often present.

2. **Computed tomography (CT)** with a **myelogram** can be used when MRI is not available or contraindicated.

3. **Radiographs** and **bone scans** are of little value in the diagnosis of cord compression (although they may be a useful initial screen in patients presenting only with back pain). Radiographs are not sensitive enough to detect vertebral metastases, and neither test evaluates the spinal cord itself.

B. Indications

1. **Absolute indications.** The following patients usually require testing:

   a. **All patients with a known cancer** accompanied by symptoms or signs of possible cord compression (e.g., back pain)

   b. **Patients with acute radiculopathy** accompanied by urinary retention, saddle anesthesia, or bilateral neurologic findings

2. **Risk stratification.** In the remaining patients who present with back pain, you can perform a simple risk stratification to assess the likelihood of possible cord compression and the appropriateness of imaging studies.

   a. **Simple back pain.** Patients with back pain who are younger than 50 years, without a history of cancer or weight loss, and with no evidence of sciatica or neurologic deficit have musculoskeletal pain approximately 99% of the time. Usually, no tests are performed, and conservative therapy is recommended.

b. Back pain with risk factors. Risk factors include pain worse at rest, history of or suspected malignancy, history of chronic infection, history of trauma, age older than 50, pain lasting for more than 1 month, history of intravenous drug use, steroid use, rapidly progressive neurologic deficit, unexplained fever or weight loss, or spine percussion tenderness. These patients have a higher incidence of an underlying malignancy or infectious process and are often initially evaluated with plain radiographs, complete blood count (CBC), and an erythrocyte sedimentation rate (ESR). If these test results are abnormal or if conservative therapy has failed, additional diagnostic testing to rule out serious causes of back pain is usually indicated.

HOT KEY

If spinal cord compression is a possibility, then imaging studies need to be performed immediately. Patients with stable symptoms may be evaluated on a less acute basis.

V TREATMENT

A. Steroids. High-dose **dexamethasone** (often 10–100 mg via an intravenous bolus) followed by 4–6 mg every 6 hours (intravenously or orally) is often administered. If cord compression is suspected, do not wait for the MRI results before initiating treatment. There is usually little harm in one dose of steroids if your clinical diagnosis proves incorrect.

B. Radiation therapy should be initiated once the diagnosis is made. Early steroid treatment is also useful in decreasing the swelling associated with radiation therapy.

C. Ketoconazole administered intravenously can reduce malignant prostatic metastases acutely; therefore, it is sometimes used in patients who have known prostate cancer associated with cord compression.

D. Chemotherapy alone is sometimes effective in patients with extremely chemosensitive tumors (e.g., small cell lung cancer, lymphoma).

E. Emergency surgery. Early consultation with a neurosurgeon is very helpful. **Surgery** for cord compression is usually indicated:
1. With rapidly progressive neurologic deficits
2. When radiation therapy is failing
3. For radio-insensitive tumors
4. When the etiology is unclear

References

Abrahm JL. Management of pain and spinal cord compression in patients with advanced cancer. ACP-ASIM End-of-life Care Consensus Panel. American College of Physicians-American Society of Internal Medicine. Ann Intern Med 1999;131 (1):37–46.

Deyo RA, Weinstein JN. Low back pain. N Engl J Med 2001;344(5):363–370.

Kirshblum SC, Groah SL, McKinley WO, Gittler MS, Stiens SA. Spinal cord injury medicine. 1. Etiology, classification, and acute medical management. Arch Phys Med Rehabil 2002;83(3 Suppl 1):S50-S57, S90-S98.

PART XI

DERMATOLOGY

90. Exanthems

INTRODUCTION

A. A vascular lesion is caused by congestion within the blood vessel and therefore usually blanches with pressure. The term **erythematous** implies that the lesion **blanches.**

> **HOT** The best way to determine blanchability is to place a glass microscope slide (or another transparent object) onto the lesion while applying pressure. You will be able to tell quickly whether
> **KEY** the lesion blanches.

B. A **purpuric lesion,** on the other hand, is caused by the escape of blood into the perivascular tissue. Purpuric lesions **do not blanch with pressure.** Purpuric lesions may be more worrisome than erythematous ones because the diseases that can cause purpura are occasionally life-threatening (e.g., meningococcemia).
  1. There are two types of purpuric lesions:
    a. Petechiae are small purpuric lesions.
    b. Ecchymoses are large purpuric lesions.
  2. When purpuric lesions become raised, they are considered **"palpable purpura"** and represent a vasculitis (see Chapter 76).
C. An **exanthem** is an **acute, generalized rash.** Exanthemas are common in hospitalized patients and in those visiting the emergency department. Most of these eruptions are benign; however, life-threatening disorders can also cause exanthemas and must be considered. Exanthemas can be **morbilliform** or **scarlatiniform** eruptions. Both morbilliform and scarlatiniform eruptions blanch.

MORBILLIFORM RASH. A morbilliform rash is an erythematous macular/papular, **nonconfluent** eruption that usually involves the torso. Morbilliform eruptions are much more common than scarlatiniform ones.

A. **Causes**
   1. **Drug reactions.** Any drug can cause a morbilliform rash; however, **penicillins** and **sulfa-containing compounds** are the most common culprits. The skin reaction is usually symmetric and involves the torso more than the appendages. In previously exposed patients, the rash appears within 3 days; in previously unexposed patients, the eruption appears 7–9 days into the course of treatment. Clinical manifestations such as fever, pruritus, lymphadenopathy, and eosinophilia are sometimes present.
   2. **Infections**
      a. **Viral infections** [e.g., **rubeola (measles), rubella, Epstein-Barr virus, echovirus, coxsackievirus, adenovirus,** and **early human immunodeficiency virus [HIV]**] are the most common infectious causes of morbilliform rashes.

HOT KEY
Viral exanthemas are usually preceded by fever and constitutional symptoms.

      b. **Bacterial** causes include **typhoid fever** and **secondary syphilis.** Early **rickettsial** and **meningococcal** disease—diseases usually associated with purpuric lesions—can initially present as morbilliform reactions and must be considered, given the mortality associated with each. **If you suspect rickettsial or meningococcal disease, begin empiric antibiotics while awaiting the definitive diagnosis** (see Chapter 50).
   3. **Acute graft versus host disease (GVHD)** is seen in allogeneic bone marrow transplant recipients when immunocompetent donor lymphocytes and macrophages are transplanted and attack the new host.
B. **Diagnosis.** If the diagnosis is unclear, skin biopsy (a safe, easy procedure) should be considered.

 SCARLATINIFORM RASH. A scarlatiniform eruption is a generalized, confluent, blanching erythema. It may be difficult to distinguish a scarlatiniform rash from a morbilliform rash, which can begin to coalesce; however, scarlatiniform eruptions are **usually confluent at the outset.**

A. Scarlet fever. Patients with a β-hemolytic streptococcal (group A) pharyngitis or tonsillitis can develop a characteristic rash caused by an erythrogenic toxin. The rash, which is confluent, papular, and sandpaper-like in texture, begins on the neck and upper chest and then spreads over the extremities and abdomen. Circumoral pallor and a strawberry tongue are characteristic; desquamation of most of the involved areas occurs in 5 days.

B. Kawasaki disease is a multisystemic disorder of unknown etiology that mainly affects children.

1. **Clinical manifestations.** Kawasaki disease is characterized by fever, conjunctivitis, mucous membrane involvement, edema, cervical lymphadenopathy, and a scarlatiniform (or sometimes a morbilliform) rash that is most prominent on the trunk.

2. **Treatment** is usually with intravenous immune globulin (IVIG) and aspirin.

3. **Complications.** Patients are at risk for coronary artery aneurysms and myocardial infarction.

H O T

KEY Kawasaki disease rarely affects adults but may occasionally occur in epidemic fashion. One theory of pathogenesis proposes that staphylococcal toxin acts as a "superantigen" that interacts with T cells.

C. Toxic shock syndrome is a life-threatening disorder caused by toxins elaborated by *Staphylococcus aureus* or group A streptococci.

1. Toxic shock syndrome is most commonly seen in tampon-using menstruating women, post-surgical patients, and in those with a site of toxin-producing staphylococcal or streptococcal infection (e.g., an abscess). **However, whenever a patient has a scarlatiniform rash, always consider toxic shock syndrome.**

2. **Clinical manifestations.** Toxic shock syndrome is characterized by **fever, hypotension,** and **multiorgan involvement:**

a. **Gastrointestinal.** Nausea, vomiting, diarrhea, elevated liver enzymes

b. **Musculoskeletal.** Myalgias, arthralgias, myositis

c. **Renal.** Acute renal failure

d. **Mucous membranes.** Nonexudative conjunctivitis, strawberry tongue

e. **Pulmonary.** Acute respiratory distress syndrome (ARDS)

f. Cutaneous. Diffuse erythematous rash that blanches very easily; desquamation occurs after 1–2 weeks

---

HOT

 The rash of toxic shock syndrome is often accentuated in the flexural folds.

KEY

References

Babu KS, Belgi G. Management of cutaneous drug reactions. Curr Allergy Asthma Rep 2002;2(1):26–33.

Sullivan JR, Shear NH. Drug eruptions and other adverse drug effects in aged skin. Clin Geriatr Med 2002;18(1):21–42.

Issa NC, Thompson RL. Staphylococcal toxic shock syndrome. Suspicion and prevention are keys to control. Postgrad Med 2001;110(4):55–56.

91. Pruritus

I **INTRODUCTION.** Itching can be caused by a variety of dermatologic and nondermatologic disorders.

A. Dermatologic disorders. Itching is a very common symptom of dermatologic disorders. Skin lesions are usually present when a dermatologic disorder is the cause of the itching.

B. Systemic disorders. When no skin lesions are present, the itching is often caused by a systemic disorder. Approximately 15% of patients with itching but without skin lesions have a systemic disorder diagnosed at initial presentation.

II **CAUSES OF PRURITUS**

A. Dermatologic disorders
1. **Xerosis (dry skin)** is a very common cause.
2. **Parasitic infestation** (e.g., scabies, pediculosis) and **insect bites** cause pruritus.
3. Other causes include **urticaria, atopic** or **contact dermatitis, superficial fungal infections, drug reactions, sunburn, dermatitis herpetiformis, fiberglass dermatitis, lichen planus,** and **folliculitis.**

B. Systemic disorders
1. **Uremia** is the most common cause of pruritus when lesions are not present.
2. **Primary biliary cirrhosis, extrahepatic biliary obstruction,** and **cholestatic drugs** cause **total bilirubin elevation,** bile salt retention, and pruritus.
3. **Cancer.** Neoplasms that can cause pruritus include lymphoma (especially **Hodgkin's disease**) and **breast, lung,** and **stomach cancer.**
4. **Hematologic disorders. Polycythemia vera** (and the other myeloproliferative disorders) and **iron deficiency anemia** can cause pruritus.
5. **Endocrine disorders** (e.g., diabetes mellitus, hyperthyroidism and hypothyroidism, carcinoid syndrome) can cause pruritus.

III **APPROACH TO THE PATIENT**

A. Patient history. A detailed history focusing on medications, other medical conditions, travel, hobbies, occupation, and the

Most Common Causes of Pruritus ("ITCHED")

Infestation (e.g., scabies)
Total bilirubin elevation (e.g., primary biliary cirrhosis)
Chronic renal failure (uremia) or **C**ancer
Hematologic disorders
Endocrine disorders
Dermatologic disorders

presence of constitutional symptoms (e.g., weight loss, fever) is very useful.
  1. The itching associated with **Hodgkin's disease** is often described as a "burning" sensation, especially on the lower extremities.
  2. Patients with **scabies** usually describe worsening of their pruritus at night.
  3. **Polycythemia vera** is often associated with a "prickly" itch that usually occurs as the patient cools off after bathing.
  4. **Xerosis** is common in the elderly, especially when the heater is turned on during the winter months.
B. Physical examination
  1. A thorough dermatologic examination, focusing on the presence of burrows (due to scabies), plate-like scaling (due to xerosis), and other lesions that will aid in the diagnosis should be performed.
  2. If no obvious skin cause is found, examination of the abdomen (to look for hepatosplenomegaly) and the peripheral lymph nodes is necessary.
C. Diagnostic tests. If the history and physical examination fail to reveal the likely cause of the patient's pruritus, then blood tests [e.g., a **complete blood count** (CBC) with platelets, **alkaline phosphatase, thyroid-stimulating hormone** (TSH), and **creatinine** levels] and a **chest radiograph** should be considered. Biopsy of the skin should also be considered for patients with persistent symptoms without an obvious cause.

 TREATMENT of the specific cause is, of course, the optimal management.

A. Discontinue medications, if possible, that may cause the release of histamine (e.g., opiates, nonsteroidal anti-inflammatory drugs).
B. Consider antihistamines. Hydroxyzine (25–50 mg orally every 4–6 hours) or loratadine (10 mg orally daily) may provide symptomatic relief.

C. If the cause of the pruritus is not evident, try **empirically treating for xerosis** with a 2-week course of emollients (e.g., Aquaphor) and the use of a mild soap (e.g., Dove).

References

Braun M, Lowitt MH. Pruritus. Adv Dermatol 2001;17:1–27.

Jones EA, Bergasa NV. Evolving concepts of the pathogenesis and treatment of the pruritus of cholestasis. Can J Gastroenterol 2000;14(1):33–40.

Urbonas A, Schwartz RA, Szepietowski JC. Uremic pruritus—an update. Am J Nephrol 2001;21(5):343–350.

92. Clubbing

I **INTRODUCTION.** A curious relationship exists between certain systemic disorders and the shape of the fingertips: some diseases cause the tips of the phalanges to become enlarged, or "clubbed."

A. **Clubbing** is a bulbous enlargement of the connective tissue in the distal phalanges of the fingers and toes.

B. **Hypertrophic osteoarthropathy** is a more advanced stage of clubbing that is characterized by:
1. Periosteal new bone formation (especially of the long bones)
2. Symmetric arthritis-like changes in various joints
3. Neurovascular changes of the hands and feet (leading to paresthesias, erythema, or sweating)

II **CLINICAL MANIFESTATIONS OF CLUBBING**

A. The **thumb** and **index finger** are typically affected first.

B. Clubbing is **usually symmetrical;** however, it may be unilateral in certain vascular disorders (e.g., aortic arch anomalies, subclavian artery aneurysms, patent ductus arteriosus).

C. Clubbing is usually a **gradual, painless process;** however, some patients will complain of a **dull aching** in the fingertips. In general, there are **three stages** in clubbing:
1. During the initial stage, the most difficult stage to appreciate, the nail bed becomes spongy.

HOT KEY

The best way to assess whether a patient's nail bed is spongy is to compare it with your own nail of the same finger.

2. During the next stage, the angle made by the nail and the dorsum of the distal phalanx increases (when viewed from the side). Normally, this angle is less than 180°, but in patients with clubbed fingers, the angle exceeds 180°. **Schamroth's sign** can be helpful in confirming this increased angle. In patients without clubbing, when the dorsal surfaces of distal digits of similar fingers are placed together, a diamond-shaped opening appears at the bases of the nails. Schamroth noted that in patients who have mild clubbing, this opening is obliterated.

3. During the final stage, the overall shape of the digit is visibly altered.

III COMMON CAUSES OF CLUBBING

A. **Acquired**
1. **Pulmonary disease.** Approximately 75% of patients with acquired clubbing have pulmonary disease.
   a. **Lung abscess**
   b. **Bronchiectasis**
   c. **Cancer** (usually primary lung cancer)
2. **Cardiac disease.** Approximately 10% of patients with acquired clubbing have cardiac disease.
   a. **Congenital cyanotic heart disease**
   b. **Subacute bacterial endocarditis**
3. **Gastrointestinal disease.** Approximately 10% of patients with acquired clubbing have gastrointestinal disease.
   a. **Inflammatory bowel disease**
   b. **Cirrhosis**
   c. **Colon** or **esophageal cancer**
4. **Miscellaneous causes**
   a. **Hyperthyroidism**
   b. **Hemoglobinopathies**
   c. **Local vascular diseases** (leading to unilateral clubbing)
B. **Hereditary.** Clubbing caused by hereditary factors is indistinguishable morphologically from clubbing caused by acquired disease. However, hereditary clubbing generally **develops during childhood** and persists for life. There is usually a family history of clubbing.

IV APPROACH TO THE PATIENT. For patients with **acquired clubbing,** an exhaustive search for the underlying causes is unnecessary; however, looking for potentially treatable and reversible diseases is worthwhile. If the patient gives a history compatible with hereditary clubbing, no further evaluation is usually necessary.

A. **Patient history.** The history should focus on eliciting information about pulmonary symptoms, constitutional symptoms (e.g., fever, weight loss, night sweats), signs (e.g., bloody diarrhea, jaundice, nervousness, tremulousness), alcohol and tobacco use, and family history.
B. **Physical examination.** The examination should be focused on finding evidence of pulmonary, cardiac, gastrointestinal, or thyroid disease.
C. **Diagnostic tests.** A complete blood count (CBC), a chest radiograph, an electrocardiogram (ECG), blood gas analysis, serum

thyroid-stimulating hormone (TSH) levels, and stool samples (to search for occult blood) may be useful. Additional tests may also be necessary.

 TREATMENT usually entails treatment of the underlying cause and pain relief with nonsteroidal anti-inflammatory medications if necessary.

References

Martinez-Lavin M. Hypertrophic osteoarthropathy. Curr Opin Rheumatol 1997;9(1): 83–86.

Myers KA, Farquhar DR. The rational clinical examination. Does this patient have clubbing?. JAMA 2001;286(3):341–347.

PART XII

TOXICOLOGY

93. Alcohol Intoxication and Withdrawal

I **INTRODUCTION.** Alcohol use is important to consider in hospitalized patients for many reasons:

A. Although modest alcohol intake (i.e., up to one 14-g drink daily) may have cardioprotective effects, heavier use contributes to multiple medical conditions including hypertension, cardiac arrhythmias, stroke, gastritis, pancreatitis, cirrhosis, and nutritional deficiency.

B. Alcohol has a potent immunosuppressive effect. Its use increases the frequency and mortality of infectious diseases such as bacterial pneumonia.

C. Patients with severe withdrawal (delirium tremens) are at a significant risk of death if not treated properly.

II **ALCOHOL INTOXICATION.** Tolerance occurs with chronic alcohol consumption. Thus, higher serum alcohol levels are needed to cause intoxication in long-term, heavy drinkers compared with first-time drinkers.

A. Clinical manifestations of alcohol intoxication. Alcohol is a central nervous system (CNS) depressant. Alcohol intoxication results in a wide variety of responses that may include slurred speech, euphoria, disinhibition, uncontrolled mood swings, violence, nausea, ataxia, stupor, altered mental status, and respiratory depression.

B. Approach to the patient

1. Supportive care. The clinical approach depends on the degree of CNS and respiratory depression. Supportive care may mean as little as observation until the patient is clinically sober or as much as intubation in a comatose patient. The cervical spine should be protected if there is any history of trauma.

Physical restraints should be used cautiously and only with frequent re-evaluation. Chemical restraints may worsen respiratory depression.

2. **Glucose.** Alcohol use without glucose intake may result in hypoglycemia. Rapid blood glucose assessment should be undertaken in all acutely intoxicated patients.

3. A **blood alcohol level** (BAL) of 500 mg/dl is fatal to 50% of adults. Tolerant individuals may, however, present with significantly higher levels. An altered mental status with a low alcohol level or one that fails to improve with time should prompt further evaluation, which may include a head computed tomography (CT) scan, lumbar puncture, or further toxicologic assessment (see Chapter 82).

4. A toxic alcohol ingestion (e.g., methanol or ethylene glycol) should always be considered if an anion gap acidosis (see Chapter 42) is accompanied by an osmolar gap.

5. Patients with isolated alcohol intoxication typically do not require admission to the hospital unless they have a comorbid condition or develop concerning signs of withdrawal.

III ALCOHOL WITHDRAWAL

A. **Pathogenesis.** Alcoholics may drink continually to avoid the discomfort of alcohol withdrawal. As physiologic tolerance develops, more alcohol is needed to avoid withdrawal. When something occurs to keep the alcoholic from drinking, such as an illness or hospitalization, withdrawal may develop.

B. **Clinical manifestations of alcohol withdrawal.** As the blood alcohol level decreases, symptoms and signs develop that are generally opposite in nature to the primary CNS depressant effects of the drug (i.e., generalized CNS arousal and hyperactivity). Withdrawal may begin while the BAL is still above zero. There are **four alcohol withdrawal syndromes** that may have differing time courses and clinical manifestations; however, substantial overlap may occur. If only one sign of withdrawal appears, consider other diagnoses.

1. **"The shakes."** Symptoms may appear within 3–12 hours of the patient's last drink. Early symptoms include jitters or shakes, an intense craving for alcohol, anxiety, weakness, diaphoresis, nausea, and myalgias. The patient is often agitated, irritable, and hypervigilant. Common signs also include tachycardia, hypertension, and a coarse tremor of the hands or tongue.

2. **Hallucinations.** Hallucinations are classically auditory, although they may also be visual (e.g., bugs crawling on the wall). Patients may become fearful or paranoid, which may

further increase agitation. Hallucinations typically occur in the first 2 days after the last drink.

3. **Seizures.** Withdrawal seizures are typically diffuse tonic-clonic seizures that peak 12–24 hours after the patient's last drink. Single seizures occur 50% of the time, with short bursts being most common when multiple seizures occur. The postictal period is often short, and status epilepticus is rare. Many alcoholics, however, have other reasons for seizing, and it is important to look for these, especially if the patient is febrile, has head trauma, has prolonged seizure activity, or if the seizures begin more than 48 hours after the last drink.

4. **Delirium tremens** is characterized by hallucinations, profound confusion, fever, and tachycardia. Typically, delirium tremens begin 2–3 days after the patient's last drink, peak on day 4, and may last 1-2 weeks.

5. **Other illnesses** to consider in the setting of the autonomic hyperactivity that defines alcohol withdrawal are sepsis, thyrotoxicosis, heat stroke, hypoglycemia, intracranial hemorrhage, and cocaine intoxication.

HOT

When managing a patient who appears to be withdrawing from alcohol, always ask yourself: is this patient septic?

KEY

C. **Approach to the patient**
   1. **Alleviate withdrawal symptoms**
      a. **Supportive measures.** Keep the patient in a quiet room. Restraining the patient may increase paranoia and agitation. Restraints should be used only when necessary. The patient's status must be monitored frequently.
      b. **Pharmacologic therapy**
         (1) **Benzodiazepines** are the drugs of choice. They act at the same receptor as alcohol, the γ-aminobutyric acid (GABA) receptor, to sedate the patient. Lorazepam (1-2 mg intravenously every 30 minutes until symptoms resolve) is the preferred agent, especially in the elderly, because of its short half-life and fast onset of action. The **barbiturate** phenobarbital is another possibility. If outpatient treatment is desired, lorazepam, diazepam, or chlordiazepoxide may be used in a tapering dose over 3 days.
         (2) β **blockers** and **central** α_2 **agonists** (e.g., clonidine) block the hypertension and tachycardia of withdrawal

but do not treat the underlying autonomic derangement and so may mask developing delirium tremens.

(3) Phenytoin should be used only to treat seizures not entirely attributable to alcohol.

2. **Correct metabolic deficiencies**

   a. **Fluid deficit** should be replaced initially with normal saline, with appropriate adjustment in volume for renal insufficiency or heart failure.

   b. **Thiamine** (100 mg intravenously) and other **vitamins** should be administered before infusing glucose to prevent the development of Wernicke's encephalopathy.

   c. **Glucose** may be infused as 50% dextrose or as part of the intravenous fluid rehydration (D5 normal saline), or as a good meal.

   d. **Potassium, magnesium,** and **phosphorus** should be replaced if serum levels are low.

   e. **Vitamin K** is administered if the prothrombin time (PT) is prolonged.

3. **Manage associated medical conditions.** Perform a complete history and physical examination to look for associated medical conditions and to rule out other causes of altered mental status. A head CT, chest radiograph, and lumbar puncture are often necessary in patients with fever, persistent altered mental status, seizures, or abnormal neurologic examination findings.

4. **Attempt rehabilitation.** The patient should be referred to an alcohol rehabilitation center, Alcoholics Anonymous, or an outpatient mental health center.

IV **ALCOHOLISM.** Alcohol plays a roll in 100,000 deaths and costs the U.S. economy approximately $170 billion annually. Every $1 invested in treatment saves an estimated $7. Men at risk for alcohol abuse are defined as individuals consuming 14 drinks/week or 4 drinks/occasion. Women at risk are those consuming 7 drinks/week or 3/occasion.

A. **Detection.** Screening recommendations include asking patients about whether they drink beer, wine, liquor, or distilled spirits. The CAGE questions—In the last 12 months, have you ever felt that you should *c*ut down on your drinking? Have people ever *a*nnoyed you by criticizing your drinking? Have you ever felt bad or *g*uilty about your drinking? Have you ever had a drink first thing in the morning to steady your nerves or get rid of a hangover (an *e*ye-opener)?—have a sensitivity of 75% and specificity of 88% for at-risk drinkers when one or more responses are positive for women and two or more are positive for men.

B. Approach to the patient
  1. Brief negotiated interview (BNI). The BNI is a short method by which the practitioner attempts to facilitate awareness and change in the drinker. The process consists of **five steps.**
    a. Establish rapport with the patient.
    b. Ask the patient's permission and then discuss the pros and cons of alcohol use.
    c. Summarize what the patient has said.
    d. Ask the patient to describe (e.g., from 1 to 10) his or her readiness to change.
    e. Negotiate with the patient based on the perception of readiness. If the patient is ready, approaches to quitting might be brainstormed; if the patient is unsure, then pros and cons might be further explored.
  2. Medications used in alcohol treatment include disulfiram, which promotes vomiting when ingested before drinking alcohol, and naltrexone, which curbs the urge to drink.
  3. In all cases, the patient should be provided a list of **resources and referrals.** If the patient is ready to accept referral, a hospital staff member may be able to assist in arranging an appointment or entry into a treatment program.

V. ALCOHOLIC KETOACIDOSIS (AKA)

A. Pathogenesis. AKA typically occurs after a period of heavy drinking associated with "relative starvation" when vomiting or limited food intake has reduced the amount of glucose available to drive the Krebs cycle.
B. Clinical manifestations. No physical findings point definitively to AKA. Most commonly, patients complain of nausea, vomiting, and abdominal pain and are found to be tachycardic, tachypneic, and with mild, diffuse abdominal tenderness. An **increased anion gap** must be present to diagnose AKA. Other simultaneous conditions such as fever or contraction alkalosis may produce a mixed acid-base disorder and thus may mask acidosis. Testing for **ketosis** may be of limited value as β-hydroxybutyrate, which the most common tests do not demonstrate, is far more abundant than acetoacetate. **Blood glucose** is often slightly elevated but less than 300 mg/dl.
C. Approach to the patient
  1. Fluid rehydration and glucose administration. Patients typically are not hyperosmolar, and fluid resuscitation can be undertaken with less concern for cerebral edema than exists with diabetic ketoacidosis.
  2. Vitamin repletion. Thiamine (100 mg) should be given before glucose-containing fluids. A multivitamin, magnesium, or phosphorous may be indicated.

3. Search for concurrent illness. The development of AKA may be associated with an underlying illness that led the patient to stop drinking. Pancreatitis, gastrointestinal bleeding, withdrawal, and infection should all be considered.

References

Nelson S, Kolls JK. Alcohol, host defense and society. Nat Rev Immunol 2002;2:205-209.

Olmedo R, Hoffman RS. Withdrawal syndromes. Emerg Med Clin North Am 2000; 18:273-288.

www.niaaa.nih.gov. The National Institutes of Health, National Institute on Alcohol Abuse and Alcoholism.

94. Toxicologic Emergencies

I **INTRODUCTION.** Drug overdose is common in medical practice and, if not managed expediently and appropriately, can be lethal. More than 2,000,000 cases of poisoning were reported to U.S. poison control centers in 1999, accounting for more than 775 deaths. Analgesics, antidepressants, stimulants (including many street drugs), and cardiovascular medications are the most commonly fatal.

II **GENERAL APPROACH TO THE OVERDOSE PATIENT**

A. **ABCs.** Initial attention should focus on airway, breathing, and circulatory system management. Intravenous catheterization, supplemental oxygen, and cardiac monitoring are usually required. Serial monitoring of vital signs and respiratory and mental status allows one to follow the progress of intoxication.

B. **Patient history.** The patient history is of critical importance and should be obtained from the patient, friends, caregivers, and paramedics. Pill counts and attention to empty bottles found at the site are useful.

C. **Physical examination.** Areas of focus include the patient's vital signs with pulse oximetry, mental status, pupillary size and responsiveness, skin moisture, and bowel sounds. Table 94-1 summarizes physical examination findings for four of the major types of overdoses.

D. **Testing**
1. **Electrocardiography.** An electrocardiogram (ECG) is indicated for all patients with ingestion to rule out any potential cardiac effects of ingested drugs. Particularly notable are dysrhythmias and widening of the QRS.
2. **A chest radiograph, complete blood count (CBC), serum electrolytes, blood glucose,** and **renal panel** are useful for evaluating possible concomitant disease or toxicologic effects.
3. **Drug levels** and **toxicologic screens.** Drug-specific urine and serum analysis may be useful in the management of ingestion patients. A positive qualitative screen, which can remain positive for days and provides no quantitative information, should not be relied on to explain a change in mental status.

E. **Gut decontamination**
1. **Activated charcoal** (50 g by mouth or nasogastric tube, typically with sorbitol) is the preferred agent for limiting ab-

TABLE 94-1. Clinical Manifestations of Common Overdoses

Type of Overdose	Vital Signs	Mental Status	Pupils	Bowel Sounds
Opioid	↓ RR, ↓ BP	Varies from euphoria to obtundation	Constricted	Decreased
Adrenergic agonist (stimulant)	↑ HR, ↑ RR, ↑ BP	Hypervigilance	Dilated	Variable
Cholinergic agonist	↓↑ HR	Restless, confused	Constricted	Increased
Cholinergic antagonist*	↑↓ HR, ↑ temperature	Irritability, delusions	Dilated	Decreased

BP = blood pressure; HR = heart rate; RR = respiratory rate.
*In patients with clinical manifestations of an anticholinergic syndrome, tricyclic overdose should be considered.

sorption of acute ingestions. It works best when **given within 1 hour of ingestion.** It should never be given to a patient who cannot protect his or her airway unless that patient is intubated. Some toxins (e.g., theophylline, phenobarbital) may require multiple intermittent doses of activated charcoal.

2. **Gastric lavage** has no clear evidence supporting a clinical benefit, has concerning risks including aspiration and esophageal injury, and should only be considered within 1 hour of a massive or life-threatening ingestion.

3. **Emetics** (e.g., syrup of ipecac) are of no benefit compared with activated charcoal alone and are best **avoided.**

4. **Whole bowel irrigation** with polyethylene glycol (2 L/hr until stools run clear) may be indicated for some ingestions such as iron, lithium, or sustained-release preparations.

F. **Antidotes.** The first goal in clinical toxicology is treating the patient symptomatically, providing respiratory and cardiovascular support as needed. There are occasions, however, when an antidote may be both indicated and available (e.g., N-acetylcysteine in the setting of acetaminophen overdose, glucagon for β blocker overdose, or digoxin Fab for digoxin overdose).

III. SPECIFIC TOXIC SYNDROMES ("TOXIDROMES")

A. **Opioid receptor agonists** include **morphine** and related narcotic substances such as heroin and oxycodone. Acute toxicity can result from both clinical overdose in the hospitalized patient and from accidental overdose in the intravenous drug user.

1. **Clinical manifestations of opioid overdose.** These patients are typically lethargic and have constricted pupils. There may be needle marks or other suggestions of intravenous drug use. A memory aid for the opioid toxidrome may be derived from the street term for heroin, "DOPE."

Clinical Manifestations of Opioid Agonist Overdose ("DOPE")

Decreased respiratory drive
Obtundation
Pinpoint pupils
Euphoria

---

2. **Major concerns**
   a. **Respiratory depression** is the major clinical concern and may lead to hypoventilation, hypoxemia, and death. In the

setting of persistent hypoxemia, consider non-cardiogenic pulmonary edema. **Seizures** may occur with some opioid compounds including meperidine.

  b. Hypotension may also complicate opioid overdose.

  3. Treatment. The establishment of a patent airway and adequate ventilation are critical first steps. The opioid antagonist **naloxone** (0.2–2 mg IV repeated every 2–3 minutes if no response, up to a total dose of 10–20 mg; lasts 20–60 minutes) may produce dramatic reversal of some of the acute symptoms of opioid overdose including respiratory depression.

B. Stimulants include **cocaine** and **amphetamines** (e.g., **ecstasy, speed**).

  1. Clinical manifestations of stimulant overdose. The clinical syndrome results primarily from stimulation of adrenergic receptors, leading to tachypnea, tachycardia, vasoconstriction, and psychostimulation including hyperactivity.

  2. Major concerns include **tachycardia, hypertension,** and **vasospasm of the coronary arteries.** The last may lead to myocardial infarction even with otherwise normal coronary arteries.

  3. Treatment in the acute setting is primarily supportive.

    a. Benzodiazepines reduce agitation and often effectively treat hypertension and tachycardia. Persistent hypertension may be treated with a peripheral vasodilator such as nitroprusside.

    b. Chest pain should be treated as any acute coronary syndrome with aspirin, nitrates, and oxygen. Benzodiazepine use should be liberal, but β **blockers should be avoided** as they may generate unopposed α-adrenergic effects and actually worsen hypertension.

C. Cholinergic agonists. Organophosphate and carbamate **insecticides** inhibit acetylcholinesterase and are a common cause of a pure cholinergic syndrome. They may be ingested, inhaled, or absorbed through the skin. The resulting toxidrome is primarily seen in farm workers. The chemical warfare agents Sarin and VX work through the same mechanism.

  1. Clinical manifestations of cholinergic agonist toxicity typically begin within 1-2 hours. Sustained stimulation of acetylcholine (ACh) receptors causes muscarinic effects (nausea, vomiting, urinary incontinence, diarrhea, sweating, bradycardia), nicotinic effects (tremor, respiratory muscle paralysis), and central nervous system (CNS) effects (agitation to seizure or coma). Many of the important features can be remembered using the mnemonic "SLUDGE" (see next page).

  2. Major concerns include **respiratory muscle paralysis** with subsequent **hypoxemia, bronchospasm, seizures,** and **hypotension** secondary to **dehydration.**

Clinical Manifestations of Cholinergic Agonist Toxicity ("SLUDGE")

Salivation
Lacrimation
Urination
Defecation
Grimacing
Erection

3. **Treatment**
   a. **Supportive measures.** Contaminated clothing should be removed and the patient washed thoroughly with soapy water. Respiration and blood pressure should be maintained. Intubation may be needed. Benzodiazepines should be given for seizures.
   b. **Atropine,** repeated frequently, is administered to block the action of ACh at the receptor.
   c. **Pralidoxime (2-PAM)** is the specific antidote to organophosphates, reversing effects at all receptors. Ideally, it is given within 24–36 hours.
D. **Anticholinergic agents** antagonize the activity of ACh at muscarinic and CNS receptors. Many common drugs including atropine, antihistamines, phenothiazines, and tricyclic antidepressants produce anticholinergic effects. Exposure to deadly nightshade (*Atropa belladonna*) or jimsonweed may also cause toxicity.
   1. **Clinical manifestations of cholinergic antagonist toxicity** include the following:
      a. Restlessness, irritability, and delusions ("mad as a hatter")
      b. Dilation of cutaneous blood vessels ("red as a beet")
      c. Decreased apocrine and salivary gland secretion, most easily checked at the axilla ("dry as a bone")
      d. Mydriasis and cycloplegia ("blind as a bat")
      e. Tachycardia ("fast as a rabbit")
      f. Decreased gastrointestinal motility with decreased bowel sounds ("slow as a mule")
      g. Increased bladder sphincter tone ("tight as a drum")
   2. **Treatment**
      a. **Supportive treatment.** Respiratory and circulatory support may be necessary. Cardiac monitoring will provide warning of arrhythmias. Benzodiazepines can be used for agitation.
      b. **Decontamination** with activated charcoal is appropriate. Hemodialysis and hemoperfusion are not effective.

    c. Physostigmine may be used in the setting of pure anticholinergic toxicity, but it carries the risks of cardiac arrhythmias and seizures.

E. Acetaminophen is the most commonly reported drug overdose.

  1. Clinical manifestations of acetaminophen toxicity can be divided into four stages.

    a. In the first 24 hours, patients may be asymptomatic or have mild nausea and malaise.

    b. From 24–48 hours, hepatic necrosis begins and patients develop right upper quadrant pain and tenderness.

    c. Fulminant hepatic failure with coagulopathy and encephalopathy occurs by days 3–4.

    d. Recovery, if the patient survives, takes place over the ensuing week.

  2. Treatment is based on acetaminophen serum levels with the first level drawn at 4 hours.

    a. N-acetylcysteine works by replenishing glutathione, an essential component in the metabolism of acetaminophen. It is best given early but has beneficial effects out to 24 hours from ingestion, and possibly longer.

    b. Supportive care includes monitoring for coagulopathy, renal failure, and hepatic encephalopathy. These may indicate a need for liver transplantation.

    c. Activated charcoal should be given for decontamination.

F. Tricyclic antidepressants (TCAs)

  1. Clinical manifestations. TCA overdose may produce any of **three syndromes.** Symptoms often begin within 30 minutes of ingestion.

    a. Anticholinergic effects include dry skin, dilated pupils, urinary retention, tachycardia, and myoclonic jerking.

    b. Cardiovascular effects result from both TCA blockade of the myocardial fast sodium channel (similar to a type Ia antiarrhythmic) and blockade of α_1 adrenergic receptors. Effects include decreased myocardial contractility, bradycardia, and hypotension.

    c. Seizures may result in rhabdomyolysis, brain damage, and death.

  2. Approach to the patient. Rapid diagnosis is imperative and is made on the basis of the patient history, physical examination findings, and ECG findings (e.g., QRS prolongation > 100 ms, rightward shift of the terminal 40 ms of the QRS complex).

  3. Treatment

    a. Supportive measures include supporting respiration and circulation as needed.

    b. Activated charcoal should be given for gut decontamination. Hemoperfusion and hemodialysis are ineffective.

    c. Seizures should be treated with benzodiazepines.

    d. Cardiac effects as demonstrated by hypotension or QRS prolongation may be reversed through **sodium bicarbonate** infusion with a goal arterial pH of 7.45–7.55.

G. Phenothiazines include both antipsychotics (clozapine, haloperidol) and antiemetics (prochlorperazine, promethazine).

  1. Clinical manifestations of phenothiazine overdose. Like tricyclic antidepressants, phenothiazines have multiple pharmacologic effects and produce a similar clinical syndrome.

    a. At low doses, **anticholinergic effects** may predominate including dry mouth, tachycardia, and urinary retention.

    b. Cardiac effects may include QRS or QT interval prolongation.

    c. Extrapyramidal dystonic effects from dopamine receptor antagonism include torticollis, jaw muscle spasm, and oculogyric crisis. Akathisia is a condition of motor restlessness.

    d. Neuroleptic malignant syndrome (NMS) is an idiosyncratic and occasionally fatal reaction comprising lead-pipe rigidity, altered mental status, and autonomic instability including high fever, diaphoresis, and tachycardia.

  2. Treatment

    a. Supportive care includes respiratory and cardiovascular support as well as cooling of fever.

    b. Decontamination with **multiple dose activated charcoal** may be beneficial.

    c. Diphenhydramine can be used to treat dystonic reactions.

    d. Benzodiazepines can be used to treat seizures and musculoskeletal rigidity.

    e. Dantrolene, a skeletal muscle relaxant, and **bromocriptine** can be used in the management of NMS.

References

Bond GR. The role of activated charcoal and gastric emptying in gastrointestinal decontamination: a state-of-the-art review. Ann Emerg Med 2002;39:273-286.

Chu J, Wang RY, Hill NS. Update in clinical toxicology. Am J Respir Crit Care Med 2002;166:9-15.

toxnet.nlm.nih.gov. The National Library of Medicine's easily searched cluster of toxicology databases.

Appendix: Procedures

....

Procedures are an essential part of taking care of a patient. This section provides an overview of the most common procedures a clinician is likely to perform as a student or house officer. Table A-1 describes some essential steps that apply to the majority of the procedures described in this section.

▮ THORACENTESIS

A. Definition: removal of pleural fluid
B. Indications
  1. Diagnostic: to determine the etiology of a pleural effusion
  2. Therapeutic: to relieve dyspnea due to a pleural effusion
C. Contraindications: none
D. Complications: pneumothorax, hemothorax
E. Before the procedure
  1. Obtain decubitus chest radiographs to confirm that fluid is free-flowing (i.e., forms a layer along the lateral chest wall) and is not loculated.
  2. Consider ultrasound localization of the pleural fluid.
F. Patient positioning: seated at the edge of the bed, with arms resting on a bedside table
G. Locating the point of entry
  1. Identify the highest point of the effusion by percussion and move one or two interspaces below.
  2. Mark the skin at the superior aspect of the inferior rib of the interspace. Use a pen or the indentation of a needle hub.
  3. Alternatively, mark the location of the pleural effusion with ultrasound guidance.
H. Technique
  1. Clean the entry point with povidone—iodine solution.
  2. Feel the lower rib of the interspace (i.e., inferior to the mark).
  3. Anesthetize the skin at the mark with 1% lidocaine, using a 25-gauge needle.
  4. Anesthetize the subcutaneous tissue and the periosteum of the rib (superior aspect) using a 22-gauge needle. Note that the planned trajectory is above the rib, avoiding the neurovascular bundle that courses *below* the rib.
  5. Advance the needle over the rib, first withdrawing, and then injecting anesthetic if there is no return of fluid. Appearance of pleural fluid in the syringe signifies entry into

---

TABLE A-1: Essential Steps to Consider While Performing Procedures

Before the Procedure
Obtain informed consent from the patient.
Inform the nurse of the procedure and enlist his or her assistance.
Prepare all equipment. An extra set of equipment is often helpful.
Remove your pager, stethoscope, and "lab" coat.
Comfortably position yourself and the patient.
Always wash hands and observe universal precautions.
Wear a mask for all procedures.

After the Procedure
Dispose of all sharps in the sharps container.
Carry important or hard-to-obtain specimens to the laboratory
yourself.
Write a procedure note, which should include the names of the
operators (including supervisors); the procedure name and
indication; a one-line description of the technique; complications and
blood loss; and follow-up (e.g., chest radiograph pending,
specimens sent to lab). Peripheral intravenous lines and arterial
blood gas sampling generally do not require a procedure note.

---

the pleural space (i.e., between the visceral and parietal pleura).

6. Remove the needle, noting the site of insertion and trajectory.
7. Insert a 14- or 16-gauge catheter-over-needle apparatus along the same (anesthetized) path, carefully advancing over the rib.
8. Use the nondominant hand to stabilize the needle. Use the dominant hand to apply negative pressure to the syringe as you slowly advance.
9. With the return of pleural fluid into the syringe, stop advancing and withdraw 30–60 ml of fluid (for diagnostic studies). (See figure A-1.)
10. If therapeutic drainage is anticipated, advance the catheter-over-needle apparatus slightly further inward.
11. While maintaining the position of the syringe and needle with the dominant hand, use the nondominant hand to advance the catheter into the pleural space; then pull the needle out.
12. Quickly attach the end of the catheter to the extension tubing, which is then connected to vacuum drainage bottles. Alternatively, the catheter-over-needle apparatus can be attached to a three-way stopcock, initially opening

Neurovascular bundle

Pleural fluid

FIGURE A-1

To specimen collection bottle or tubes

to the syringe and then switching over to preattached extension tubing connected to vacuum drainage bottles. (See figure A-2.)

13. Once all fluid is removed, remove the catheter and quickly apply a bandage.

14. Consider performing a chest radiograph, which is recommended to rule out a pneumothorax but is not always necessary if thoracentesis has proceeded smoothly (i.e., without excessive pain or shortness of breath during fluid removal).

I. Fluid analysis (see Chapter 24)

II PARACENTESIS

A. Definition: removal of peritoneal fluid
B. Indications
    1. Diagnostic: to determine the cause of ascites, to diagnose or exclude peritonitis
    2. Therapeutic: to relieve abdominal pain or dyspnea due to ascites
C. Contraindications: surgical scar or hernia at the site of needle entry. Note that **coagulopathy is not a contraindication.**
D. Complications
    1. Bowel perforation, persistent leakage of peritoneal fluid, abdominal wall hematoma
    2. Hypotension (after large-volume paracentesis)
E. Before the procedure
    1. Have the patient empty his or her bladder; alternatively, insert a Foley catheter. (This step avoids the very rare complication of puncture of the bladder.)

FIGURE A-2

F. Patient positioning: semirecumbent

G. Locating the point of entry

1. Choose one of the following entry sites (the preferred site is not universally agreed on):
   a. At the midline, 2–3 cm below the umbilicus
   b. In either of the lower quadrants, lateral to the rectus abdominus muscle and below the level of the umbilicus (i.e., at the anterior superior iliac spine)
2. Localize the fluid by percussion or by ultrasound.
3. Mark the skin here with a pen or the indentation of a needle hub.

H. Technique

1. Clean the entry site with povidone–iodine and apply the sterile drape.
2. Anesthetize the skin at the mark with 1% lidocaine, using a 25-gauge needle.
3. Inject additional anesthetic into the subcutaneous tissue and anterior abdominal wall.
4. Keep the needle perpendicular to the skin and aspirate before each advancement, both to avoid entry into a vessel and to detect peritoneal fluid (typically straw-colored).
5. With the return of peritoneal fluid, withdraw the needle, noting the site of insertion and trajectory.
6. Choose the needle for the next puncture.
   a. For **diagnostic paracentesis:** 22-gauge 1.5-inch needle attached to a 30-ml or 60-ml syringe
   b. For **therapeutic paracentesis:** 16-gauge catheter-over-needle apparatus (or 15-gauge multihole blunt needle with removable trocar) with an attached syringe
7. For large-volume (therapeutic) paracentesis, a "Z" technique is recommended. Before insertion, pull the skin 1 inch to the side and then insert the needle. (When the procedure is completed and the needle is withdrawn, the intact skin will slide back over the hole created in the abdominal wall, preventing a persistent track that can leak.)
8. Slowly advance the needle along the same track. Aspirate after each small advancement. If there is no fluid (or blood), release negative pressure on the syringe and advance further.
9. Withdraw 30–60 ml of peritoneal fluid into the syringe (for diagnostic studies).
10. After diagnostic paracentesis, withdraw the needle and apply a bandage.
11. For therapeutic paracentesis, use the nondominant hand to stabilize the catheter position, and use the dominant hand to slowly pull back and remove the syringe and attached needle.

12. Quickly attach tubing to the end of the catheter.
13. Insert the needle attached at the other end of tubing into vacuum drainage bottles.
14. Drain up to 6 L of peritoneal fluid.
15. If fluid return decreases unexpectedly, gently manipulate the position of catheter, turn the patient, or both.
16. Once all fluid is removed, remove the catheter and apply a bandage.

I. **Fluid analysis** (see Table 32-1)

III LUMBAR PUNCTURE

A. **Definition:** removal of cerebrospinal fluid (CSF)
B. **Indications:** diagnosis of various neurologic diseases (e.g., meningitis, subarachnoid hemorrhage, tertiary syphilis)
C. **Contraindications**
   1. Infection at the site of lumbar puncture
   2. Increased intracranial pressure secondary to a mass lesion
   3. Coagulopathy or platelets < 50,000/ml
D. **Complications:** postprocedure headache, local hematoma (rare), infection (rare), tonsillar herniation (rare)
E. **Before the procedure**
   1. Rule out elevated intracranial pressure with funduscopic and neurologic examinations.
   2. If papilledema or a focal neurologic deficit is present, obtain a computed tomography (CT) scan of the brain to rule out a mass lesion.
F. **Patient positioning**
   1. Lateral decubitus position, with the neck, back, hips, and knees all maximally flexed, putting the patient into the "fetal position."
   2. Alternatively, the patient can be seated leaning over a bedstand. With this technique, opening pressure measurements are not accurate.
G. **Locating the point of entry**
   1. Find the intersection of a line formed by the spinous processes and a line formed between the superior iliac crests; this marks the L3–L4 interspace. (See figure A-3).
   2. Feel between the spinous processes for the site of entry, and mark the skin here with a pen or the indentation of a needle hub.
H. **Technique**
   1. Clean the area with povidone–iodine solution (this is often provided in the lumbar puncture tray) and then apply the sterile drape.
   2. Anesthetize the skin at the mark with 1% lidocaine, using a 25-gauge needle.

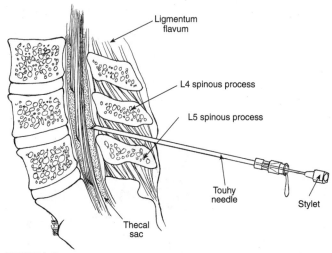

FIGURE A-3

3. Anesthetize the subcutaneous tissues with 1% lidocaine, using a 22-gauge needle, injecting in the intended track of the lumbar puncture (i.e., slightly toward the head and parallel to the midline).

4. Introduce the spinal needle (with the bevel upward, facing the ceiling) in the interspace along the same track.

5. Slowly advance the needle, frequently stopping to remove the stylet and check for the return of CSF.

6. If there is no CSF, replace the stylet and advance the needle slightly, then check again; a "pop" or giving-way is felt as the needle penetrates the dura.

7. With the return of fluid, attach the pressure manometer and measure the opening pressure. The patient must be relaxed and in the lateral decubitus position in order to obtain an accurate measurement.

8. Collect 2–3 ml in each of the four collecting tubes (see figure A-4, bottom).

9. Replace the stylet in the needle and withdraw the needle.

10. Apply a bandage over the entry site.

I. **Fluid analysis** (see Chapter 88)

IV ARTHROCENTESIS

A. Definition: removal of synovial fluid from a joint

FIGURE A-4

B. Indications
   1. Diagnostic: to determine the etiology of a joint effusion or arthritis
   2. Therapeutic: to drain large, hemorrhagic, or purulent effusions; or inject medication into a joint
C. Contraindications
   1. Infection overlying the arthrocentesis site
   2. Prosthetic joint (procedure should be performed by an orthopedic surgeon)
D. Complications: septic joint (very rare), bleeding at injection site or into joint (very rare)
E. Patient positioning (knee): supine with the knee slightly flexed; place a roll under the knee
F. Locating the point of entry (knee)
   1. Confirm the presence of an effusion (ballottable patella, lateral or medial fluid bulge around the patella).
   2. The needle will be injected midway between the top (rostral) and bottom (caudal) of the patella, just under the inferior aspect of the patella (figure A-5).
G. Technique (knee)
   1. OPTIONAL: use sterile gloves instead of standard gloves.
   2. Clean the entry point with povidone–iodine solution.
   3. OPTIONAL: anesthetize the entry site with 1% lidocaine.

FIGURE A-5

    4. Advance a 1.5-inch 18-gauge needle (attached to a 30–60-ml syringe) rapidly through the entry point, directed at the center of the joint.

    5. Apply negative pressure on the syringe as you advance the needle.

    6. Once synovial fluid enters the syringe, do not advance any further.

    7. Stabilize the position of the needle with the nondominant hand and continue to withdraw fluid by applying negative pressure on the syringe with the dominant hand.

    8. To attach another syringe to either withdraw more fluid or inject a medication, secure the position of the needle with a sterile hemostat.

        a. Remove the first syringe and carefully attach a second syringe to the needle.

        b. Inject or withdraw.

    9. Withdraw the needle and apply a bandage

H. Fluid analysis (see Table 74-1)

V CENTRAL LINE PLACEMENT (femoral line). Note that femoral vein cannulation is the easiest central venous procedure to learn and perform. More often, internal jugular and subclavian vein cannulation are preferred; however, these procedures have a higher risk with different anatomic considerations and are not outlined here.

A. Definition: catheterization of the central venous circulation via the femoral vein
B. Indications
  1. Administration of multiple intravenous medications or medications that require central venous delivery
  2. Frequent blood draws
  3. Inability to place a peripheral intravenous catheter
C. Contraindications
  1. Overlying skin infection
  2. Inability to leave a leg in the extended position
D. Complications
  1. Arterial puncture with or without local hematoma
  2. Retroperitoneal hemorrhage
  3. Infection and thrombosis of the line
E. Patient positioning: recumbent
F. Locating the point of entry
  1. Palpate the femoral pulse
  2. Locate the point of entry into the femoral vein, 2–3 cm below the inguinal ligament and 1 cm medial to the femoral arterial pulsation (figure A-6).
  3. Alternatively may use bedside ultrasonographic localization of femoral artery and vein.
G. Technique
  1. Sterilize the entry site and a wide field with chlorhexidine gluconate solution.
  2. Anesthetize the overlying skin with 1% lidocaine using a 25-gauge needle.
  3. Anesthetize the underlying subcutaneous tissue with 1% lidocaine using a 20-gauge needle.
  4. With the nondominant hand palpating the femoral artery, use the dominant hand to insert a 18-gauge needle on a syringe at a 45-degree angle aiming cephalad and slightly medially (figure A-7).
  5. While applying negative pressure to the syringe, slowly advance the needle forward until blood enters the syringe.
  6. If there is no blood return, slowly withdraw the needle, watching for a flash of blood that may occur if the vein was completely punctured on the first pass.
  7. When good blood flow is achieved, maintain the position of the needle with the nondominant hand, which is braced on the patient's skin.
  8. Lower the angle of the needle and aspirate to confirm good flow (i.e., that the needle remains in the vessel).
  9. With the position of the needle secured with the nondominant hand, remove the syringe from the needle with the dominant hand.

FIGURE A-6

FIGURE A-7

10. Assess the flow of blood (via the needle), which should be dark and steady but not bright red or pulsatile (which would suggest femoral artery puncture).
11. Feed the guidewire through the needle. Be sure to have control of the guidewire at all times.
12. Remove the needle over the guidewire.
13. Make an incision in the skin at the entry of the guidewire. The scalpel should penetrate both the skin and the subcutaneous tissue.
14. Pass the dilator over the guidewire, dilating down to the subcutaneous tissue.
15. With the dominant hand, pass the triple-lumen catheter (distal port uncapped) over the guidewire.
16. When the end of the catheter nearly reaches the skin, advance the guidewire **backward,** until it just exits the distal port.

17. Grab this end of the guidewire, and then advance the entire catheter over the guidewire into the vein.
18. Remove the guidewire.
19. Aspirate blood from each port, and flush with saline.
20. Sew the catheter into place, and apply a sterile dressing.

VI ARTERIAL LINE PLACEMENT

A. **Definition:** introduction of catheter into the (radial) artery
B. **Indications**
    1. Continuous monitoring of heart rate and blood pressure
    2. Frequent arterial blood gas measurement
C. **Contraindication:** digital ischemia
D. **Complications**
    1. Hematoma at the insertion site
    2. Arterial pseudoaneurysm
    3. Thrombosis or infection of the arterial line
    4. Hand or digit ischemia or infarction
E. **Technique**
    1. Place a roll under the dorsal surface of the wrist, leaving it in dorsiflexion (i.e., hyperextended). (See figure A-8.)
    2. Secure the fingers and forearm to an armboard.
    3. Localize the radial artery pulsation proximal to the wrist crease.
    4. Sterilize the entry site with povidone–iodine or chlorhexidine gluconate solution.

FIGURE A-8

5. OPTIONAL: anesthetize the skin at the entry site with 1% lidocaine.
6. Advance a 20-gauge catheter-over-needle apparatus at a 45-degree angle while gently palpating the radial artery proximal to the site of insertion (too much pressure will occlude the pulse).
7. Stop when bright red blood appears in the hub of the needle; this signifies entry of the **needle** into the artery.
8. Slowly lower the entire apparatus, making a more acute angle with the skin.
9. Advance the entire apparatus approximately 2 mm; this places **the catheter,** as well as the needle, into the lumen of the artery.
10. While resting the dominant hand against the skin to stabilize the position of the needle (i.e., do not pull back on the needle), slowly advance the catheter with the nondominant hand until the hub is at the skin (figure A-9).
11. With compression applied proximal to the catheter insertion site, remove the needle with the dominant hand.
12. Release compression; the return of pulsatile, bright blood signifies the presence of successful arterial cannulation
13. If there is no blood return, then the catheter is not within the artery lumen.
    a. Remove the catheter and apply pressure for 5 minutes.
    b. Repeat the process at a more proximal entry site.
14. Attach the catheter to the flush system and sensors, and check for an adequate arterial waveform on the monitor.
15. Secure the catheter with a suture and/or sterile dressing and remove the arm board.

VII ARTERIAL BLOOD GAS

A. **Definition:** sampling of (radial) arterial blood
B. **Indications**
   1. Measurement of pH
   2. Measurement of partial pressures of oxygen and carbon dioxide (PO_2, PCO_2)
   3. Assessment of methemoglobinemia and carboxyhemoglobinemia
C. **Contraindications:** none
D. **Complications:** insertion point hematoma, arterial thrombosis
E. **Patient positioning:** Patient seated or recumbent with the wrist in a slightly hyperextended position.
F. **Locating the point of entry:** Palpate the radial artery at the proximal wrist crease.
G. **Technique:**
   1. Clean the overlying skin with an alcohol swab.

FIGURE A-9

2. OPTIONAL: anesthetize the skin with 1% lidocaine using a 25-gauge needle.
3. Flush the blood gas needle and syringe with heparin, and leave 1 ml of air in the syringe.
4. With your nondominant hand lightly palpating the artery,

enter the artery at a 45 degree angle. The return of briskly flowing bright red blood signifies arterial puncture.

5. Keep the needle in the same position, collecting 2–3 ml of blood.
6. Remove the needle, and quickly apply pressure.
7. Cover the puncture site with a bandage.
8. Remove the needle from the syringe.
9. Place a cap on the syringe.
10. Ensure that the specimen remains anaerobic by advancing the blood in the syringe up to the point of the cap.
11. Transport the sample immediately to the laboratory.

VIII PERIPHERAL INTRAVENOUS LINE

A. **Definition:** introduction of a catheter into a peripheral vein
B. **Indication:** administration of intravenous medications or fluids
C. **Contraindication:** infection overlying the insertion site
D. **Complications:** infection, bleeding or hematoma
E. **Technique**
   1. Locate the vein with inspection and palpation, preferably in the upper extremity at a point of vein bifurcation.
   2. Apply a tourniquet proximal to insertion point, allowing the vein to engorge.
   3. Clean the overlying skin at the puncture site with alcohol or chlorhexidine gluconate solution.
   4. Apply slight pressure distal to the insertion site, securing the vein position.
   5. Insert a 20-gauge catheter-over-needle apparatus into the vein at an acute angle (as flat as possible), with the bevel facing upward.
   6. Stop when blood enters the flashback chamber.
   7. Advance the apparatus 1 mm further into the vessel.
   8. Maintain the position of the needle with the dominant hand.
   9. Slowly advance the catheter into the lumen of the vessel with the nondominant hand.
   10. Remove the tourniquet.
   11. Withdraw the needle.
   12. Quickly apply pressure to the vein proximal to the catheter, interrupting the return of blood.
   13. Attach tubing and fluids to the catheter.
   14. Apply a sterile dressing.

Index

519